Current Concepts in the Treatment of Distal Radius Fractures

Guest Editor

KEVIN C. CHUNG, MD, MS

HAND CLINICS

www.hand.theclinics.com

May 2012 • Volume 28 • Number 2

SAUNDERS an imprint of ELSEVIER, Inc.

W.B. SAUNDERS COMPANY
A Division of Elsevier Inc.

1600 John F. Kennedy Blvd. • Suite 1800 • Philadelphia, Pennsylvania 19103

http://www.theclinics.com

HAND CLINICS Volume 28, Number 2
May 2012 ISSN 0749-0712, ISBN-13: 978-1-4557-4562-3

Editor: David Parsons

Hand Clinics (ISSN 0749-0712) is published quarterly by Elsevier Inc., 360 Park Avenue South, New York, NY 10010-1710. Months of publication are February, May, August, and November. Business and Editorial Offices: 1600 John F. Kennedy Blvd., Ste. 1800, Philadelphia, PA 19103-2899. Customer Service Office: 3251 Riverport Lane, Maryland Heights, MO 63043. Periodicals postage paid at New York, NY and at additional mailing offices. Subscription price is $368.00 per year (domestic individuals), $583.00 per year (domestic institutions), $184.00 per year (domestic students/residents), $420.00 per year (Canadian individuals), $666.00 per year (Canadian institutions), $500.00 per year (international individuals), $666.00 per year (international institutions), and $243.00 per year (international and Canadian students/residents). Foreign air speed delivery is included in all *Clinics* subscription prices. All prices are subject to change without notice. **POSTMASTER:** Send address changes to *Hand Clinics*, Elsevier Health Sciences Division, Subscription Customer Service, 3251 Riverport Lane, Maryland Heights, MO 63043. Customer Service (orders, claims, online, change of address): Elsevier Health Sciences Division, Subscription Customer Service, 3251 Riverport Lane, Maryland Heights, MO 63043. Tel: 1-800-654-2452 (U.S. and Canada); 314-447-8871 (outside U.S. and Canada). Fax: 314-447-8029. E-mail: journalscustomerservice-usa@elsevier.com (for print support); journalsonlinesupport-usa@elsevier.com (for online support).

Reprints. For copies of 100 or more of articles in this publication, please contact the Commercial Reprints Department, Elsevier Inc., 360 Park Avenue South, New York, New York 10010-1710. Tel.: 212-633-3812; Fax: 212-462-1935; E-mail: reprints@elsevier.com.

Hand Clinics is covered in *MEDLINE/PubMed (Index Medicus), Current Contents/Clinical Medicine, EMBASE/Excerpta Medica,* and *ISI/BIOMED.*

Printed and bound by CPI Group (UK) Ltd, Croydon, CR0 4YY

Transferred to Digital Print 2012

Contributors

GUEST EDITOR

KEVIN C. CHUNG, MD, MS
Charles B.G. de Nancrede Professor of
Surgery, Section of Plastic Surgery,
Department of Surgery; Assistant Dean for
Faculty Affairs, University of Michigan Medical
School, Ann Arbor, Michigan

AUTHORS

JOSHUA G. BALES, MD
Hand Surgery Specialists, Inc, Cincinnati, Ohio

ARJAN G.J. BOT, MD
Research Fellow, Orthopaedic Hand and
Upper Extremity Service, Massachusetts
General Hospital, Boston, Massachusetts

KEVIN C. CHUNG, MD, MS
Charles B.G. de Nancrede Professor of
Surgery, Section of Plastic Surgery,
Department of Surgery; Assistant Dean for
Faculty Affairs, University of Michigan Medical
School, Ann Arbor, Michigan

T.R.C. DAVIS, FRCS
Professor, Consultant Hand Surgeon,
University Department of Trauma and
Orthopaedics, Nottingham University
Hospitals, Nottingham, United Kingdom

DAVID G. DENNISON, MD
Assistant Professor of Orthopedic Surgery,
Division of Hand and Microvascular Surgery,
Department of Orthopedic Surgery, Mayo
Clinic, Rochester, Minnesota

RAFAEL J. DIAZ-GARCIA, MD
House Officer, Section of Plastic Surgery,
Department of Surgery, The University of
Michigan Hospital and Health System,
Ann Arbor, Michigan

RUBY GREWAL, MD, MSc
Assistant Professor, Division of Orthopedic
Surgery, University of Western Ontario, The
Hand and Upper Limb Centre, St. Joseph's
Health Centre, London, Ontario, Canada

STEVEN C. HAASE, MD
Associate Professor of Surgery, Section of
Plastic Surgery, University of Michigan Medical
School, Ann Arbor, Michigan

DOUGLAS P. HANEL, MD
Professor, Department of Orthopaedics and
Sports Medicine, University of Washington
Medical Center, Seattle, Washington

JERRY I. HUANG, MD
Assistant Professor, Department of
Orthopaedics and Sports Medicine, University
of Washington Medical Center, Seattle,
Washington

JESSE JUPITER, MD
Hansjorg Wyss/AO Professor, Orthopaedic
Surgery, Harvard Medical School; Visiting
Surgeon, Massachusetts General Hospital,
Boston, Massachusetts

SANJEEV KAKAR, MD, MRCS
Assistant Professor of Orthopedic Surgery,
Division of Hand and Microvascular Surgery,
Department of Orthopedic Surgery, Mayo
Clinic, Rochester, Minnesota

A. KARANTANA, FRCS (Orth)
Specialist Registrar in Trauma and
Orthopaedics, University Department of
Trauma and Orthopaedics, Nottingham
University Hospitals, Nottingham,
United Kingdom

EVAN KOWALSKI, BS
Research Associate, Section of Plastic
Surgery, University of Michigan Health System,
Ann Arbor, Michigan

FRASER J. LEVERSEDGE, MD
Assistant Professor, Department of
Orthopaedic Surgery, Duke University,
Durham, North Carolina

KATE W. NELLANS, MD, MPH
Hand Fellow, Section of Plastic Surgery,
University of Michigan Health System,
Ann Arbor, Michigan

KAGAN OZER, MD
Associate Professor of Orthopaedic Surgery,
University of Michigan Health System,
Ann Arbor, Michigan

PETER C. RHEE, DO
Department of Orthopedic Surgery, Mayo
Clinic, Rochester, Minnesota

DAVID C. RING, MD, PhD
Orthopaedic Hand and Upper Extremity
Service, Yawkey Center, Massachusetts
General Hospital; Associate Professor of
Orthopaedic Surgery, Harvard Medical School,
Boston, Massachusetts

ANDREW W. RITTING, MD
Chief Resident, Department of Orthopaedic
Surgery, New England Musculoskeletal
Institute, University of Connecticut Health
Center, Farmington, Connecticut

DOUGLAS M. SAMMER, MD
Assistant Professor, Department of Plastic
Surgery, Program Director Hand Surgery
Fellowship, UT Southwestern Medical Center,
Dallas, Texas

SANDEEP J. SEBASTIN, MCh (Plastic)
Consultant, Department of Hand and
Reconstructive Microsurgery, National
University Hospital, Singapore

RAMESH C. SRINIVASAN, MD
Department of Orthopaedic Surgery, Duke
University, Durham, North Carolina

PETER J. STERN, MD
Hand Surgery Specialists, Inc, Cincinnati, Ohio

JENNIFER M. WOLF, MD
Associate Professor, Department of
Orthopaedic Surgery, New England
Musculoskeletal Institute, University of
Connecticut Health Center, Farmington,
Connecticut

ALBERT YOON, MBChB
Clinical Fellow, The Hand and Upper Limb
Centre, St. Joseph's Health Centre, London,
Ontario, Canada

Contents

Distal radius fractures (DRFs) have been a common affliction for millennia, but their treatment is a more recent development resulting from human erudition. Although immobilization has served as the only available treatment for most of our history, many advances have been made in the management of DRFs over the last century as orthopedics has grown. Yet the topic remains hotly contested in the literature and, given the frequency of the injury, research continues to focus on it. This article traces the evolution of DRF treatment to provide a context for the future.

Distal radius fractures are one of the most common types of fractures. Although the pediatric and elderly populations are at greatest risk for this injury, distal radius fractures still have a significant impact on the health and well-being of young adults. Data from the past 40 years have documented a trend toward an overall increase in the prevalence of this injury in both the pediatric and elderly populations. Understanding the epidemiology of this fracture is an important step toward the improvement of treatment strategies and the development of preventive measures with which to target this debilitating injury.

Distal radius fractures (DRFs) are the most common fracture treated by physicians, but questions remain regarding optimal management. Fracture patterns, biomechanics, and treatment strategies have been debated for more than 200 years, and research shows many controversies regarding long-held beliefs. Although these common myths have been propagated and considered fact, they are not based on the best-available evidence. This article illustrates some of the major controversies regarding the management of DRFs. To provide optimal care in a world of evidence-based medicine, clinicians must shift their thinking and accept that some of the indoctrinated ideas may represent a flawed heuristic approach.

In North America, the rate of nonoperative management of displaced distal radius fractures has declined as the rate of internal fixation has increased. Volar locking plate fixation has increased in popularity despite a lack of supportive level 1 evidence. Issues of cost-effectiveness are relevant because there is no best-practice treatment at this stage. Clinicians should be aware of the goals of treatment and challenges, particularly in managing elderly patients with distal radius fractures. Large, randomized controlled trials or meta-analyses may provide answers about when operative intervention is favored over nonoperative management and which operative intervention provides the best outcomes.

There has been a surge in the operative management of distal radius fractures. Closed reduction, external fixation, and open reduction with internal fixation each have advantages and disadvantages. The purpose of this review is not to provide the clinician with an algorithm for treatment of distal radius fractures. These fractures span an extensive spectrum of severity across age groups and demographics. Fortunately, the surgeon holds a vast array of options to provide care for patients with distal radius fractures. The choice of fixation or conservative care resides in the personality of the fracture and the needs of the patients.

Numerous methods of treatment are available for the management of distal radius fractures, with modern trends favoring volar fixed-angle distal radius plates. Whatever the method of fixation, recognition, management, and prevention of the known associated complications are essential to achieve a good outcome. This article reviews the common preventable complications that are associated with operative treatment of distal radius fractures, including tendon injuries, inadequate reduction, subsidence or collapse, intra-articular placement of pegs or screws, nerve injuries, complex regional pain syndrome, carpal tunnel syndrome, and compartment syndrome.

Fractures of the distal radius and ulnar styloid have the potential to disturb the normal function of the distal radioulnar joint (DRUJ), resulting in loss of motion, pain, arthritis, or instability. The DRUJ can be adversely affected by several mechanisms, including intra-articular injury with step-off, shortening, and angulation of an extra-articular fracture; injury to the radioulnar ligaments; ulnar styloid avulsion fracture; and injury of secondary soft tissue stabilizers. This article discusses the management of the DRUJ and ulnar styloid fracture in the presence of a distal radius fracture.

Despite encouraging results from small case series, correction of distal radius malunion remains a challenging procedure with uncertain outcomes. The most appropriate treatment for a distal radius malunion is prevention. If a symptomatic malunion is discovered, correction should be undertaken as early as possible. It is recommended that action be taken within six months of the primary injury to decrease the negative impact of soft-tissue contracture on the eventual reconstruction. Although some patients complain about residual problems after malunion surgery, corrective surgery has been shown to improve both radiographic and functional outcomes, and may prevent future secondary problems.

The interest in developing biomaterials to augment fracture healing continues to grow. New products promise early return to function with minimal morbidity;

however, indications to use these products remain unclear. An ideal bone graft material stimulates bone healing and provides structural stability while being biocompatible, bioresorbable, easy to use, and cost-effective. This article reviews the biology of bone grafts and the clinical evidence in the use of bone graft substitutes for the treatment of distal radius fractures.

HAND CLINICS

Preface

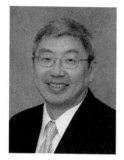

Kevin C. Chung, MD, MS
Guest Editor

In this era of evidence-based medicine, long cherished beliefs and myths are constantly challenged by critically examining available data to form a scientific basis for treatment selection. Despite over 200 years of treating distal radius fractures, and many thousands of publications on this topic, surgeons and patients alike are still vexed that we have not arrived at a consensus regarding the most optimal treatment option for a particular injury type and for a unique patient characteristic. This *Hand Clinics* volume strives to synthesize the best available evidence by providing a comprehensive analysis of the current treatments for distal radius fractures. The majority of the authors for this volume hail from the Wrist and Radius Injury Surgical Trial (WRIST) study group. This group is the largest collaboration of hand surgeons in the world, consisting of 19 sites and over 50 hand surgeons who will be participating in this clinical trial. For the first time, the WRIST study group will randomize patients over 60 years of age into K-wire fixation, external fixation, or volar locking plating fixation to identify the most optimal treatment for this prevalent injury. At the same time, an observational group of subjects with similar fracture types will be treated with casting to exam the outcomes of casting treatment and compare them to the outcomes of surgical treatment. This ambitious 5-year study supported by the National Institutes of Health is entitled, "A Clinical Trial for the Surgical Treatment of Distal Radius Fractures in the Elderly."

This project is currently underway and should provide robust level 1 data that will help to guide future treatment decisions for distal radius fractures.

The uniqueness of this *Hand Clinics* volume is that it traces the genesis of treatment for distal radius fractures from a historical perspective all the way to current treatment options. This collection engages experts from three different regions of the world, including North America, Europe, and Asia, culminating in an article on the future research and treatment directions in the care of this fracture. The growing interest in the use of large database analysis enables investigators to look at this common injury from a population standpoint, and the continued refinement of surgical techniques and implant technology will surely change the approach to treating this fracture. The question now is not whether these fractures can heal, but how we can enable patients to recover their hand function much quicker with less morbidity when compared to the past. Additionally, in the current era of cost constraints, how can we provide the most effective care at the lowest cost? For example, can we save resources by avoiding routine prescription of hand therapy or by being more selective in advocating therapy, when a substantial subset of the subjects may recover uneventfully without these expensive and time-consuming treatments? These are issues that this particular volume will address to present critical viewpoints of the

Hand Clin 28 (2012) xi–xii
doi:10.1016/j.hcl.2012.03.009

hand.theclinics.com

various subjects I have assigned. I very much appreciate the contributions of my colleagues who generously shared their expertise to this volume. All of the articles are meticulously written and well researched. There is no doubt that this *Hand Clinics* issue represents an authoritative treatise on an injury that continues to challenge and stimulate all of us to deliver the most optimal care to our patients.

Kevin C. Chung, MD, MS
Section of Plastic Surgery, Department of Surgery
The University of Michigan Health System
2130 Taubman Center
1500 East Medical Center Drive
Ann Arbor, MI 48109, USA

E-mail address:
kecchung@med.umich.edu

Dedication

To the members of the WRIST study group for your continued support to advance our knowledge on the treatment of distal radius fractures.

Hand Clin 28 (2012) xiii
doi:10.1016/j.hcl.2012.03.010
0749-0712/12/$ – see front matter © 2012 Elsevier Inc. All rights reserved.

The Evolution of Distal Radius Fracture Management: A Historical Treatise

Rafael J. Diaz-Garcia, MD, Kevin C. Chung, MD, MS*

KEYWORDS

- Distal radius fracture • Orthopedics • X-ray
- Internal fixation

The distal radius fracture (DRF) is an injury that predates our species, with a significant milestone in our evolution being the transition to bipedal ambulation by Australopithecus. This elevated posture likely represents a significant risk factor that has played a role in DRFs being the most common fracture treated by physicians.[1] This possibility is echoed by the paucity of the injury in our closest evolutionary relative, the chimpanzee.[2] As humans gained sophistication, they began to develop treatments of maladies, such as fractures, to minimize morbidity. Although the exploration in the precursors of medicine likely predates the written word, the advances in the treatment of DRFs have a more abbreviated history. There are accounts of fracture splinting that stem back to ancient Egypt, but most of the contributions into the DRF management have been made in the past century.

Nowadays a better understanding of radiocarpal anatomy, wrist biomechanics, and bone physiology is available than ever before, and there is continuous effort to refine surgical techniques to optimize outcomes. Understanding the advances that have been made in DRF treatment provides an appreciation for the past, and a keen perspective of the progress toward the future. Based on the history of DRF management, the contributions made can be loosely divided into 3 eras with seemingly different goals. In the first era, physicians struggled with the ability to diagnose fractures in the distal radius. In the second, they had a grasp of the diagnosis but lacked good therapeutic options to address every injury. In the most recent period, surgeons aim to improve their surgical technique and better delineate treatment protocols to maximize functional outcomes and minimize morbidity.

ERA OF NAIVETÉ (PRE-1895)

The first era in the management of DRF fractures is by far the longest, spanning back much further than the records that remain for any interpretation and understanding. The oldest surviving descriptions regarding the management of fractures stem back at least 5000 years to ancient Egyptian case reports within the Edwin Smith Papyrus.[3] The translation of the hieroglyphics among these ancient scrolls describes manipulating a fractured arm until it is straight, then applying splints of wood and rolls of linen, which were subsequently hardened with grease and honey to maintain their position. This ancient work represents one of the first surgical texts: an early preliterate civilization's attempt to preserve medical knowledge for the sake of posterity. Few cases in these works remain fully enough preserved to allow substantial insight

Supported in part by a grant from the National Institute on Aging and National Institute of Arthritis and Musculoskeletal and Skin Diseases (R01 AR062066) and a Midcareer Investigator Award in Patient-Oriented Research (K24 AR053120) to Dr Kevin C. Chung.

Section of Plastic Surgery, Department of Surgery, The University of Michigan Health System, 2130 Taubman Center, 1500 East Medical Center Drive, Ann Arbor, MI 48109, USA
* Corresponding author.
E-mail address: kecchung@umich.edu

Hand Clin 28 (2012) 105–111
doi:10.1016/j.hcl.2012.02.007

into the methods of diagnosis and treatment by the ancient Egyptians.[4] Thus, most of the credit regarding the earliest roots of medicine goes to the ancient Greeks.

Often viewed as the father of Western medicine, Hippocrates is ascribed with most of the medical knowledge acquired during the Golden Age of Greece. However, most of the works credited to him are actually an anonymous collection of Greek medical manuscripts from the library of Alexandria.[5] Nonetheless, the Hippocratic Corpus represents an aggregate of the medical knowledge of the ancient world, and contains significant discussion of dislocations and subluxations of the radiocarpal joint along with the prescribed treatment: manual reduction and gentle bandaging.[6] However, given the rarity of this injury and the high frequency with which the ancient Greeks described it, it is likely that they misdiagnosed DRFs as radiocarpal dislocations. Millennia of misdiagnosis passed until the eighteenth century, when Petit and Pouteau first theorized that Hippocrates had failed to fully conceptualize the injury he was describing and treating.[7] Their theories, unfortunately, largely failed to disseminate out of France, leaving them with little recognition.

In 1814, Abraham Colles[8] published his landmark treatise on DRF that led to his eponymous reward. In "On the Fracture of the Carpal Extremity of the Radius," Colles questions those who describe all wrist injuries as dislocations, and offers an explanation as to why this may have been so. He postulates that "the absence of crepitus, and of the other common symptoms of fracture, together with the swelling which instantly arises in this, as in other injuries of the wrist, render the difficulty of ascertaining the real nature of the case very considerable." He also describes how to reduce the injury and notes the importance of immobilization with a wooden splint to prevent the wrist from falling into dorsal displacement. However, this article would also receive little attention, and it was the work of Guillaume Dupuytren that brought these fractures to the interest of the surgical world at large.[7]

Throughout this era, treatment of DRFs changed very little. Casting and splinting was mostly unchanged from the times of the ancient Egyptians and Greeks. Glues, resins, and waxes were used to harden bandages to immobilize the wrist and forearm (**Fig. 1**). In the 1850s, plaster of Paris gained popularity in Europe as the solidifying agent in casting techniques.[9] Results were mixed but deemed reasonable overall, because of the physicians' inability to follow up the anatomic alignment with anything other than physical examination (**Fig. 2**). In 1895, Wilhelm Röntgen made

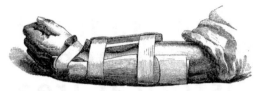

Fig. 1. An example of functional splinting created to prevent the dorsal collapse of the distal fragment in a Colles fracture by flexing the wrist and applying pressure to the metacarpal bases and carpal rows. (*Reprinted from* Gordon A. A treatise on the fractures of the lower end of the radius on fractures of the clavicle and on the reduction of the recent inward dislocations of the shoulder joint. London: Churchill; 1875.)

a discovery that forever changed the landscape of medicine.[4] Owing to his Nobel Prize–winning work on x-rays, the conservative management of DRFs would be called into question for the first time.

ERA OF INVENTION (1895–1965)

The advent of roentgenography marked a significant milestone in the evaluation and management of fractures. The information about x-rays disseminated so quickly that within 2 months of Röntgen's discovery, the first case of using x-rays for clinical diagnosis was published in *The Lancet*,[10] which sparked a significant increase in the literature about fractures and their management. For the first time, physicians were able to discuss fractures based on the degree of displacement and articular involvement in the live patient, rather than the autopsy specimen. Several investigators began publishing on the radiographic findings of DRFs in the late nineteenth and early twentieth centuries,[11–15] questioned the results that had previously been thought adequate, and started postulating how to address their concerns.

Throughout this era, management of DRFs remained predominantly nonoperative. Although advances in imaging did allow for better assessment of initial fracture reduction and follow-up, cast immobilization resulted in frequent malunions and residual deformity (**Fig. 3**). That DRF frequently resulted in shortening and loss of volar tilt was well established; however, treatment options were limited. Physicians developed complex splints in a wide variety of wrist positions in an attempt to prevent the collapse of the fracture fragments over time. Although surgeons began to discuss surgical options to address difficult fractures, it remained a risky endeavor that exposed the patient to infection. The pivotal works in antisepsis by Lister paved the way to make primary surgical fixation a safe and prudent option in the management of

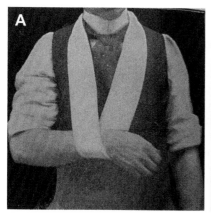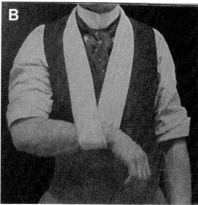

Fig. 2. Images of how to properly (*A*) and improperly (*B*) don a cravat sling as treatment of a distal radius fracture. Note how in the proper position (*A*), the wrist is held in slight flexion, slight supination, and ulnar deviation to maintain radial length. (*Reprinted from* Scudder CL. The treatment of fractures. Philadelphia: WB Saunders; 1902.)

fractures.[16,17] Albin Lambotte was the first to attempt controlling the fragments in a DRF by surgical means, building on his experience in other bones of the body.[18] In 1908, he described the use of a percutaneously placed wire through the radial styloid to maintain reduction. However, it took more than 40 years to publish a case series with results using K-wires.[19]

Comminuted DRFs remained a significant problem for the treating physician equipped with only cast immobilization (**Fig. 4**). Reduction was impossible to maintain, and shortening of the radius would inevitably develop. The principles of ligamentotaxis were understood in terms of fracture reduction, but in the early twentieth century attempts were made to extend that to definitive treatment. Lorenz Böhler[20] introduced the use of pins with plaster to treat DRFs much like he had treated lower extremity fractures with

traction. Donald Murray[21] described the use of an adhesive traction device to maintain radial length during the consolidation phase of bony union (**Fig. 5**). This elaborate contraption distracted the fracture out to length via the radial digits and maintained that alignment while the fracture healed. Skeletal traction via pins and plaster led to formal external fixators as we know them today, when Anderson and O'Neil[22] introduced their initial design in 1944 (**Fig. 6**). Pins were placed in the radius proximally and the index metacarpal distally, and were kept at a length with a simple bar. Thus, surgeons were able to predictably prevent what had previously been considered inevitable radial shortening.

Internal fixation had its earliest proponents in the early nineteenth century with pioneers such as J.K. Rodgers,[23] who introduced internal fixation of the skeleton as a treatment for nonunions

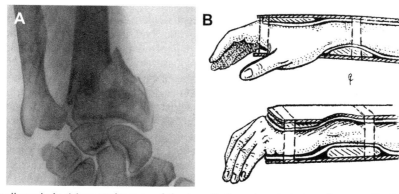

Fig. 3. X-rays allowed physicians at the turn of the twentieth century to better diagnose distal radius fractures, but treatment options were still limited. Even comminuted fractures (*A*) were treated with splinting (*B*). (*Reprinted from* Cotton FJ. The pathology of fracture of the lower extremity of the radius. Ann Surg 1900;32:194–218; and Cotton F. Dislocations and joint fractures. Philadelphia: W.B. Saunders; 1910.)

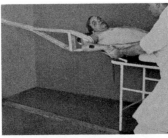
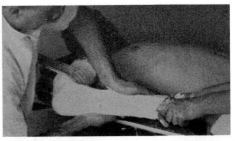

Fig. 4. Reduction and plaster immobilization of shortened fractures often required multiple hands to maintain reduction and place a well-fitted cast. Nevertheless, reduction was often lost, leaving suboptimal results. (*Reprinted from* Böhler L. Treatment of fractures. Vienna (Austria): Wilhelm Maudrich; 1929; with permission.)

and pseudoarthroses. The only fixation instrument available at the time was surgical wire, which was tightened down after passing it through drill holes in an early cerclage technique. With the dissemination of Lister's advances in antisepsis, surgical management was becoming a safer option, and internal fixation had its first vocal and effective advocates in the early twentieth century with men such as Sir Arbuthnot Lane and Albin Lambotte.[4] Lane's interest in the field was a direct result of his experience with postmortem dissections, in which he observed the frequency of malunions and the effect they had on the skeleton and articular surfaces.[24] Lane and Lambotte began to treat fresh closed fractures with internal fixation, thus developing the early principles of osteosynthesis.[25–28]

Even with some promising results in other long bones, the literature is devoid of any report of

a primary open reduction and internal fixation of a DRF before 1960, which may be because the early attempts at open reduction internal fixation (ORIF) were so poor that they never made it into the literature, or possibly the functional outcomes in DRF at the time were deemed good enough that a new surgical option was not explored. Regardless of the cause, there was a significant lag in using plates and screws in DRF in comparison with fractures of other long bones. However, a significant milestone occurred in 1958 when more than a dozen Swiss surgeons met to discuss their dissatisfaction with results in fracture management. This group of visionaries would later serve as the nucleus of the organization presently known as Arbeitsgemeinschaft für Osteosynthesefragen, or AO.[29] Soon afterward, the first 2 case reports using internal fixation in the distal radius were published in the literature because of this growing interest in operative management of fractures.[30,31] Nevertheless, ORIF of DRFs remained a rarely used option in the orthopedic surgeon's armamentarium for decades.

ERA OF REFINEMENT (1965 THROUGH PRESENT)

By the mid 1960s, the forefathers of modern orthopedics had developed the foundations of DRF management that is known today. Operative techniques were introduced because of the frequent malunions that resulted from the conservative management of fractures, yet as this era began almost all DRFs continued to be treated nonoperatively.[32] The operative indications and benefits were poorly understood by the average practitioner and were thus rarely advocated. However, there were some who were dissatisfied with their end results, and many surgeons continued to experiment with new techniques and apply them to their most difficult cases. Thus, this most recent era has experienced a refinement of the available techniques and a continuing search to better

Fig. 5. Adhesive traction, advanced by surgeons, such as Murray, was a precursor to external fixation for comminuted distal radius fractures that was based on the principle of ligamentotaxis. (*Reprinted from* Murray DA. Treatment of fractures of the carpal end of the radius by traction. Am J Surg 1939;44:135–8; with permission.)

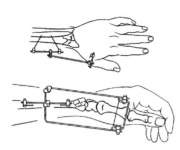
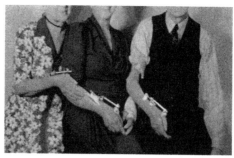

Fig. 6. Anderson and O'Neil were the first to use external fixators on the distal radius in the 1940s, finally providing a surgical option for comminuted intra-articular fractures. (*Reprinted from* Anderson R, O'Neil G. Comminuted fractures of the distal end of the radius. Surg Gynecol Obstet 1944;78:434–40; with permission.)

understand the appropriate indications for each intervention.

Each operative technique has had its proponents over the last several decades: surgeons who innovated the previously described procedures to improve their results as well as the manufacturers who have improved implant design and materials. Percutaneous pinning was most notably revolutionized by Kapandji,[33] who introduced the concept of intrafocal pinning of the fracture site in the 1970s as a means to buttress the distal segment.[33–35] Difficulty with the pins and plaster techniques led to an increase in the use of external fixators in the 1980s.[36–38] External fixation devices have been designed to provide surgeons with more options: multiple degrees of freedom to position the wrist in space as well as the choice of whether to bridge the radiocarpal joint or not.[39,40] However, the use of internal fixation in DRF has probably seen the greatest change in interest and largest increase in operative options over the past 2 decades. With a better understanding of DRF fracture patterns and wrist biomechanics, a multitude of implant systems with a wide variety of designs have been developed. Internal fixation devices have transitioned from stainless steel to titanium alloys, which are lighter and more biocompatible.[41,42] Dorsally applied Pi and Forte plates were popularized in the 1990s, but fell quickly out of favor because of the frequent tendon irritations.[43–45] Over the last decade, volar locking plates have taken hold as the implant of choice, and operative fixation of DRF is at an all-time high.[46–50]

Most recently, the *Journal of the American Medical Association* introduced the concept of evidence-based medicine into the lexicon of the medical literature, and with it gave new impetus to research on treatment algorithms for the management of DRFs.[51,52] The notion is that clinical decision making should reflect the best available evidence from clinical research, rather than heuristics and unsystematic experience.[53] However, this concept has had difficulty gaining momentum in the surgical specialties in which clinical questions have a paucity of high-quality evidence, and randomized controlled trials are few and far between. Often, the surgeon's clinical experience leads to changes in treatment patterns not as yet proven to be superior in the literature. A prime example is the dramatic increase in the use of volar locking plate for operative fixation over the last decade, with little in the way of comparative studies.[46,47] Ultimately outcomes should be used to further elucidate the indications for operative management of DRFs, particularly as medicine is practiced in this cost-conscious climate going forward.

SUMMARY

Although the injury is older than even our species, most of the advances regarding DRF management have been made over the past century since the advent of x-rays. DRF remains a common ailment, and there are more options regarding treatment today than at any previous point in history. Cast immobilization is often used for definitive treatment, but operative management continues to take hold of a larger share of DRFs each year. By reviewing the history of the evolution of DRF management, one gains appreciation for the contributions made thus far in a relatively small window of time. The future in DRF management sees an evolving discussion about the outcomes each treatment option affords and a better understanding of an evidence-based system of practice.

REFERENCES

1. Chung KC, Spilson SV. The frequency and epidemiology of hand and forearm fractures in the United States. J Hand Surg Am 2001;26(5):908–15.

2. Jurmain R. Trauma, degenerative disease, and other pathologies among the Gombe chimpanzees. Am J Phys Anthropol 1989;80(2):229–37.

3. Breasted JH. The Edwin Smith surgical papyrus. Special edition. Birmingham (AL): The Classics of Medicine Library; 1984.

4. Peltier LF. Fractures: a history and iconography of their treatment. San Francisco (CA): Norman Publishing; 1990.

5. Garrison FH, Wantz GE. An introduction to the history of medicine: with medical chronology, suggestions for study and bibliographic data. 4th edition. Philadelphia, London: WB Saunders; 1929. reprinted.

6. Hippocrates, Adams F, Sydenham Society. The genuine works of Hippocrates. London: Printed for the Sydenham Society; 1849.

7. Peltier LF. Fractures of the distal end of the radius. An historical account. Clin Orthop Relat Res 1983;(187):18–22.

8. Colles A. On the fracture of the carpal extremity of the radius. Edinb Med Surg J 1814;10:181.

9. Rang M. The story of orthopaedics. Philadelphia: WB Saunders; 2000. p. 587.

10. Jones R, Lodge O. The discovery of a bullet lost in the wrist by the means of Roentgen rays. Lancet 1896;1:476–7.

11. Codman E. A study of the x-ray plates of one hundred and forty cases of fracture of the lower end of the radius. Boston Med Surg J 1900;143:305–9.

12. Cotton F. The pathology of fracture of the lower extremity of the radius. Ann Surg 1900;32:194–218.

13. Pilcher LS. Fractures of the lower extremity or base of the radius. Ann Surg 1917;65:1–27.

14. Destot E. La poignet et les accidents du travail: Étude radiographique et clinique. Paris: Vitot Freres; 1905.

15. Beck C. Colle's fracture and the Roentgen-rays. Med News 1898;72:230.

16. Lister J. Illustrations of the antiseptic system of treatment in surgery. Lancet 1867;2:668–9.

17. Lister J. On a new method of treating compound fracture, abscess, with observations on the conditions of suppuration. Lancet 1867;1:326–9.

18. Rayhack JM. The history and evolution of percutaneous pinning of displaced distal radius fractures. Orthop Clin North Am 1993;24:287–300.

19. Depalma A. Comminuted fractures of the distal end of the radius treat by ulnar pinning. J Bone Joint Surg 1952;34:651.

20. Bohler L. Treatment of fractures. Vienna (Austria): Wilhelm Maudrich; 1929.

21. Murray D. Treatment of fractures of the carpal end of the radius by traction. Am J Surg 1938;44:135–8.

22. Anderson R, O'Neil G. Comminuted fractures of the distal end of the radius. Surg Gynecol Obstet 1944; 78:434–40.

23. Rodgers JK. Case of ununited fracture of the os brachii, successfully treated. New York Med Phys J 1827;6:521.

24. Lane W. Some clinical observations on the principles involved in the surgery of fractures. Clin J 1894;5: 392.

25. Lambotte A. Notes sur l'ostéo-synthèse dans les fractures du poignet. Ann Soc de méd d'Anvers 1904;lxvi:321–6, 3 pl [in French].

26. Lane W. The operative treatment of simple fractures. Br Med J 1905;2:1325.

27. Lane W. The operative treatment of fractures. Ann Surg 1909;50:1106.

28. Vrebos J, Dupuis C. From circumferential wiring to miniaturized plates and screws: the history of osteosynthesis of the mandible. Eur J Plast Surg 2005;28: 170–8.

29. Allgower M, Spiegel PG. Internal fixation of fractures: evolution of concepts. Clin Orthop Relat Res 1979;(138):26–9.

30. Cauchoix J, Duparc J, Poral M. Les fractures-luxations marginales anterieures du radius. Revue de Chirurgie Orthopedique 1960;46:233 [in French].

31. Ellis J. Smith's and Barton's fractures. A method of treatment. J Bone Joint Surg Br 1965;47:724–7.

32. Older T, Stabler E, Cassebaum W. Colles fracture: evaluation and selection of therapy. J Trauma 1965;5:469–76.

33. Kapandji A. Internal fixation by double intrafocal plate. Functional treatment of non articular fractures of the lower end of the radius (author's transl). Ann Chir 1976;30:903–8 [in French].

34. Greatting MD, Bishop AT. Intrafocal (Kapandji) pinning of unstable fractures of the distal radius. Orthop Clin North Am 1993;24:301–7.

35. Peyroux LM, Dunaud JL, Caron M, et al. The Kapandji technique and its evolution in the treatment of fractures of the distal end of the radius. Report on a series of 159 cases. Ann Chir Main 1987;6: 109–22.

36. Carrozzella J, Stern PJ. Treatment of comminuted distal radius fractures with pins and plaster. Hand Clin 1988;4:391–7.

37. Green DP. Pins and plaster treatment of comminuted fractures of the distal end of the radius. J Bone Joint Surg Am 1975;57:304–10.

38. Seitz WH Jr, Froimson AI, Leb R, et al. Augmented external fixation of unstable distal radius fractures. J Hand Surg Am 1991;16:1010–6.

39. Zanotti RM, Louis DS. Intra-articular fractures of the distal end of the radius treated with an adjustable fixator system. J Hand Surg Am 1997;22:428–40.

40. Atroshi I, Brogren E, Larsson GU, et al. Wrist-bridging versus non-bridging external fixation for displaced distal radius fractures: a randomized assessor-blind clinical trial of 38 patients followed for 1 year. Acta Orthop 2006;77:445–53.

41. Pennekamp PH, Wimmer MA, Eschbach L, et al. Microvasculatory reaction of skeletal muscle to Ti-15Mo in comparison to well-established titanium alloys. J Mater Sci Mater Med 2007;18:2053–60.

42. Dennison DG. Distal radius fractures and titanium volar plates: should we take the plates out? J Hand Surg Am 2010;35:141–3.

43. Ring D, Jupiter JB, Brennwald J, et al. Prospective multicenter trial of a plate for dorsal fixation of distal radius fractures. J Hand Surg Am 1997;22:777–84.

44. Carter PR, Frederick HA, Laseter GF. Open reduction and internal fixation of unstable distal radius fractures with a low-profile plate: a multicenter study of 73 fractures. J Hand Surg Am 1998;23:300–7.

45. Rozental TD, Beredjiklian PK, Bozentka DJ. Functional outcome and complications following two types of dorsal plating for unstable fractures of the distal part of the radius. J Bone Joint Surg Am 2003;85:1956–60.

46. Chung KC, Shauver MJ, Birkmeyer JD. Trends in the United States in the treatment of distal radial fractures in the elderly. J Bone Joint Surg Am 2009;91: 1868–73.

47. Koval KJ, Harrast JJ, Anglen JO, et al. Fractures of the distal part of the radius. The evolution of practice over time. Where's the evidence? J Bone Joint Surg Am 2008;90:1855–61.

48. Orbay JL, Fernandez DL. Volar fixed-angle plate fixation for unstable distal radius fractures in the elderly patient. J Hand Surg Am 2004;29:96–102.

49. Sammer DM, Fuller DS, Kim HM, et al. A comparative study of fragment-specific versus volar plate fixation of distal radius fractures. Plast Reconstr Surg 2008; 122:1441–50.

50. Chung KC, Squitieri L, Kim HM. Comparative outcomes study using the volar locking plating system for distal radius fractures in both young adults and adults older than 60 years. J Hand Surg Am 2008; 33:809–19.

51. Handoll HH, Madhok R. From evidence to best practice in the management of fractures of the distal radius in adults: working towards a research agenda. BMC Musculoskelet Disord 2003;4:27.

52. Lichtman DM, Bindra RR, Boyer MI, et al. American Academy of Orthopaedic Surgeons clinical practice guideline on: the treatment of distal radius fractures. J Bone Joint Surg Am 2011;93:775–8.

53. Evidence-Based Medicine Working Group. Evidence-based medicine. A new approach to teaching the practice of medicine. J Am Med Assoc 1992;268:2420–5.

The Epidemiology of Distal Radius Fractures

Kate W. Nellans, MD, MPH[a], Evan Kowalski, BS[a],
Kevin C. Chung, MD, MS[b],*

KEYWORDS

- Distal radius fracture • Epidemiology • Incidence
- Fragility fracture

Distal radius fractures are one of the most common types of fractures, with more than 640,000 cases reported during 2001 in the United States alone.[1] For reasons not fully understood, and likely multifactorial, the incidence of this fracture is on the increase in the United States and abroad.[2–5] Many of the societal effects of these fractures extend beyond the significant medical costs, including decreased school attendance, lost work hours, loss of independence, and lasting disability. Fragmented care and coding discrepancies can make accounting for the true number of these fractures difficult, likely underestimating the rates typically quoted in the literature. When analyzing the incidence of distal radius fractures, there are 3 major populations to consider: children and adolescents, young adults, and the elderly. The pediatric and elderly populations are both considered at high risk for this injury, and the contributing factors are examined in this article. In addition to the 3 main age groups, gender and ethnicity may also be considered distinct risk factors within each of these populations. Understanding the epidemiology of distal radius fractures can help physicians choose the most appropriate treatment options for the fracture, as well as effectively target at-risk populations with preventive measures.

POPULATION INCIDENCE
Overall

Chung and Spilson[1] used data from the National Hospital Ambulatory Medical Care Survey (NHAMCS) database, and determined that 1.5% of all emergency department visits were due to hand and wrist fractures. Radius and ulna fractures consisted of 44% of these fractures. This data corresponds to a study by Larsen and Lauritsen[6] showing that distal radius fractures accounted for 2.5% of all emergency department visits. These numbers vary more widely in earlier reports, but still represent a high incidence rate. In 1962, an analysis of fractures in Sweden documented the number of distal radius and ulna fractures to be as high as 75% of all forearm fractures.[7] A study by Knowelden and colleagues[8] in 1964 found 32% of all fractures seen in women older than 35 years in the distal end of the radius.

Trends of Increasing Incidence

Current and past clinical data point to an increase in the incidence of distal radius fractures for the pediatric, adult, and elderly populations in recent years. This phenomenon has been a subject of debate as early as the 1960s, when Alffram and Bauer[7] published their report on the increasing

Supported in part by grants from the National Institute on Aging and National Institute of Arthritis and Musculoskeletal and Skin Diseases (R01 AR062066) and the National Institute of Arthritis and Musculoskeletal and Skin Diseases (2R01 AR047328-06), and a Midcareer Investigator Award in Patient-Oriented Research (K24 AR053120) (to Dr Chung).

[a] Section of Plastic Surgery, University of Michigan Health System, Ann Arbor, MI, USA
[b] Section of Plastic Surgery, Department of Surgery, The University of Michigan Health System, 2130 Taubman Center, 1500 East Medical Center Drive, Ann Arbor, MI 48109, USA
* Corresponding author.
E-mail address: kecchung@umich.edu

hand.theclinics.com

occurrence of distal radius fractures in a large Swedish city. A study from Rochester, Minnesota found a 17% increase in the incidence of this injury over a 40-year period.[2] The incidence in Sweden almost doubled for the elderly population over a 30-year time span when compared with previous data from the same location. During the same study period as this increase, the incidence rates of shaft fractures of the radius and ulna remained the same, lending further validity to the increase in the incidence of distal radius fractures as a legitimate trend.[9] Although there is no single factor responsible for this phenomenon, any individual contributing factor is bound to have confounding variables.

Many theories have been proposed to determine the source of the increasing rates of distal radius fractures, but studies correlating a specific cause to the incidence of this injury must be carefully evaluated. The influence of lifestyle and environmental factors on the risk and incidence of distal radius fractures has recently been assessed to further examine the causes for the increasing rates. One study found a 30% greater risk for a distal radius fracture in urban women than in rural women.[10] Although the data indicated a significant difference between risk factors, they were unable to determine the cause of this discrepancy, even after analysis of lifestyle and health factors. Other investigators point to the impact of epigenetic influences on the development of diseases such as childhood obesity and osteoporosis as a basis for the increasing incidence of this fracture in different populations.[11,12] It is possible that changing cultural dietary habits may be altering bone metabolism, affecting the overall incidence of distal radius fractures. In addition, as the population ages and individuals strive to remain active, fractures caused by relatively minor traumas have increased.[7] Other theories are discussed in further detail in the following sections.

Costs

As the incidence of distal radius fractures increases, the short-term and long-term costs become apparent. Each year, fractures account for more than half of the days patients spend in hospitals receiving treatment and care for upper extremity injuries.[1,13] The costs of treating distal radius fractures in the pediatric population of the United States has been cited to be in upward of $2 billion per year.[12] Considering the overall prevalence of this injury, this is not surprising. Shauver and colleagues[14] recently evaluated the costs that accompany this injury with respect to the elderly community. In 2007, Medicare paid $170 million

in distal radius fracture–related payments. The investigators projected that the future burden of Medicare could be $240 million if the current trend in the use of internal fixation continues. These costs did not include any secondary expenses associated with this injury such as prescription drugs, lost time at work, and loss of independence, which may be more significant than the direct costs. These data reveal the significant socioeconomic costs incurred as a direct result of distal radius fractures, and highlights the importance of analyzing preventive measures and treatment protocols for individuals who are at a high risk for or suffer from this injury.

PEDIATRIC INCIDENCE

Children and adolescents are at a particularly high risk for distal radius fractures, in part because of a rapidly developing skeletal structure. Studies have documented that up to 25% of fractures in children involve the distal end of the radius.[15–18] A study by Landin[15] estimated that up to the age of 16 years, the risk of incurring a fracture is 42% in boys and 27% in girls. In this analysis, fractures of the distal forearm accounted for approximately 21% of all fractures in the pediatric population. The indirect costs of this injury are incalculable in terms of medical costs, lost time from school, and even future work potential.

Increasing Overall Incidence

The incidence of distal radius fractures in children appears to be rising, but it is difficult to explain the exact cause of this steady increase over the past 40 years (**Fig. 1**).[3,19,20] Some studies suggest this could be the result of an overall increase in the participation of sports-related activities in the pediatric population.[3,12,19,21] A study by de Putter et al[3] found that an increase in sports-related activities correlated with an increase in sports-related distal radius fractures (**Fig. 2**). In another study, 23% of all sports fractures occurred in the distal part of the radius.[22] However, Mathison and Agrawal[21] attest that this increase may be due to improved access to care and better detection of fractures.

Age and Bone Biology

Studies have revealed the average fracture incidence related to age to be higher in boys than in girls.[12,15] In the 1960s, the peak rate of fractures of the distal radius was found to occur during the start of puberty, between the ages of 10 and 14 years.[7] A study in 1989 found the peak age to be specifically between 11.5 and 12.5 years for girls

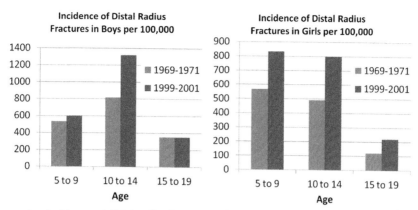

Fig. 1. The increasing incidence of distal radius fractures in boys and girls younger than 20 years. The increase in incidence was statistically significant for both boys and girls. (*Data from* Khosla S, Melton LJ 3rd, Dekutoski MB, et al. Incidence of childhood distal forearm fractures over 30 years: a population-based study. JAMA 2003;290:1479–85.)

and 13.5 and 14.5 years for boys,[23] whereas more recent data suggest that for girls the peak age is anywhere from 8 to 11 and for boys from 11 to 14.[19] Using current data from the NHAMCS, Chung and Spilson[1] recently documented this peak for the pediatric population, and noted a similar trend (**Fig. 3**). After this peak rate of occurrence, the frequency of distal radius fractures decreases, and is then only exceeded by the incidence rates in women 50 years of age and older.[23] Although it might seem logical to attribute the causes of this peak rate during puberty to an increase in physical activity, it is known that activity levels tend to decrease as children progress through puberty.[24] Rather, the peak rate of fractures appears to be closely correlated to the bone mineral density and bone mineral content

of the distal radius during the pubescent growth spurt.

Studies have confirmed a large dissociation between skeletal growth and mineralization during puberty, which may account for the increased fragility of bones seen during this stage of development.[23,25–28] In an early study on the subject, Krabbe and colleagues[25] found that during the pubescent growth spurt children experience large, sudden advances in linear development, or bone lengthening, concurrent with very small increases in bone mineral content. The process of bone mineralization cannot keep up with the abrupt increase in new bone development, resulting in bones that are particularly susceptible to fracture. After puberty, linear development begins to slow and bone mineral content begins to increase

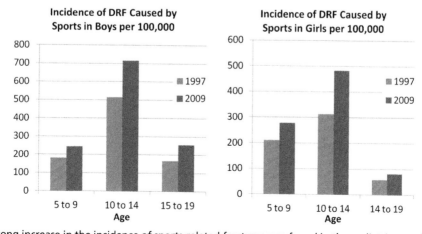

Fig. 2. A strong increase in the incidence of sports-related fractures was found in the pediatric population, which may account for the increase in the overall incidence rates of distal radius fractures. (*Data from* de Putter CE, van Beeck EF, Looman CW, et al. Trends in wrist fractures in children and adolescents, 1997–2009. J Hand Surg Am 2011;36:1810–5.e2.)

Rate by Age of Pediatric Distal Radius Fractures

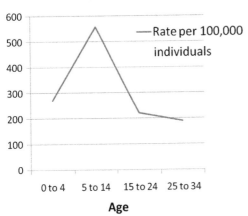

Fig. 3. The combined peak rate of fractures of both boys and girls shown here occurs around 10 years old, corresponding to peak rates documented in other studies. (*Data from* Chung KC, Spilson SV. The frequency and epidemiology of hand and forearm fractures in the United States. J Hand Surg Am 2001; 26:908–15.)

rapidly, creating stronger bones that are more resistant to trauma. Ryan and colleagues[12] found a statistically significant higher proportion of injuries caused by minor trauma in the 10- to 14-year age group in comparison with the 5- to 9-year age group. This finding may suggest that a weakened skeletal structure caused by low rates of bone mineralization during the adolescent growth spurt leaves even a minor trauma with the potential to cause a distal radius fracture.

In addition, some suggest there may be a brief period of increased cortical porosity during the adolescent growth spurt to allow for efficient absorption of calcium required by the bones during this rapid stage of growth.[29] Before mineralization, the increased bone porosity may contribute to the peak rate of distal radius fractures seen during this period of rapid physiologic development.

Gender and Ethnicity

The incidence rate of distal radius fractures is known to be higher in boys than in girls. A study by Ryan and colleagues[12] demonstrated a statistically significant difference between the incidence rates of boys and girls, with 64% of all fractures occurring in boys. Other studies have shown similar results.[3,15,20,23] There is no evidence suggesting significant ethnic differences in the rates of pediatric distal radius fractures. One large study found no significant difference in the rate between urban and rural pediatric populations.[19]

Mechanism of Injury

The mechanism of injury in distal radius fractures in the pediatric population has been well documented. The main types of activities causing distal radius fractures in children are sports, car accidents, and playing. Khosla and colleagues[19] found that from 1999 to 2001, 10% of all pediatric distal radius fractures in Olmsted County occurred while children were using playground equipment. Data from Ryan and colleagues[12,30] documented 30% of distal radius fractures resulting from sports-related injuries in the 10- to 14-year age group, whereas sports were responsible for 47% of these fractures in the 15- to 17-year age group. The most common mechanism of injury was fall related, with studies showing around 80% of injuries occurring in this fashion.

INCIDENCE IN YOUNG ADULTS

The incidence of distal radius fractures in the adult population is significantly lower than in other age groups.[31] As a result of this lower incidence, and the apparent random occurrence of fractures in this low-risk group, few data are available on this population regarding the epidemiology of this injury. However, even at a low rate, the complications following such an injury can result in lasting disability in previously young, healthy individuals. Although infrequent, this injury is still the most common fracture seen in the young adult population.[32] Sports and car accidents are known to be one of the most common causes of distal radius fractures in young adults.

Gender and Ethnic Differences

Research has shown that white women have higher rates of distal radius fractures in individuals older than 65 years, a trend not apparent in younger adults.[33,34] Brogren and colleagues[31] found that in the age group of 19 to 49 years, men and women had almost identical incidence rates. However, in the 19- to 65-year age group, women had almost double the rate compared with men, likely owing to the onset of osteoporosis in women older than 50 years. A study by Chung and Spilson[1] found that Caucasians represented 83% of all fractures but also had the largest proportion of visits to the emergency department. If other ethnic minorities are less likely than Caucasians to present themselves to the emergency room after an injury, this may account for the discrepancy in the published rates of ethnic differences in distal forearm fractures.

INCIDENCE IN THE ELDERLY

Distal radius fractures account for up to 18% of all fractures in the over-65-year age group.[35] Numerous factors contribute to this risk, including architectural changes in the bone, increased activity levels, and metabolic bone disease. This fracture will prove to be a strain on the medical system over the next several decades due to the explosive growth of the elderly population.[14]

Most fractures occurring in the elderly are the result of trauma caused by a low-energy force, with a fall from a standing height the leading cause of injury.[36,37] Many of the accidents causing these low-energy fractures occur as an individual tries to stop a fall with a dorsally outstretched hand. Evidence has also shown that distal radius fractures seem to occur more often in cognitively intact individuals as opposed to those with significant dementia. Women with good neuromuscular control and faster walking speeds were found to be at higher risk for distal radius fracture, as they tend to "reach out" to break a fall rather than fall onto the side of their arm or leg, which would result in a proximal humerus or hip fracture.[13,38]

Age and Gender

Age and gender have a pronounced effect on the incidence rates of distal radius fractures in the elderly community. Women are known to have a significantly greater risk for this injury than men in this age group, compared with the opposite trend found in the pediatric population. Baron and colleagues[35] found that one of the largest gender discrepancies occurred in the distal forearm, when looking at fracture rates in the over-65 age group. According to their data, women were approximately 4.88 times more likely than men to obtain a distal forearm fracture. This finding is in direct contrast to rate ratios in other regions of the upper extremity, where women had a risk factor of around only 3 times that of men. Brogren and colleagues[31] also documented comparable differences between elderly men and women, finding that women had a higher overall incidence, with almost 5 times more fractures in women than in men. The incidence for women increased rapidly from 50 years of age and older, almost doubling every 10 years until 90 years of age (**Fig. 4**). The incidence in men remained low until 80 years of age, but despite this increase still remained significantly lower than the rates observed in women. Flinkkila and colleagues[36] took a closer look at this trend, breaking the age groups into 5-year increments, and found a similar trend (**Fig. 5**).

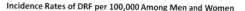

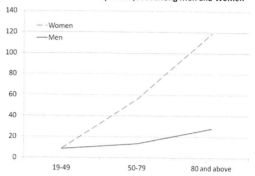

Fig. 4. Incidence rate of distal radius fractures per 10,000 people in men and women aged 19 to 80 years. The increasing incidence was statistically significant in both men and women on comparison of the 3 age groups. (*Data from* Brogren E, Petranek M, Atroshi I. Incidence and characteristics of distal radius fractures in a southern Swedish region. BMC Musculoskelet Disord 2007;8:48.)

Osteoporosis

Osteoporosis and osteopenia are common degenerative bone diseases that plague the elderly population. These injuries are caused by a reduced capacity to build and remodel bone. The World Health Organization defines osteoporosis as occurring in an individual with a bone mineral density −2.5 standard deviations or less than that of a matched adult, whereas osteopenia falls between osteoporosis and normal bone density for age-matched controls.[39] Low bone mineral density

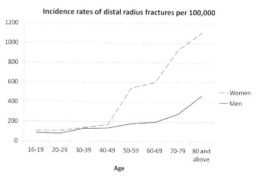

Fig. 5. Incidence rate of distal radius fractures per 100,000 people in men and women aged 16 to 80 years. A statistically significant difference was documented between the overall incidence in men and women, with women having a higher rate of fracture. (*Data from* Flinkkila T, Sirnio K, Hippi M, et al. Epidemiology and seasonal variation of distal radius fractures in Oulu, Finland. Osteoporos Int 2011;22: 2307–12.)

has been well documented in elderly women who suffer a distal radius fracture.[40–45] A recent study by Oyen and colleagues[43] found that decreased bone mineral density was a better predictor of the risk of distal radius fractures in women than in men, but a significant predictor in both men and women once osteoporosis was diagnosed.

Clayton and colleagues[46] recently documented the relationship between osteoporosis and the severity of distal radius fractures. This study indicated that less bone mineral density was correlated with more severe, intra-articular fractures. It also revealed that a decrease in bone mineral density is related to an increase in the probability of early instability after closed reduction, with a 66% chance in the osteoporosis group compared with only a 48% chance in the normal group. In addition, the probability of late carpal malalignment was 35% in the osteoporosis group but only 25% in the normal group.

PEDIATRIC OUTCOMES
Age

In skeletally immature individuals, anatomic reduction of distal radius fractures is usually not required because of the potential for growth and remodeling, and operative intervention is seldom warranted. This fracture is rarely intra-articular, allowing for initial imperfect reductions to be well tolerated. It is accepted that distal fractures have a more favorable prognosis than those in a more proximal aspect of an extremity. Observational studies indicate displacement of very distal fractures in patients of all ages is better tolerated than more proximal malunions in even very young children.[47,48]

Based on long-term functional outcomes of malunions in pediatric forearm fractures, Noonan and Price[49] made a series of recommendations for reduction in pediatric patients presenting with this injury. For patients younger than 9 years, reduction could be accepted with complete displacement (bayonet apposition) and up to 1 cm of shortening, 15° of angulation, and 45° of malrotation, without resulting in functional deficits. In children 9 years and older, 30° of malrotation would be acceptable, with 10° of angulation for proximal fractures and 15° for more distal fractures. Complete bayonet apposition was acceptable, especially for distal radius fractures, as long as angulation did not exceed 20° and 2 years of growth remained.[49]

Complications

Children with distal radius fractures have particularly low rates of complications,[3,50] often attaining superior outcomes with casting alone, because the developing bone in children has a remarkable ability to remodel itself back into the correct anatomic orientation after trauma, even with an injury as severe as a fracture. A recent study showed that only 17 of 305 distal radius fractures in children had a complication.[50] The tendency of surgeons to strive for perfect anatomic reduction in patients with distal radius fractures has caused debate about the appropriate treatment protocol for children with these injuries. A study by Do and colleagues[51] compared the functional outcomes of children with distal radius fractures who underwent closed reduction and those who had only splint stabilization. The 34 children who had no attempted reduction had the same functional results at their follow-up visits as the 34 children who underwent reduction. In addition, the total cost for patients with attempted reduction was 50% more than those without reduction, even though both groups achieved the same functional outcomes with no complications at their follow-up visits. A more recent study by Al-Ansari and colleagues[30] showed that none of 124 children with minimally angulated distal radius fractures required surgical intervention or manipulation of any type before a cast was applied.

On occasion, pediatric distal radius fractures are accompanied by distal ulna fractures. Most studies to date have not separated outcomes for isolated distal radius fractures from those that include a distal ulna fracture (complete or incomplete).[47] Synostosis is a rare complication, but is difficult to treat in this type of injury. Those most at risk are individuals with high-energy trauma or those with a concomitant head injury.[52] Refracture at the same site following a distal radius fracture is not infrequent if the immobilization is removed too early and the child returns to activities before the lamellar bone has fully remodeled. Outcomes following refracture have been documented as having worse clinical outcomes than fractures that have healed primarily.[47,53] Specifically for girls with low bone mass density and a previous distal forearm fracture, the risk of another distal radius fracture was shown to be 4 times greater than for controls, because bone mineral deposition lags behind increases in body weight and bone length.[54]

OUTCOMES IN YOUNG ADULTS

Once patients have reached skeletal maturity, most extra-articular distal radius fractures have good long-term functional results with conservative treatment if initially reduced to restore anatomic height and inclination. In a 30-year follow-up study in Sweden of young adults with distal radius fractures, of the 28% of study participants who had extra-articular fractures (average age of 31 years at time of fracture, range 18–40), only 37% had even minor complaints of pain, decreased mobility, or cosmetic deformity.[55]

It is difficult to obtain satisfactory results with intra-articular distal radius fractures in young adults. This difficulty is attributable to the development of symptomatic post-traumatic arthritis if treated nonoperatively, with rates reported as high as 40%.[55–57] In a 1986 study by Knirk and Jupiter[58] of intra-articular fractures in young adults (average age at fracture of 28 years) treated either with cast immobilization or pins and plaster, there was radiographic evidence of arthritis in 65% of patients at 7 years' follow-up. Ninety-three percent of those with radiographic arthritis were symptomatic, which the investigators asserted were most commonly the result of a malreduced die-punch fragment. Catalano and colleagues[59] studied 21 patients younger than 45 years who had undergone internal fixation of displaced intra-articular fractures. At an average of 7 years, osteoarthrosis of the radiocarpal joint was radiographically apparent in 76% of wrists.

The ability of young adults to return to work following a distal radius fracture may be one of the most objective parameters by which to assess the epidemiologic impact of these injuries on this population. In the study by Knirk and Jupiter,[58] only 1 of the 40 patients was unable to return to their prior occupation, owing to the residual effects of the distal radius fracture. In the study by Catalano and colleagues,[59] only 1 of 21 patients was unable to continue her current profession as a nurse. Although rates of posttraumatic arthritis may be high in these younger adults, data suggest that these reported symptoms may not significantly affect the livelihood of these patients.

OUTCOMES IN THE ELDERLY

Over the past decade, a multitude of studies have attempted to discover and understand the factors that define treatment options and optimize outcomes in the active elderly patient following a distal radius fracture. However, these factors are often interconnected and are difficult to isolate for evaluation from an epidemiologic perspective. One of the major limiting factors in examining these outcomes is that few studies designate whether the fracture has intra-articular extension. This factor is emerging as an important one in regaining functional motion and strength, rather than absolute measures of fracture alignment and malunion.

Mortality and Functional Decline

Distal radius fractures can be a significant source of mortality and loss of independence in the elderly. In examining the functional status of a prospective cohort of 9000 older women followed through the Study for Osteoporotic Fractures, women with a wrist fracture were 50% more likely than those without fractures to have a clinically important functional decline. This decline was practically defined by worsening ability to prepare meals, perform heavy housekeeping, climb 10 stairs, go shopping, and get out of a car.[60] Mortality rates gathered from the Centers for Disease Control and the National Death Index in patients with a distal radius fracture, compared with a standard United States matched control group, were shown to be significantly higher than those of the standard United States elderly population, an average of a 14% increase 7 years after the fracture.[61] In this study, men with a distal radius fracture were found to be 2.65 times more likely than women with this fracture to die during this time period, likely in part because the largest increase in incidence in men occurred in the over-80-year age group. In practice, this information can provide insight to the patient and family that a distal radius fracture in an elderly man portends worse outcomes than the same fracture in a woman.

Age

Previous radiographic parameters for acceptable reductions in displaced distal radius fractures had been developed using a subset of younger, more active patients. In a 2007 study by Jaremko and colleagues,[62] it was asserted that these factors had not been appropriately validated for the "elderly" in their study (average age 68.5 years), and had little effect on self-reported functional outcomes in short-term follow-up in nonoperative cases. In a retrospective study of 114 patients (average age 79 years) who met operative criteria for unstable distal radius fracture, but for whom 63 declined surgery, Mattila and colleagues[63] found no significant differences in functional outcomes or pain at 5 years. A recent meta-analysis of more than 1000 distal radius fractures comparing cast immobilization with any operative treatment in patients older than 60 years has shown that despite worse radiographic outcomes associated with casting, functional outcomes were no different from those of surgically treated groups.

Increasing Rates of Operative Interventions

Over the past 10 years there has been an increase in the use of surgical interventions for the treatment of distal radius fractures.[63,64] Although this might appear to be directly correlated with the increased incidence of these fractures seen in recent years, no evidence is available to support such a claim. Mattila and colleagues[63] found that between 1998 and 2008, the use of surgical intervention for the treatment of distal radius fractures doubled. There was also an increase in the use of internal fixation over other techniques, which more than doubled over the 11-year period of the study.

A recent 10-year review of Medicare data conducted by Chung and colleagues[64] documented trends in the treatment of distal radius fractures in the elderly. Closed fixation was found to be the most prevalent form of fracture fixation, but the use of this treatment protocol has decreased from 82% to 70% over the past 10 years. It was also documented that distal radius fractures are increasingly being treated by hand surgeons, with rates increasing from 0.8% to 3.9% during the study period. In addition, hand surgeons were shown to be more likely to use internal fixation in the treatment of these fractures. In contrast, orthopedic surgeons were found to be 5.7 times more likely than hand surgeons to use closed treatment. This finding coincides with that of a study by Koval and colleagues[65] showing hand surgeons leaning toward the use of internal fixation in preference to closed treatment. There is evidence that more than 50% of fractures treated with closed reduction are plagued by malunion, which highlights why it is important that distal radius fractures should be evaluated on a case-by-case basis.[66,67]

The increased tendency for surgical manipulation in recent years has been coupled with a shift in favor of open reduction and internal fixation over other treatment options. Although this new treatment is exciting, no conclusive evidence has shown it to be more effective than any other treatment protocol. It is not clear why this increase is occurring, but it may be due to the fact that more distal radius fractures are being treated by hand surgeons. It also may be the result of increasingly successful marketing schemes directed toward surgeons, or even just the excitement that comes with the novelty of a new technology. Whatever the case, numerous studies have made it clear that there is no significant difference between the long-term functional outcomes of open reduction and internal fixation and available other therapeutic options for these fractures.[68-71] Although some of these studies found that the volar locking plate did provide better short-term outcomes, the long-term results remained the same.

Seeking to answer some of these difficult surgical treatment questions in the elderly, the WRIST (Wrist and Radius Injury Surgical Trial) study group was formed in 2009, comprising 19 centers across North America with participation from both plastic and orthopedic hand surgeons.[72] The group collaborated on the study design and pilot trials, and obtained funding from the National Institutes of Health to investigate the outcomes of volar locking plates in comparison with other forms of surgical fixation through a multicenter clinical trial (MCCT). This MCCT design, obtained through consensus, structures a rigorous study protocol, collects a diverse patient sample, and recruits a large number of patients to detect smaller treatment effects.

A Dartmouth study of more than 100,000 Medicare patients between 1998 and 2004 showed internal fixation rates close to doubling, from 5% to 8% nationally across all ages. More interestingly, the type of operative fixation was extremely variable between hospital referral regions, with internal fixation ranging from 0.4% to 25% in some areas.[73] These major differences in treatment rates are not unexpected given the variability in fracture patterns at the distal radius, numerous treatment options available, and the lack of consensus in the literature regarding treatment outcomes.

The most recent article to explore the use of internal fixation for distal radius fractures in the Medicare population examined regional variations, ethnic variability, and treating-physician characteristics to better understand the factors contributing to the changing trends.[74] In 2007, the investigators found that nearly 86,000 Medicare patients suffered a closed distal radius fracture, of whom 17% were treated with internal fixation. This rate is over 2 times that of internal fixation from a 6-year time period ending just 3 years before the study. It was also found that men were significantly less likely to receive internal fixation than were women, as were blacks in comparison with whites. Like the Dartmouth study, there was also a nearly 10-fold difference in the rates of internal fixation across different hospital referral regions. The study then examined these differences by region based on whether the patient was treated by a hand surgeon, finding significant positive correlations between the rates of internal fixation and the percentage of patients treated by a hand surgeon in each area.

Osteoporosis Treatment and Risk of Future Fracture

Distal radius fractures in the active elderly population can be one of the first indicators of underlying osteoporosis, and the event represents a prime point for intervention. In the year following a distal radius fracture, studies have shown 5 and 10 times greater rates of vertebral fractures in women and men, respectively, in accordance with a 60% increase in the rates of hip fractures for women older than 70 years.[75] It can be argued that the easiest distal radius fracture to treat is the one that does not happen, and several fall-prevention initiatives in the active elderly have been both successful and cost effective in preventing distal radius fractures.[76,77] Other simple preventive measures include warnings for dangerous weather conditions and clearing or preventing accumulation of snow and ice to decrease the incidence of falls resulting in this injury.[36]

The elderly population has several options to aid in the prevention of distal radius fractures. One of the most important preventive measures is the proper diagnosis and treatment of bone diseases such as osteoporosis and osteopenia. However, in a study of 111 patients in the military medical system to determine rates of osteoporosis follow-up in the year following a distal radius fracture, it was discovered that only 66% received some sort of intervention for osteoporosis. One-quarter of the patients were referred to endocrinology, 20% had a dual-emission x-ray absorptiometry scan, and only 47% had been taking some sort of medication to treat their osteoporosis.[78]

The use of bisphosphonates (BPs) in combination with supplements such as calcium and vitamin D has been shown to help decrease the risk of fractures caused by osteopenia and osteoporosis. BPs are the most common therapy protocol for the treatment of bone resorption resulting from the effects of osteoporosis and other bone diseases.[79–85] Osteoporosis is a leading risk factor for distal radius fractures, and the use of BPs has played an important role in reducing this risk. Research is currently providing new insights into the exact mechanism of action that gives BPs their antiresorptive properties.[86]

BPs are able to increase bone mineral density through the inhibition of osteoclastic bone resorption by altering upstream differentiation of osteocytes in addition to promoting the apoptosis of these osteoclasts.[87] Because of the suppressive actions they have on bone remodeling, it was originally theorized that BPs would disrupt the healing process of fractures. It has been shown that this is not the case, and in fact BPs stimulate bone remodeling by promoting the recruitment and activity of osteoblasts and osteocytes while decreasing apoptosis of these cells.[88] This activity causes an increase in bone mineral density, which can result in up to a 50% decrease in the risk of future fractures.[89] A recent study found less than a 1-week difference in the rate of distal radius fracture healing for those taking BPs and those not taking them (55 days vs 49 days), a difference thought to be not clinically significant.[90]

Recent reports have highlighted that BP treatment is not without risk, despite an estimated 30 million individuals prescribed BP therapy per year in the United States alone.[91] Known esophageal irritation is common, but atypical subtrochanteric femur fractures are increasingly being reported, primarily in the setting of long-term bisphosphonate use.[92–94] Osteonecrosis of the jaw has also been reported to occur in up to 0.04% of osteoporotic patients on bisphosphonate therapy.[95] The dose-dependency effect is now more clearly defined, but the exact pathogenic role of bisphosphonates in these atypical bone events remains unclear. The physician must weigh the risks and benefits with the patient, but the absolute risk of atypical fracture associated with bisphosphonate use compared with the high risk of osteoporotic fractures is small when compared with the beneficial effects of the drug.

The ability to efficiently and accurately diagnose osteoporosis is another important step that could help decrease medical costs and morbidity of those afflicted by this disease. It would not be cost effective to diagnose and treat everyone, so it is essential that only those at high risk for osteoporosis should be evaluated and treated.

SUMMARY

Possessing knowledge of the incidence and outcomes of distal radius fractures allows the physician to better counsel individual patients and determine the best management to optimize treatment. Although treatment outcomes for pediatric patients and young adults are fairly well defined for distal radius fractures, recent research in the elderly population has made decision making for the patient and surgeon more complex. It is becoming increasingly difficult to define the difference between the active older adult who will continue to place high demands on an injured wrist, and the true elderly patient who may better adapt to an imperfect outcome. Large multicenter studies, such as the WRIST study, with long-term follow-up may be the only way to accurately delineate the best treatment options for an individual based on outcomes for a similar patient population.

REFERENCES

1. Chung KC, Spilson SV. The frequency and epidemiology of hand and forearm fractures in the United States. J Hand Surg Am 2001;26:908–15.
2. Melton L III, Amadio P, Crowson C, et al. Long-term trends in the incidence of distal forearm fractures. Osteoporos Int 1998;8:341–8.
3. de Putter CE, van Beeck EF, Looman CW, et al. Trends in wrist fractures in children and adolescents, 1997-2009. J Hand Surg Am 2011;36:1810–5.e2.
4. Hagino H, Yamamoto K, Ohshiro H, et al. Changing incidence of hip, distal radius, and proximal humerus fractures in Tottori Prefecture, Japan. Bone 1999;24: 265–70.
5. Thompson PW, Taylor J, Dawson A. The annual incidence and seasonal variation of fractures of the distal radius in men and women over 25 years in Dorset, UK. Injury 2004;35:462–6.
6. Larsen CF, Lauritsen J. Epidemiology of acute wrist trauma. Int J Epidemiol 1993;22:911–6.
7. Alffram PA, Bauer GC. Epidemiology of fractures of the forearm. A biomechanical investigation of bone strength. J Bone Joint Surg Am 1962;44:105–14.
8. Knowelden J, Buhr AJ, Dunbar O. Incidence of fractures in persons over 35 years of age. A report to the M.R.C. Working Party on Fractures in the Elderly. Br J Prev Soc Med 1964;18:130–41.
9. Bengner U, Johnell O. Increasing incidence of forearm fractures. A comparison of epidemiologic patterns 25 years apart. Acta Orthop Scand 1985; 56:158–60.
10. Omsland TK, Ahmed LA, Gronskag A, et al. More forearm fractures among urban than rural women: the NOREPOS study based on the Tromso study and the HUNT study. J Bone Miner Res 2011;26: 850–6.
11. Holroyd C, Harvey N, Dennison E, et al. Epigenetic influences in the developmental origins of osteoporosis. Osteoporos Int 2012;23(2):401–10.
12. Ryan LM, Teach SJ, Searcy K, et al. Epidemiology of pediatric forearm fractures in Washington, DC. J Trauma 2010;69:S200–5.
13. Kelsey J, Praemer A, Nelson L, et al. Upper extremity disorders: frequency, impact, and cost. New York: Churchill Livingstone; 1997.
14. Shauver MJ, Yin H, Banerjee M, et al. Current and future national costs to Medicare for the treatment of distal radius fracture in the elderly. J Hand Surg Am 2011;36:1282–7.
15. Landin LA. Fracture patterns in children. Analysis of 8,682 fractures with special reference to incidence, etiology and secular changes in a Swedish urban population 1950-1979. Acta Orthop Scand Suppl 1983;202:1–109.
16. Cooper C, Dennison EM, Leufkens HG, et al. Epidemiology of childhood fractures in Britain: a study using the general practice research database. J Bone Miner Res 2004;19:1976–81.
17. Rennie L, Court-Brown CM, Mok JY, et al. The epidemiology of fractures in children. Injury 2007;38: 913–22.
18. Ward WT, Rihn JA. The impact of trauma in an urban pediatric orthopaedic practice. J Bone Joint Surg Am 2006;88:2759–64.
19. Khosla S, Melton LJ 3rd, Dekutoski MB, et al. Incidence of childhood distal forearm fractures over 30 years: a population-based study. JAMA 2003; 290:1479–85.
20. Hagino H, Yamamoto K, Ohshiro H, et al. Increasing incidence of distal radius fractures in Japanese children and adolescents. J Orthop Sci 2000;5:356–60.
21. Mathison DJ, Agrawal D. An update on the epidemiology of pediatric fractures. Pediatr Emerg Care 2010;26:594–603 [quiz: 4–6].
22. Wood AM, Robertson GA, Rennie L, et al. The epidemiology of sports-related fractures in adolescents. Injury 2010;41:834–8.
23. Bailey DA, Wedge JH, McCulloch RG, et al. Epidemiology of fractures of the distal end of the radius in children as associated with growth. J Bone Joint Surg Am 1989;71:1225–31.
24. Caspersen CJ, Pereira MA, Curran KM. Changes in physical activity patterns in the United States, by sex and cross-sectional age. Med Sci Sports Exerc 2000;32:1601–9.
25. Krabbe S, Christiansen C, Rodbro P, et al. Effect of puberty on rates of bone growth and mineralisation: with observations in male delayed puberty. Arch Dis Child 1979;54:950–3.
26. Rizzoli R, Bonjour JP, Ferrari SL. Osteoporosis, genetics and hormones. J Mol Endocrinol 2001;26: 79–94.
27. Henry YM, Fatayerji D, Eastell R. Attainment of peak bone mass at the lumbar spine, femoral neck and radius in men and women: relative contributions of bone size and volumetric bone mineral density. Osteoporos Int 2004;15:263–73.
28. Faulkner RA, Davison KS, Bailey DA, et al. Size-corrected BMD decreases during peak linear growth: implications for fracture incidence during adolescence. J Bone Miner Res 2006;21:1864–70.
29. Parfitt AM. The two faces of growth: benefits and risks to bone integrity. Osteoporos Int 1994;4:382–98.
30. Al-Ansari K, Howard A, Seeto B, et al. Minimally angulated pediatric wrist fractures: is immobilization without manipulation enough? CJEM 2007;9: 9–15.
31. Brogren E, Petranek M, Atroshi I. Incidence and characteristics of distal radius fractures in a southern Swedish region. BMC Musculoskelet Disord 2007;8:48.
32. Court-Brown CM, Caesar B. Epidemiology of adult fractures: A review. Injury 2006;37:691–7.

33. Griffin MR, Ray WA, Fought RL, et al. Black-white differences in fracture rates. Am J Epidemiol 1992; 136:1378–85.

34. Baron JA, Barrett J, Malenka D, et al. Racial differences in fracture risk. Epidemiology 1994;5:42–7.

35. Baron JA, Karagas M, Barrett J, et al. Basic epidemiology of fractures of the upper and lower limb among Americans over 65 years of age. Epidemiology 1996;7:612–8.

36. Flinkkila T, Sirnio K, Hippi M, et al. Epidemiology and seasonal variation of distal radius fractures in Oulu, Finland. Osteoporos Int 2011;22:2307–12.

37. Sigurdardottir K, Halldorsson S, Robertsson J. Epidemiology and treatment of distal radius fractures in Reykjavik, Iceland, in 2004. Comparison with an Icelandic study from 1985. Acta Orthop 2011;82:494–8.

38. Vogt MT, Cauley JA, Tomaino MM, et al. Distal radius fractures in older women: a 10-year follow-up study of descriptive characteristics and risk factors. The study of osteoporotic fractures. J Am Geriatr Soc 2002;50:97–103.

39. World Health Organization. Assessment of fracture risk and its application to screening for postmenopausal osteoporosis. Report of a WHO Study Group. World Health Organ Tech Rep Ser 1994;843:1–129.

40. Kanterewicz E, Yanez A, Perez-Pons A, et al. Association between Colles' fracture and low bone mass: age-based differences in postmenopausal women. Osteoporos Int 2002;13:824–8.

41. Lofman O, Hallberg I, Berglund K, et al. Women with low-energy fracture should be investigated for osteoporosis. Acta Orthop 2007;78:813–21.

42. Oyen J, Rohde GE, Hochberg M, et al. Low-energy distal radius fractures in middle-aged and elderly women-seasonal variations, prevalence of osteoporosis, and associates with fractures. Osteoporos Int 2010;21:1247–55.

43. Oyen J, Brudvik C, Gjesdal CG, et al. Osteoporosis as a risk factor for distal radial fractures: a case-control study. J Bone Joint Surg Am 2011;93:348–56.

44. Oyen J, Rohde G, Hochberg M, et al. Low bone mineral density is a significant risk factor for low-energy distal radius fractures in middle-aged and elderly men: a case-control study. BMC Musculoskelet Disord 2011;12:67.

45. Melton LJ 3rd, Christen D, Riggs BL, et al. Assessing forearm fracture risk in postmenopausal women. Osteoporos Int 2010;21:1161–9.

46. Clayton RA, Gaston MS, Ralston SH, et al. Association between decreased bone mineral density and severity of distal radial fractures. J Bone Joint Surg Am 2009;91:613–9.

47. Price CT, Scott DS, Kurzner ME, et al. Malunited forearm fractures in children. J Pediatr Orthop 1990;10:705.

48. Fuller D, McCullough C. Malunited fractures of the forearm in children. J Bone Joint Surg Br 1982; 64:364.

49. Noonan KJ, Price CT. Forearm and distal radius fractures in children. J Am Acad Orthop Surg 1998;6:146–56.

50. Randsborg P-H, Sivertsen EA. Distal radius fractures in children: substantial difference in stability between buckle and greenstick fractures. Acta Orthop 2009;80:585–9.

51. Do TT, Strub WM, Foad SL, et al. Reduction versus remodeling in pediatric distal forearm fractures: a preliminary cost analysis. J Pediatr Orthop B 2003;12:109–15.

52. Vince K, Miller J. Cross-union complicating fracture of the forearm. Part II: Children. J Bone Joint Surg Am 1987;69:654.

53. Arunachalam V, Griffiths J. Fracture recurrence in children. Injury 1975;7:37–40.

54. Goulding A, Grant AM, Williams SM. Bone and body composition of children and adolescents with repeated forearm fractures. J Bone Miner Res 2005;20:2090–6.

55. Kopylov P, Johnell O, Redlund-Johnell I, et al. Fractures of the distal end of the radius in young adults: a 30-year follow-up. J Hand Surg Br 1993;18:45–9.

56. Cooney WP, Linscheid RL, Dobyns JH. External pin fixation for unstable Colles' fractures. J Bone Joint Surg Am 1979;61:840–5.

57. Green DP. Pins and plaster treatment of comminuted fractures of the distal end of the radius. J Bone Joint Surg Am 1975;57:304–10.

58. Knirk JL, Jupiter JB. Intra-articular fractures of the distal end of the radius in young adults. J Bone Joint Surg Am 1986;68:647–59.

59. Catalano LJ, Cole RJ, Gelberman RH, et al. Displaced intra-articular fractures of the distal aspect of the radius. Long-term results in young adults after open reduction and internal fixation. J Bone Joint Surg Am 1997;79:1290–302.

60. Edwards BJ, Song J, Dunlop DD, et al. Functional decline after incident wrist fractures—study of osteoporotic fractures: prospective cohort study. BMJ 2010;341:c3324.

61. Rozental TD, Branas CC, Bozentka DJ, et al. Survival among elderly patients after fractures of the distal radius. J Hand Surg 2002;27:948–52.

62. Jaremko J, Lambert R, Rowe B, et al. Do radiographic indices of distal radius fracture reduction predict outcomes in older adults receiving conservative treatment? Clin Radiol 2007;62:65–72.

63. Mattila VM, Huttunen TT, Sillanpaa P, et al. Significant change in the surgical treatment of distal radius fractures: a nationwide study between 1998 and 2008 in Finland. J Trauma 2011;71:939–42.

64. Chung KC, Shauver MJ, Birkmeyer JD. Trends in the United States in the treatment of distal radial

fractures in the elderly. J Bone Joint Surg Am 2009; 91:1868–73.

65. Koval KJ, Harrast JJ, Anglen JO, et al. Fractures of the distal part of the radius. The evolution of practice over time. Where's the evidence? J Bone Joint Surg Am 2008;90:1855–61.

66. Mackenney PJ, McQueen MM, Elton R. Prediction of instability in distal radial fractures. J Bone Joint Surg Am 2006;88:1944–51.

67. Strange-Vognsen HH. Intraarticular fractures of the distal end of the radius in young adults. A 16 (2-26) year follow-up of 42 patients. Acta Orthop Scand 1991;62:527–30.

68. Xu GG, Chan SP, Puhaindran ME, et al. Prospective randomised study of intra-articular fractures of the distal radius: comparison between external fixation and plate fixation. Ann Acad Med Singapore 2009; 38:600–6.

69. Wei DH, Raizman NM, Bottino CJ, et al. Unstable distal radial fractures treated with external fixation, a radial column plate, or a volar plate. A prospective randomized trial. J Bone Joint Surg Am 2009;91: 1568–77.

70. Grewal R, Macdermid JC, King GJ, et al. Open reduction internal fixation versus percutaneous pinning with external fixation of distal radius fractures: a prospective, randomized clinical trial. J Hand Surg Am 2011;36:1899–906.

71. Belloti JC, Tamaoki MJ, Atallah AN, et al. Treatment of reducible unstable fractures of the distal radius in adults: a randomised controlled trial of De Palma percutaneous pinning versus bridging external fixation. BMC Musculoskelet Disord 2010;11:137.

72. Chung KC, Song JW. A guide on organizing a multicenter clinical trial: the WRIST study group. Plast Reconstr Surg 2010;126:515.

73. Fanuele J, Koval K, Lurie J, et al. Distal radial fracture treatment: what you get may depend on your age and address. J Bone Joint Surg Am 2009;91: 1313–9.

74. Chung KC, Shauver MJ, Yin H, et al. Variations in the use of internal fixation for distal radial fracture in the United States Medicare population. J Bone Joint Surg Am 2011;93:2154–62.

75. Cuddihy MT, Gabriel SE, Crowson CS, et al. Forearm fractures as predictors of subsequent osteoporotic fractures. Osteoporos Int 1999;9:469–75.

76. Rizzo JA, Baker DI, McAvay G, et al. The cost-effectiveness of a multifactorial targeted prevention program for falls among community elderly persons. Med Care 1996;34:954.

77. Kelsey JL, Prill MM, Keegan TH, et al. Reducing the risk for distal forearm fracture: preserve bone mass, slow down, and don't fall! Osteoporos Int 2005;16: 681–90.

78. Freedman BA, Potter BK, Nesti LJ, et al. Missed opportunities in patients with osteoporosis and distal radius fractures. Clin Orthop Relat Res 2007; 454:202.

79. Wells GA, Cranney A, Peterson J, et al. Alendronate for the primary and secondary prevention of osteoporotic fractures in postmenopausal women. Cochrane Database Syst Rev 2008;1:CD001155.

80. Wells GA, Cranney A, Peterson J, et al. Etidronate for the primary and secondary prevention of osteoporotic fractures in postmenopausal women. Cochrane Database Syst Rev 2008;1:CD003376.

81. Wells G, Cranney A, Peterson J, et al. Risedronate for the primary and secondary prevention of osteoporotic fractures in postmenopausal women. Cochrane Database Syst Rev 2008;1:CD004523.

82. Rodan GA, Fleisch HA. Bisphosphonates: mechanisms of action. J Clin Invest 1996;97:2692–6.

83. Cummings SR, Karpf DB, Harris F, et al. Improvement in spine bone density and reduction in risk of vertebral fractures during treatment with antiresorptive drugs. Am J Med 2002;112:281–9.

84. Reid IR, King AR, Alexander CJ, et al. Prevention of steroid-induced osteoporosis with (3-amino-1-hydroxypropylidene)-1, 1-bisphosphonate (APD). Lancet 1988;1:143–6.

85. Saag KG, Emkey R, Schnitzer TJ, et al. Alendronate for the prevention and treatment of glucocorticoid-induced osteoporosis. Glucocorticoid-Induced Osteoporosis Intervention Study Group. N Engl J Med 1998;339:292–9.

86. Lomashvili KA, Monier-Faugere MC, Wang X, et al. Effect of bisphosphonates on vascular calcification and bone metabolism in experimental renal failure. Kidney Int 2009;75:617–25.

87. Hughes DE, Wright KR, Uy HL, et al. Bisphosphonates promote apoptosis in murine osteoclasts in vitro and in vivo. J Bone Miner Res 1995;10: 1478–87.

88. Plotkin LI, Weinstein RS, Parfitt AM, et al. Prevention of osteocyte and osteoblast apoptosis by bisphosphonates and calcitonin. J Clin Invest 1999; 104:1363–74.

89. Harris ST, Watts NB, Genant HK, et al. Effects of risedronate treatment on vertebral and nonvertebral fractures in women with postmenopausal osteoporosis: a randomized controlled trial. Vertebral Efficacy With Risedronate Therapy (VERT) Study Group. JAMA 1999;282:1344–52.

90. Rozental TD, Vazquez MA, Chacko AT, et al. Comparison of radiographic fracture healing in the distal radius for patients on and off bisphosphonate therapy. J Hand Surg Am 2009;34:595–602.

91. Masoodi NA. Oral bisphosphonates and the risk for osteonecrosis of the jaw. Br J Med Pract 2009;2:11–5.

92. Lenart BA, Lorich DG, Lane JM. Atypical fractures of the femoral diaphysis in postmenopausal women taking alendronate. N Engl J Med 2008; 358:1304–6.

93. Rizzoli R, Åkesson K, Bouxsein M, et al. Subtro-chanteric fractures after long-term treatment with bisphosphonates: a European Society on Clinical and Economic Aspects of Osteoporosis and Osteoarthritis, and International Osteoporosis Foundation Working Group report. Osteoporos Int 2011; 22:1–18.

94. Schilcher J, Michaëlsson K, Aspenberg P. Bisphosphonate use and atypical fractures of the femoral shaft. N Engl J Med 2011;364:1728–37.

95. Cartsos VM, Zhu S, Zavras AI. Bisphosphonate use and the risk of adverse jaw outcomes: a medical claims study of 714,217 people. J Am Dent Assoc 2008;139:23–30.

Common Myths and Evidence in the Management of Distal Radius Fractures

Rafael J. Diaz-Garcia, MD, Kevin C. Chung, MD, MS*

KEYWORDS

- Distal radius fracture • Radiocarpal joint
- Open reduction internal fixation • Distal radioulnar joint
- Evidence-based medicine

Distal radius fractures (DRFs) are common injuries that have a substantial impact on health care systems. They represent the most common fracture treated by physicians, with an incidence of greater than 640,000 cases annually in the United States alone.[1] The bimodal distribution of this injury shows two peaks, one representing high-energy injuries in the young and the other representing low-impact injuries in osteoporotic elderly individuals. This latter group is expanding because the modern-day elderly generation is more active than its predecessors, and life expectancies are increasing. Thus, with a 10% incidence of DRFs in Caucasian women older than 65 years, the number of these fractures can only increase as the baby boomers enter retirement age.[2] Consequently, physicians treating patients with this injury must have a complete understanding of the effectiveness, risks, and benefits of the different management options available.

DRFs have been a topic of discussion in the medical literature since Petit and Pouteau[3] brought them to light in the early 18th century. Before their work that established the entity of DRF, upper extremity deformities at the radiocarpal joint were believed to be caused by wrist dislocations and subluxations. However, because of poor dissemination of their works outside of France, Abraham Colles[4] and the medical community at large were unaware of their theories when Colles published his seminal work, "On the Fracture of the Carpal Extremity of the Radius," in 1814, and therefore he is most often rewarded with the eponym.[4] Great strides have been made over the past 2 centuries in better understanding the biomechanics of injury patterns and the kinematics and muscle forces that influence fracture stability. Device innovation has led to a wide array of options for percutaneous fixation, external fixation, and internal fixation. Although options have greatly increased, little definitive evidence exists regarding the superiority of one technique over the others.

In the 1990s, the *Journal of the American Medical Association* ushered in a revolutionary age in the practice of medicine with the concept of evidence-based medicine. The concept seems obvious enough: that clinical decision making should be basis on evidence from clinical research, thus removing emphasis from intuition and unsystematic clinical experience.[5] However, this paradigm shift has been more difficult to realize in the surgical specialties, where clinical questions often lack high-quality evidence, and randomized controlled trials are expensive and time-consuming. Several myths regarding the management of DRFs have been dogmatic in training programs and are pervasive among clinicians at large, and may affect the outcome of treatment and value of health care investment (**Table 1**).

This work was supported in part by a grant from the National Institute of Arthritis and Musculoskeletal and Skin Diseases, and National Institute on Aging (R01 AR062066) and a Midcareer Investigator Award in Patient-Oriented Research (K24 AR053120) to Dr Kevin C. Chung.

Section of Plastic Surgery, Department of Surgery, The University of Michigan Health System, 2130 Taubman Center, 1500 East Medical Center Drive, Ann Arbor, MI 48109, USA
* Corresponding author.
E-mail address: kecchung@umich.edu

hand.theclinics.com

Table 1
Summary table of the best available evidence regarding common myths in DRF management

Common Myths of DRFs	Conclusions of Best Available Evidence
1. DRF classifications have practical value	Classification systems are complex and nonstandardized They lack intrarater and interrater reliability They lack prognostic information
2. Anatomic reduction is necessary for good outcomes	Most patients with DRFs have good functional outcomes, even with radiographic arthritis
3. Cast immobilization should include the elbow	Use of a sugar tong splint does not prevent displacement over a radial gutter splint
4. Osteoporotic DRFs require rigid fixation	Rigid fixation results in better radiographic outcomes but no significant functional benefit
5. Volar locking plates for DRF have superior outcomes to other rigid fixation	No significant benefit is seen at 1 year with volar locking plate over external fixation
6. Displaced ulnar styloid fractures require ORIF with DRF	Most displaced ulnar styloid fractures do not require ORIF, as long as the DRUJ is stable
7. Autologous bone grafting is superior to alternatives	No significant difference between autograft and substitutes except for complications at the donor site
8. Early mobilization results in better function	Early motion is safe after ORIF, but does not improve functional outcomes

Abbreviations: DRUJ, distal radioulnar joint; ORIF, open reduction internal fixation.

MYTH #1: DRF CLASSIFICATION SCHEMES HAVE PRACTICAL VALUE

The nomenclature used in the discussion of DRFs has gone through several reinventions over the past 200 years, but interestingly, the most archaic terms have withstood the test of time. The Colles eponym, which represents a metaphyseal fracture with dorsal displacement of the distal segment, represents the most commonly used extraarticular classification. Other eponyms, such as Barton and Smith fractures, are also often used, likely because of their historic significance, ease of remembering, and prevalent use. However, eponyms are not helpful in the management of fractures because they do not quantify the severity of the injury nor do they provide guidance on treatment. Furthermore, some eponyms are redundant or lack contemporary context. A prime example is the Chauffeur's fracture, which originated from the torsional injuries experienced by early chauffeurs when cars backfired as they were started with hand cranks in the early 20th century. The same fracture of the radial styloid may also be referred to as a backfire fracture or Hutchinson fracture. This redundancy in naming is confusing, and the reference to hand crank ignitions is only of historic interest.

DRF classification schemes have evolved over time from the eponymous to complex systems based on mechanism or anatomy. Some of the more commonly used schema include the Frykman, the Melone, the Mayo, and the AO classifications.[6–9] Each system has champions who tout its strengths, and detractors who point out its shortcomings, but all of the current classification schemes fail on multiple fronts. No standardized system exists, and one cannot translate easily from one system to another. Each of the classification systems lacks intrarater and interrater reliability because of its complexity.[10–12] Most importantly, these systems do not provide prognostic information or a treatment algorithm to follow when deciding management. For a DRF classification system to have great merit it should: (1) be widely adopted in the literature for research purposes, (2) describe patterns of injury with predictable outcomes, and (3) distinguish which patterns require which specific treatments to guide surgeons. Thus far, no classification system on DRFs satisfies these requirements.

MYTH #2: ANATOMIC REDUCTION IS NECESSARY FOR GOOD FUNCTIONAL OUTCOMES

Regardless of operative or nonoperative management of a fracture, anatomic reduction has been considered the goal to restore normal biomechanics to the preinjury state, particularly in intraarticular DRFs, for which the common belief is that incongruity of the radiocarpal joint must be corrected or functional limitations will result. A significant amount of the credence given to this myth stems from the seminal paper by Knirk and Jupiter[13] entitled "Intra-articular Fractures of the Distal End of the Radius in Young Adults." Although one of the most influential articles in the orthopedic literature, it is often misunderstood and inaccurately referenced.[14] In a retrospective analysis of the data, the authors found that residual intraarticular step-offs after bony union were associated with radiographic findings of arthritis. The presumption of this article is that operative reduction of articular incongruities would prevent the development of radiographic signs of osteoarthritis, and consequently lead to superior outcomes.

Haus and Jupiter[15] revisited this article in 2009, citing its flaws in methodology and limitations in its interpretations. They acknowledged their absence of controls and lack of assessment of observer reliability regarding radiologic analysis of arthritis and articular incongruity. They reviewed their original radiographs, showing that a substantial number of the patients had carpal instability that likely influenced function and promoted the progression to arthritis. Because of a lack of validated instruments at the time of publication, they did not measure patient-rated functional outcomes (eg, Michigan Hand Outcomes Questionnaire[16]; Disability of the Arm, Shoulder and Hand questionnaire [DASH][17]) and correlate them with radiographic findings.

Subsequent authors have addressed some of these questions through assessing for radiographic arthrosis with CT in patients with intraarticular incongruity after DRF, and comparing the radiographic findings with function.[18,19] Even with a 15-year follow-up and worsening radiographic arthritis, patient function remained excellent, and most patients (87.5%) were functioning at the 80th percentile or greater with the injured extremity compared to normal patients. However, even with these findings, the authors did not change their management strategies regarding displaced DRFs, and still aimed to achieve anatomic alignment at the articular surface in hopes of preventing radiographic changes, even in the presence of no discernible functional benefit.

A potential explanation for the lack of a relationship between articular integrity and patient-rated outcomes may be related to publication bias. Most of the outcomes studies published have emanated from high-volume centers that have unique expertise in treating DRFs. It is unlikely that many patients will have markedly unacceptable radiographic reductions in these series that deviate from acceptable norms. Therefore, the number of subjects with poor reductions is so low

that significant relationships are not detected. If population-type data can be obtained to evaluate a spectrum of radiographic findings, reductions that are less than satisfactory are likely to be associated with worse patient-rated outcomes, particularly in the younger population. This hypothesis remains to be tested.

MYTH #3: CAST IMMOBILIZATION AFTER REDUCTION MUST INCLUDE THE ELBOW TO PREVENT REDISPLACEMENT

Various descriptions exist on how immobilization techniques after reduction of a DRF can prevent redisplacement. Some investigators have argued that the brachioradialis is a major deforming force, and consequently, the injured forearm must be splinted in a long arm brace that maintains the forearm in supination to reduce the brachioradialis' influence.[20,21] Others have made a case that the pronator quadratus is more deformational and thus should be splinted in pronation.[22] The sugar tong splint is the most commonly used option for bracing a DRF after reduction. The classic teaching has been that this large and cumbersome splint prevents any movement of the forearm—it prevents flexion/extension at the wrist and elbow and pronation/supination at the distal radioulnar joint (DRUJ)—and that this stability is transferred to the patient's reduction. The largest prospective randomized studies, however, have found no difference in redisplacement risk with inclusion or exclusion of the elbow, and alternatives such as a radial gutter splint can lead to increased patient satisfaction and comfort compared with the sugar tong splint.[23,24]

In reality, the type of splint applied after reduction of a DRF has less impact on redisplacement than one would hope. Although surgeons feel that a sugar tong splint is a defense against losing reduction, the ability of a splint to adequately maintain the reduction of a fracture is more likely to be a product of the initial injury and the instability of the fracture pattern rather than the qualities of the splint itself. A good splint should counter the displacement of the fracture, so that a simple reduced extraarticular Colles fracture can have the reduction maintained with a radial gutter or a dorsal blocking splint with the wrist in slight flexion. More-cumbersome constructs are unlikely to keep unstable reductions from collapsing.

MYTH #4: OSTEOPOROTIC DRFs NECESSITATE RIGID FIXATION BECAUSE OF POOR BONE STOCK

DRFs are of significant concern in elderly individuals, representing a substantial public health impact given that as many as 372,000 individuals 65 years of age and older experience this type of fracture on a yearly basis.[25] Although these fractures have traditionally been treated nonoperatively with casting, a greater than fivefold increase in the use of internal fixation in this population has occurred since 1997.[26] Nonoperative management resulted in malunion in at least 50% of fractures, and with the introduction of the volar locking plate, a movement toward aggressive fixation in the elderly has been seen with the hope of speeding recovery and maximizing a patient's potential to live independently.[27,28] The osteoporotic bone of the dorsal cortex is believed to be prone to collapse, and the disuse from prolonged immobilization is thought to lead to stiffness that impacts long-term function. However, limited prospective comparative studies have evaluated the available treatment modalities.

A systematic review of all the literature over the past 30 years showed that although rigid fixation with external fixation or volar locking plates resulted in improved radiographic outcomes, no evidence of significant benefit was seen in range of motion or functional outcome scores.[25] This form of analysis is limited by the comparison of heterogenic patient groups and the aggregation of data from several case series, yet it serves as a synthesis of the best available evidence. Two ongoing multicenter, randomized, controlled trials, the Open Reduction and Internal Fixation Versus Casting for Highly Comminuted and Intra-articular Fractures of the Distal Radius (ORCHID) trial in Germany and the Wrist and Radius Injury Surgical Trial (WRIST) in the United States, will elucidate the best way to treat this increasing elderly population.[29,30]

MYTH # 5: THE UBIQUITOUS USE OF VOLAR LOCKING PLATES FOR UNSTABLE DRFs IS SUPPORTED BY SUPERIOR OUTCOMES

Since the introduction of volar fixation for unstable DRFs a decade ago, a sizable increase in the number of products available and a steady increase in the national use of the internal fixation procedure have been seen.[31,32] Medicare beneficiaries who are treated by hand surgeons undergo internal fixation at a significantly higher rate than those treated by other physicians.[33] On the surface, one would assume that this increase in the use of a new technique and implant is a reflection of superior outcomes.

Volar fixation has numerous proponents, especially because of fewer tendon complications compared with the dorsal approach.[34] However, few prospective trials have compared it with other operative techniques in the management of unstable DRFs. Evidence shows that management of a DRF with a volar locking plate leads to improved function in range of motion, grip strength, and functional outcome scores compared with external fixation for the first 3 months postoperatively.[35,36] However, those benefits decrease at 6 months and are insignificant if patients are followed out to a full year. Because these studies have been published in only the past 3 years, the dramatic rise in the use of volar locking plates for operative fixation is not a result of evidence of superior outcomes. Instead, this increase is more a manifestation of surgeon factors, such as comfort and ease of a technique, and the variation of operative management is influenced by geography and patient age.[26,37] The lack of long-term superior outcomes of open reduction internal fixation (ORIF) with volar plating reflects an early dissemination of a surgical technique that still requires comparative evidence to validate its use.

MYTH #6: DISPLACED ULNAR STYLOID FRACTURES WARRANT SURGICAL FIXATION AT THE TIME OF RADIUS ORIF

Management of an ulnar styloid fracture in the setting of DRFs is another controversial subject matter. Ulnar styloid fractures are fairly common and have been estimated to be present in more than 50% of DRFs, with approximately a quarter of those proceeding to nonunion.[38] Some authors have argued that a fracture through the base of the ulnar styloid represents a significant injury to the triangular fibrocartilage complex (TFCC) and its ligamentous attachments to the ulna, and thus can result in DRUJ instability.[39,40] Anatomic dissections supported this claim, with evidence that the TFCC and its attachments to the ulnar styloid are important in maintaining a congruous DRUJ.[41] Consequently, some authors recommend that a fracture through the base of the ulnar styloid with a 2-mm displacement or more warrants surgical fixation.[42]

In reality, most ulnar styloid fractures associated with a DRF do not warrant surgical fixation, particularly if anatomic reduction is achieved with open reduction and internal fixation of the distal radius. Nonunion of the ulnar styloid is a common result, but it is usually asymptomatic.[43,44] Even a nonunion at the base of the ulnar styloid with substantial displacement (>2 mm) does not seem to result in an appreciable loss of motion or diminished functional outcome if the concomitant DRF is treated with a volar locking plate and the DRUJ is clinically stable after distal radius fixation.[45–47] Anatomists have recently theorized that this is likely a result of the stabilizing effect of the distal oblique bundle of the interosseous membrane on the DRUJ.[48,49] Undoubtedly, some ulnar styloid fractures result in DRUJ instability, and the literature supports their treatment with operative fixation. However, this is a much smaller subset; the need for surgery cannot be determined with radiographs alone and requires clinical examination and acumen to assess stability.

MYTH #7: AUTOLOGOUS BONE GRAFTING IS SUPERIOR TO ALLOGRAFT OR BONE SUBSTITUTES IN DRF FIXATION WITH BONY LOSS

In treating unstable DRFs with significant metaphyseal comminution, surgeons have often addressed the bony loss through adding some load-bearing substance to fill the defect. Autologous iliac crest bone graft has long been deemed the standard for treating these gaps. It is readily available in both cancellous and cortical forms. It is osteoconductive, osteoinductive, and readily incorporates into the surrounding architecture of the radius. Unfortunately, many problems are associated with autologous bone graft harvest. Iliac bone harvest adds operative time, increases blood loss, has risks for complications, and can result in substantial postoperative pain. The incidence of minor complications is estimated to be 10%, whereas major complications, including hernia, vascular injury, deep infection, and fracture, have an incidence of 5.8%.[50] Furthermore, almost 20% of patients may complain of pain at their donor site as far out as 2 years from surgery.[51]

Given the morbidity of autologous bone harvest, a market is available for industry to create alternatives to meet the demand for a product with fewer side effects. The options are varied and include demineralized bone matrix, bovine collagen, coralline hydroxyapatite, and injectable cements. With such a large number of products available, few comparative data are available to guide a surgeon to choose the most appropriate bone graft material among the options. Rajan and colleagues[52] published the only prospective randomized study comparing the use of cancellous allograft and autologous bone graft in the repair of comminuted DRFs. They found no significant difference in range of wrist motion, grip strength, and radiologic parameters during follow-up of up to a year. Conversely, a sizable discrepancy was seen in operative time and complications at the donor site. Complications included hematoma, seroma, and a relatively high rate of meralgia paresthetica, which is a chronic, painful mononeuropathy caused by entrapment of the lateral femoral cutaneous nerve. Overall, they concluded that use of cancellous allograft at distal radius ORIF was not significantly different from autologous bone grafting regarding fracture union and clinical outcome at the operative wrist, but could be performed more quickly and was not associated with the complications at the iliac donor site.

MYTH #8: EARLY MOBILIZATION RESULTS IN BETTER FUNCTIONAL OUTCOMES IN DRFs

An argument has been commonly made in favor of ORIF because it afforded the patient with an opportunity to start an early motion protocol at 2 weeks rather than waiting 6 to 8 weeks with cast immobilization or external fixation.[53,54] Extrapolating from findings in other periarticular fractures, the thought has been that early mobilization would result in better motion at the wrist and thus better functional results. However, evidence does not support these claims. When other confounders are eliminated and timing of mobilization is viewed as an independent variable, early motion after internal fixation seems to have no benefit. Early wrist mobilization after internal fixation is safe, but it does not improve final arc of motion, grip strength, pain, DASH score, or radiographic measurements.[55,56]

SUMMARY

DRFs remain a public health concern, and this impact is sure to increase as the baby boomer generation enters the elder years. Even with 2 centuries of intellectual discourse regarding the pathophysiology, treatments, and outcomes of DRFs, many questions remain, necessitating further inquiry. Many of the widely held viewpoints regarding the management of DRFs are not based on the best available evidence. Although it is difficult to break practice patterns and easy to be enamored of new instrumentation, clinicians must fight the urge to follow trends indiscriminately without critically evaluating the results. To conform to evidence-based medicine standards, high-powered, randomized, multicenter studies must be designed to further elucidate optimal treatment strategies for DRFs.

REFERENCES

1. Chung KC, Spilson SV. The frequency and epidemiology of hand and forearm fractures in the United States. J Hand Surg Am 2001;26(5):908–15.
2. Cummings SR, Black DM, Rubin SM. Lifetime risks of hip, Colles', or vertebral fracture and coronary heart disease among white postmenopausal women. Arch Intern Med 1989;149(11):2445–8.

3. Peltier LF. Fractures of the distal end of the radius. An historical account. Clin Orthop Relat Res 1984; 187:18–22.

4. Colles A. On the fracture of the carpal extremity of the radius. Edinb Med Surg J 1814;10:182–6.

5. Evidence-Based Medicine Working Group. Evidence-based medicine. A new approach to teaching the practice of medicine. J Am Med Assoc 1992;268: 2420–5.

6. Frykman G. Fracture of the distal radius including sequelae–shoulder-hand-finger syndrome, disturbance in the distal radio-ulnar joint and impairment of nerve function. A clinical and experimental study. Acta Orthop Scand 1967;(Suppl 108):1–155.

7. Melone CP Jr. Articular fractures of the distal radius. Orthop Clin North Am 1984;15(2):217–36.

8. Cooney WP. Fractures of the distal radius. A modern treatment-based classification. Orthop Clin North Am 1993;24(2):211–6.

9. Newey ML, Ricketts D, Roberts L. The AO classification of long bone fractures: an early study of its use in clinical practice. Injury 1993;24(5):309–12.

10. Naqvi SG, Reynolds T, Kitsis C. Interobserver reliability and intraobserver reproducibility of the Fernandez classification for distal radius fractures. J Hand Surg Eur Vol 2009;34(4):483–5.

11. Andersen DJ, Blair WF, Steyers CM Jr, et al. Classification of distal radius fractures: an analysis of interobserver reliability and intraobserver reproducibility. J Hand Surg Am 1996;21(4):574–82.

12. Flikkila T, Nikkola-Sihto A, Kaarela O, et al. Poor interobserver reliability of AO classification of fractures of the distal radius. Additional computed tomography is of minor value. J Bone Joint Surg Br 1998;80(40): 670–2.

13. Knirk JL, Jupiter JB. Intra-articular fractures of the distal end of the radius in young adults. J Bone Joint Surg Am 1986;68(5):647–59.

14. Porrino JA Jr, Tan V, Daluiski A. Misquotation of a commonly referenced hand surgery study. J Hand Surg Am 2008;33(1):2–7.

15. Haus BM, Jupiter JB. Intra-articular fractures of the distal end of the radius in young adults: reexamined as evidence-based and outcomes medicine. J Bone Joint Surg Am 2009;91(12):2984–91.

16. Chung KC, Pillsbury MS, Walters MR, et al. Reliability and validity testing of the Michigan Hand Outcomes Questionnaire. J Hand Surg Am 1998; 23(4):575–87.

17. Gummesson C, Atroshi I, Ekdahl C. The disabilities of the arm, shoulder and hand (DASH) outcome questionnaire: longitudinal construct validity and measuring self-rated health change after surgery. BMC Musculoskelet Disord 2003;4:11.

18. Catalano LW III, Cole RJ, Gelberman RH, et al. Displaced intra-articular fractures of the distal aspect of the radius. Long-term results in young adults after open reduction and internal fixation. J Bone Joint Surg Am 1997;79(9):1290–302.

19. Goldfarb CA, Rudzki JR, Catalano LW, et al. Fifteen-year outcome of displaced intra-articular fractures of the distal radius. J Hand Surg Am 2006;31(4):633–9.

20. Sarmiento A, Pratt GW, Berry NC, et al. Colles' fractures. Functional bracing in supination. J Bone Joint Surg Am 1975;57(3):311–7.

21. Bunger C, Solund K, Rasmussen P. Early results after Colles' fracture: functional bracing in supination vs dorsal plaster immobilization. Arch Orthop Trauma Surg 1984;103(4):251–6.

22. Wahlstrom O. Treatment of Colles' fracture. A prospective comparison of three different positions of immobilization. Acta Orthop Scand 1982;53(2):225–8.

23. Pool C. Colles's fracture. A prospective study of treatment. J Bone Joint Surg Br 1973;55(3):540–4.

24. Bong MR, Egol KA, Leibman M, et al. A comparison of immediate postreduction splinting constructs for controlling initial displacement of fractures of the distal radius: a prospective randomized study of long-arm versus short-arm splinting. J Hand Surg Am 2006;31(5):766–70.

25. Diaz-Garcia RJ, Oda T, Shauver MJ, et al. A systematic review of outcomes and complications of treating unstable distal radius fractures in the elderly. J Hand Surg Am 2011;36(5):824–35 e2.

26. Chung KC, Shauver MJ, Birkmeyer JD. Trends in the United States in the treatment of distal radial fractures in the elderly. J Bone Joint Surg Am 2009; 91(8):1868–73.

27. Mackenney PJ, McQueen MM, Elton R. Prediction of instability in distal radial fractures. J Bone Joint Surg Am 2006;88(9):1944–51.

28. Beharrie AW, Beredjiklian PK, Bozentka DJ. Functional outcomes after open reduction and internal fixation for treatment of displaced distal radius fractures in patients over 60 years of age. J Orthop Trauma 2004;18(10):680–6.

29. Bartl C, Stengel D, Bruckner T, et al. Open reduction and internal fixation versus casting for highly comminuted and intra-articular fractures of the distal radius (ORCHID): protocol for a randomized clinical multicenter trial. Trials 2011;12:84.

30. Chung KC, Song JW. A guide to organizing a multicenter clinical trial. Plast Reconstr Surg 2010;126(2): 515–23.

31. Orbay JL. The treatment of unstable distal radius fractures with volar fixation. Hand Surg 2000;5(2): 103–12.

32. Koval KJ, Harrast JJ, Anglen JO, et al. Fractures of the distal part of the radius. The evolution of practice over time. Where's the evidence? J Bone Joint Surg Am 2008;90(9):1855–61.

33. Chung KC, Shauver MJ, Yin H. The relationship between ASSH membership and the treatment of distal radius fracture in the United States Medicare population. J Hand Surg Am 2011;36(8):1288–93.

34. Lucas G, Fejfar ST. Complications in internal fixation of the distal radius. J Hand Surg Am 1998;23(6):1117.

35. Wilcke MK, Abbaszadegan H, Adolphson PY. Wrist function recovers more rapidly after volar locked plating than after external fixation but the outcomes are similar after 1 year. Acta Orthop 2011;82(1): 76–81.

36. Egol K, Walsh M, Tejwani N, et al. Bridging external fixation and supplementary Kirschner-wire fixation versus volar locked plating for unstable fractures of the distal radius: a randomised, prospective trial. J Bone Joint Surg Br 2008;90(9):1214–21.

37. Fanuele J, Koval KJ, Lurie J, et al. Distal radial fracture treatment: what you get may depend on your age and address. J Bone Joint Surg Am 2009; 91(6):1313–9.

38. Bacorn RW, Kurtzke JF. Colles' fracture; a study of two thousand cases from the New York State Workmen's Compensation Board. J Bone Joint Surg Am 1953;35(3):643–58.

39. Hauck RM, Skahen J III, Palmer AK. Classification and treatment of ulnar styloid nonunion. J Hand Surg Am 1996;21(3):418–22.

40. May MM, Lawton JN, Blazar PE. Ulnar styloid fractures associated with distal radius fractures: incidence and implications for distal radioulnar joint instability. J Hand Surg Am 2002;27(6):965–71.

41. Haugstvedt JR, Berger RA, Nakamura T, et al. Relative contributions of the ulnar attachments of the triangular fibrocartilage complex to the dynamic stability of the distal radioulnar joint. J Hand Surg Am 2006;31(3):445–51.

42. Mikic ZD. Treatment of acute injuries of the triangular fibrocartilage complex associated with distal radioulnar joint instability. J Hand Surg Am 1995;20(2): 319–23.

43. Zenke Y, Sakai A, Oshige T, et al. The effect of an associated ulnar styloid fracture on the outcome after fixation of a fracture of the distal radius. J Bone Joint Surg Br 2009;91(1):102–7.

44. Kim JK, Yun YH, Kim DJ, et al. Comparison of united and nonunited fractures of the ulnar styloid following volar-plate fixation of distal radius fractures. Injury 2011;42(4):371–5.

45. Buijze GA, Ring D. Clinical impact of United versus nonunited fractures of the proximal half of the ulnar styloid following volar plate fixation of the distal radius. J Hand Surg Am 2010;35(2):223–7.

46. Kim JK, Koh YD, Do NH. Should an ulnar styloid fracture be fixed following volar plate fixation of a distal radial fracture? J Bone Joint Surg Am 2010;92(1):1–6.

47. Sammer DM, Shah HM, Shauver MJ, et al. The effect of ulnar styloid fractures on patient-rated outcomes after volar locking plating of distal radius fractures. J Hand Surg Am 2009;34(9):1595–602.

48. Kihara H, Short WH, Werner FW, et al. The stabilizing mechanism of the distal radioulnar joint during pronation and supination. J Hand Surg Am 1995; 20(6):930–6.

49. Noda K, Goto A, Murase T, et al. Interosseous membrane of the forearm: an anatomical study of ligament attachment locations. J Hand Surg Am 2009;34(3):415–22.

50. Arrington ED, Smith WJ, Chambers HG, et al. Complications of iliac crest bone graft harvesting. Clin Orthop Relat Res 1996;329:300–9.

51. Goulet JA, Senunas LE, DeSilva GL, et al. Autogenous iliac crest bone graft. Complications and functional assessment. Clin Orthop Relat Res 1997;339: 76–81.

52. Rajan GP, Fornaro J, Trentz O, et al. Cancellous allograft versus autologous bone grafting for repair of comminuted distal radius fractures: a prospective, randomized trial. J Trauma 2006;60(6): 1322–9.

53. Wright TW, Horodyski M, Smith DW. Functional outcome of unstable distal radius fractures: ORIF with a volar fixed-angle tine plate versus external fixation. J Hand Surg Am 2005;30(2):289–99.

54. Smith DW, Brou KE, Henry MH. Early active rehabilitation for operatively stabilized distal radius fractures. J Hand Ther 2004;17(1):43–9.

55. Lozano-Calderon SA, Souer S, Mudgal C, et al. Wrist mobilization following volar plate fixation of fractures of the distal part of the radius. J Bone Joint Surg Am 2008;90(6):1297–304.

56. Allain J, le Guilloux P, Le Mouel S, et al. Trans-styloid fixation of fractures of the distal radius. A prospective randomized comparison between 6- and 1-week postoperative immobilization in 60 fractures. Acta Orthop Scand 1999;70(2):119–23.

Management of Distal Radius Fractures from the North American Perspective

Albert Yoon, MBChB, Ruby Grewal, MD, MSc*

KEYWORDS

- Distal radius • Fracture • North America • Management

At the time of the last update on distal radius fractures in this journal in 2005, dorsal plating, external fixation, k wiring, volar plating, or combinations of the these were all well-accepted means of operative treatment of displaced distal radius fractures. In the last 5 years, the rate of nonoperative treatment has declined[1] just as the rate of internal fixation has increased, particularly the use of volar locked plates (VLP).[1,2] It is, therefore, no surprise that there has been an abundance of scientific investigation into the costs, outcomes, and complications of the new and old treatment methods for distal radius fractures. Since 2005, more than 140 publications on distal radius fracture management have been produced in North America alone. Most of these have investigated the optimal surgical treatment means, with a particular emphasis on volar plating. This article provides an overview of the scientific investigations originating from North America since 2005 and highlights areas where further research is needed before evidence-based treatment recommendations can be made.

OPERATIVE VERSUS NONOPERATIVE TREATMENT

In North America, the American Academy of Orthopaedic Surgeons (AAOS) approved an evidence-based clinical practice guideline in 2009 regarding the treatment of distal radius fractures.[3] The quality of the evidence behind the recommendations was graded; however, none of the supporting evidence

received a strong recommendation. Only 5 were graded as moderate, whereas 7 were weak and the remainder were inconclusive or based on consensus only. In regard to the role of operative versus nonoperative management, the AAOS suggests surgical fixation for distal radius fractures with postreduction shortening of more than 3 mm, dorsal tilt more than 10°, or intraarticular displacement or step more than 2 mm. In deriving these recommendations, complications of treatment were considered, among other factors. Given that malunion is a commonly reported complication, further research may be able to fine tune these recommendations, especially in some age groups in which radiographic malunion may not always translate into functional disability to patients.[4,5]

The recommendation for surgical fixation for fractures with an intraarticular step of more than 2 mm is based on the original article by Knirk and Jupiter.[6] Their work has been cited in more than 330 articles,[7] and the 2-mm threshold is well accepted. They reported that an intraarticular incongruity of 2 mm or more resulted in radiographic arthrosis in 100% of patients. However, less attention has been paid to the fact that 91% of patients with any degree of incongruity whatsoever also developed arthrosis. Indeed, a recent review of articles that have cited the Knirk and Jupiter article found that a significant number misquoted the importance of a 2-mm incongruity.[8] A recent review of the original article highlighted several methodological flaws related to the

Disclosures: None.

Division of Orthopedic Surgery, University of Western Ontario, Hand and Upper Limb Center, St Joseph's Health Center, Suite D0-217, 268 Grosvenor Street, London, ON N6A 4L6, Canada
* Corresponding author.
E-mail address: rgrewa@uwo.ca

Hand Clin 28 (2012) 135–144
doi:10.1016/j.hcl.2012.02.002
0749-0712/12/$ – see front matter © 2012 Elsevier Inc. All rights reserved.

radiological assessment used in this study.[7] However, the main message of the original article relating to the development of radiographic arthrosis with articular incongruity has been supported by subsequent articles. What has not been proven, however, is the link between a poor radiological outcome following distal radius fracture and poor functional outcome for patients in the long term. Over the last 5 years, treating surgeons have become more aware that it is not yet fully clear which patients with displaced distal radius fractures require surgical intervention, particularly when dealing with older patients.

Goldfarb and colleagues[4] retrospectively reevaluated 16 of their original 21 young adults who had surgical treatment of a displaced intraarticular fracture of the distal radius between 1986 and 1990. They compared their most recent evaluation (at an average of 15 years after surgery) with a previous intermediate evaluation at an average of 7 years after surgery. Patients were assessed functionally with the Musculoskeletal Functional Assessment (MSKFA) and the Hand Function Sort (validated outcomes instrument designed to classify occupations and physical demands in the United States), radiologically with a computed tomography (CT) scan, and with a physical examination to record grip strength and range of motion. The investigators found that although there was progression of radiocarpal arthrosis on CT (arthrosis noted in 13 of 16 patients), grip strength and range of motion were essentially unchanged, and patients continued to function at a high level based on the MSKFA and the Hand Function Sort. Souer and colleagues[9] also found a lack of correlation between radiographic measures and physician-rated or patient-rated outcomes at an average of 22 months. The authors of both of these articles, however, cautioned against complacency regarding the aim of anatomic reduction.

Prospectively, Chung and colleagues[10] found that articular incongruity following VLP fixation of a displaced distal radius fracture was associated with poor functional outcome at 3 months (n = 66), but no association was observed at 1 year (n = 49). It will be interesting to see if a long-term follow-up of this prospective group shows a correlation with articular reduction and functional outcome.

One randomized controlled trial published in 2006 compared closed reduction and casting to external fixation (± percutaneous k wiring) in extraarticular fractures.[11] The trial took place in 3 teaching institutions with 113 patients enrolled between 1994 and 1998. Rather than accepting predetermined levels of radiographic displacement in the nonoperative group, the treatment algorithm for this trial stipulated either repeat closed reduction as necessary (with hematoma block or regional or general anesthesia as required) or crossing over to external fixation at the discretion of the treating surgeon (intention-to-treat analysis performed). As a result, all patients in this trial were deemed to have near anatomic radiographic outcome, and it was not possible to investigate the association between malunion and function. The investigators found no statistical difference between the 2 treatment methods with the Musculoskeletal Functional Assessment, 36-Item Short Form Health Survey (SF-36), Jebsen-Taylor hand function test, or range of motion. The investigators state that a trend to better results with external fixation was seen but admit the trial was underpowered and would require 1200 patients to accurately investigate this difference. A recent Cochrane review came to the similar conclusion that although external fixation prevented collapse and malunion compared with cast immobilization, there is insufficient evidence to suggest a better functional outcome, and there are higher rates of complications, albeit mostly mild.[12] Although there is some interest in early volar plate fixation of initially well-reduced but unstable distal radius fractures,[13] the AAOS is currently unable to recommend for or against surgery in these patients.[3]

Operative Versus Nonoperative Treatment in the Elderly

Regarding the elderly population, the role of operative versus nonoperative treatment of distal radius fractures is unclear. Jaremko and colleagues[14] report on a prospective cohort of 74 patients older than 50 years of age who were managed nonoperatively for a distal radius fracture. There was no statistically significant correlation between the acceptability of radiographic alignment and patient outcome (based on Disabilities of Hand Shoulder and Arm Questionnaire [DASH] and SF-12) in this group. Grewal and MacDermid prospectively followed 216 patients with extraarticular fractures of the distal radius to determine the relationship between alignment and 1-year outcomes (based on the DASH and Patient Rated Wrist Evaluation [PRWE]).[15] The overall alignment was deemed unacceptable if the dorsal angulation was more than 10°, if radial inclination was less than 15°, or if there was 3 mm or more of ulnar positive variance. In patients younger than 65 years of age, malalignment was associated with pain and disability. Although there was no such statistically significant relationship in patients aged 65 years or older, relative risk data did show a higher risk of poor outcome with malalignment at all ages, albeit heavily mitigated in the older age group.

Synn and colleagues[5] retrospectively reviewed 53 patients older than 55 years of age (mean 69 years) with either an intraarticular or extraarticular distal radius fracture. The investigators observed no effect of radiographic displacement on patient outcome. Although surgical treatment reduced the likelihood of dorsal angulation and radial shortening, it did not alter functional outcome. Amarosa and colleagues[16] recently performed a retrospective review of 58 patients who were at least 70 years of age with a distal radius fracture treated either nonoperatively or operatively by a variety of means. The only radiographic parameter that was found to affect DASH or SF-8 scores (at mean 33 month follow-up) was the presence of an ulnar styloid fracture. Egol and colleagues[17] recently performed a retrospective case controlled study comparing operative with nonoperative treatment in patients older than 65 years of age. At 1-year follow-up, there was a significantly better grip strength and radiographic alignment in the operative group, but no difference in DASH or pain scores was seen, and the rate of complications was similar (n = 90).

WHICH OPERATIVE INTERVENTION

There has been much research generated in North America relating to specific surgical techniques and implants for fixation of distal radius fractures since 2005. Although volar plating has received the most attention, reports on experience with dorsal plating, fragment specific fixation, external fixation (both spanning and nonspanning), percutaneous pinning, bridge plating, intramedullary nail fixation, and combinations thereof are numerous. The AAOS has not been able to recommend for or against any one specific surgical method after evaluation of trials directly comparing different methods.[3] An outline of recent North American research regarding some of the available treatment options follows.

Volar Plating

Because VLP is a newer treatment option for distal radius fractures, there have been many studies looking at the patient outcomes with this technique and the specific complications that have arisen. The main proposed advantage of VLP systems is that the implant acts as a fixed-angle device. Cadaveric and synthetic bone models have shown VLP to be as good as or better than dorsal constructs for dorsally unstable distal radius fractures[18–21] and more stable than k-wire fixation.[22]

There have been several prospective studies reporting favorable outcomes with VLP. Jupiter and colleagues[23] prospectively followed 150 patients treated with 2.4-mm VLP for distal radius fractures in a multicenter study. Although dorsal and combined approaches were included, most patients (75%) had a volar-only approach for plating. A participation dropout rate of 22% at 2 years was seen. Of the patients who were assessed, the mean DASH score was 7 and the Gartland and Werley score was 2, indicating little pain and disability. Chung and colleagues[24] also prospectively followed 87 patients at 3, 6, and 12 months after surgery. Fifty-one percent were classed as having AO type C fractures of the distal radius. In this series, there was no loss of reduction radiographically despite hand therapy being initiated within 1 week after surgery. At 12 months, the mean grip strength was 18 kg compared with 21 kg on the contralateral side. At 6 months, Michigan Hand Outcomes Questionnaire domains approached normal scores, with significant functionality evident as early as 3 months. Chung[25] also prospectively compared outcomes of VLP for distal radius fractures in patients aged 20 to 40 years, and those aged 60 years or greater, to assess the use of VLP in older patients. Thirty younger and 25 older patients were enrolled and evaluated up to 12 months after surgery. They found VLP to be equally successful in older patients, with no increase in complication rates.

A retrospective review by Rozental and Blazar[26] also reported favorable outcomes with VLP. They retrospectively reviewed 41 distal radius fracture (AO type A = 18, B = 4, C = 19) at a mean of 17 months. The final average DASH score was 14, and all patients achieved an excellent or good result according to the Gartland and Werley score. Souer and colleagues[27] reported equally good outcomes for volar plating with either a 2.4-mm titanium precontoured locking plate or a 3.5-mm stainless steel locking plate according to the Gartland and Werley score, DASH, and SF-36 in a retrospective review. There was, however, a trend toward better motion at 1 and 2 years with the VLP in this retrospective review.

Complications with VLP

Flexor pollicus longus (FPL) tendon rupture following volar plate fixation of distal radius fractures was initially detailed in case reports[28,29] and is now a well-recognized complication. Prominence of the volar plate at the watershed line, where the flexor tendons lie closest to the bone and plate, has been implicated as a cause of flexor tendon rupture from abrasion.[30] Extensor tendon rupture from distal screws and retention of angled drill guides with volar plating has also been reported.[31,32] In the prospective series by Jupiter and colleagues,[23] 28 complications were reported, including 9 cases of flexor tendonitis after volar plating and 2 tendon ruptures from volar plating. Chung[24] reported 9 surgical complications (5 suture abscess, 2 incision blisters, 1 acute carpal tunnel syndrome, 1 hematoma) and 2 anesthetic complications related to intubation, with no reports of flexor tendon problems. Rozental and Blazar[26] reported 9 complications, including 4 cases of loss of reduction, 3 hardware removals for tendon irritation, 1 case of metacarpal phalangeal joint stiffness, and 1 early wound dehiscence in a patient with severe burns.

Soong and colleagues[33] retrospectively reviewed complications associated with VLP at 2 trauma centers. Early (<1 month) complications (24/594) included 8 intraarticular screws and 7 cases of loss of reduction. Late complications (>6 months) were found in 23 of 321 patients and included flexor or extensor tendon irritation (n = 14), with 1 FPL tendon rupture and 5 cases of subsequent distal radioulnar joint surgery for malunion, synostosis, or stiffness. Plate type and treatment by high-volume surgeons were found to be predictive of late complications. The investigators speculate that high-volume surgeons may have been more likely to detect tendon irritation in later follow-up.

Dorsal Plating

Two outcome assessments of distal radius fractures treated with low-profile dorsal plates were published in 2006. Simic and colleagues[34] retrospectively reviewed the outcomes of 51 distal radius fractures (including 8 AO type C) treated with a precontoured, low-profile stainless steel dorsal plate at a mean of 24 months (minimum 12 months). Thirty-one patients had an excellent Gartland and Werley score and the remainders were good. The average DASH score was 11.9, and there were no cases of extensor tendon irritation or rupture. The mean range of motion was greater than 80% of the contralateral side, and grip strength averaged 90% of the contralateral side. Kamath and colleagues[35] retrospectively reviewed their experience with the same implant in 30 patients at a minimum of 12 months (median 18). A high proportion (70%) were type C fractures, with 16 fractures having a displaced intraarticular step or gap that was corrected by the operation. The mean DASH score was 15, and 28 patients had an excellent or good outcome according to the Gartland and Werley score. One patient required extensor pollicus longus (EPL) tenolysis, but no tendon ruptures were found. Grip strength was 78% of the contralateral side and range of motion was between 81% and 89% of the contralateral side.

External Fixation

Results for bridging and nonbridging external fixation have been previously published. Since 2005, 2 variations of nonbridging external fixation, using supplemental k wires, have been described.[36,37] Good outcomes and a low rate of complications were reported, but a significant benefit in functional outcome over other available treatment options has not yet been described. A 2008 Cochrane review was unable to differentiate the effects of the various methods and materials used in the external fixation of the distal radius.[38]

A randomized prospective trial investigated 3 methods of pin-site wound care and the rate of infection in distal radius fractures treated with external fixation.[39] A power analysis was performed, and a total of 120 patients were enrolled. The investigators found a 19% rate of pin-track complications but no significant difference in the rate of infection with either weekly dry dressing changes, daily pin-site care with a solution of half normal saline and half hydrogen peroxide, or chlorhexidine impregnated discs around the pins that were changed weekly by the surgeon. Increased age was found to be associated with an increased risk of infection. The investigators recommend the use of dry sterile dressings for pin-track care following external fixation.

Pins

K-wire fixation of distal radius fractures has long been used in a variety of techniques. Ebraheim and colleagues[40] report on their experience with 121 patients treated with intrafocal pins and trans-styloid augmentation. It should be noted that comminuted intra-articular fractures treated during this time period were excluded from this retrospective review. Using their modification of the Mayo Wrist Score, 86% of patients younger than 65 years and 81% of patients older than 65 years had an excellent or good result, although the timing of the assessment after surgery is not stated. There were 5 superficial infections, 3 radial nerve neuromas, 2 entrapped EPL tendons, and 2 cases of reflex sympathetic dystrophy. Glickel and colleagues[41] retrospectively reviewed 54 patients at a mean of 59 months after closed reduction and percutaneous pinning. Radial styloid wires were introduced after the identification of the superficial radial nerve and first dorsal compartment, and all wires were aimed across the relevant fracture line as opposed to being intrafocal. It should be noted that all AO type B and AO type C3 fractures were excluded from this retrospective review. At the final review (minimum 22 months), the average DASH score was the same as the normal population and range of motion was close to the uninjured side. A total of 4 complications were seen, including the need for one reoperation after a fall. The investigators concluded that k wiring was an efficacious and cost-efficient treatment option for 2- and 3-part distal radius fractures.

The AAOS currently cannot make a recommendation regarding the number of k wires, or the method of use, when treating displaced distal radius fractures with pinning.[3]

Bridge Plate

The use of an internal spanning plate applied to the dorsum of the radius and the index or middle finger metacarpal has been described previously, but recently 2 further articles confirmed the usefulness of this technique in patients with metaphyseal and diaphyseal comminution. Ruch and colleagues[42] report on 22 patients with high-energy injuries of the distal radius followed prospectively after treatment with a 3.5-mm compression plate applied from the radius to middle finger metacarpal with 3 limited incisions. Ligamentotaxis supplemented with k wire or interfragmentary screw or bone grafting achieved the reduction that was held by the plate for an average of 110 days. Flexion and extension averaged 57° and 65° respectively, and pronation and supination averaged 77° and 76° respectively. The time to removal of the plate did not affect the range of motion or DASH scores at 1 year, and according to the Gartland and Werley rating system, 14 patients had an excellent result, 6 had good results, and 2 had fair results. Hanel and colleagues[43] reported on the Harborview variation of bridge plating that uses a combination of locking and nonlocking 2.4-mm screws to span the dorsum of the index finger to the radius. In their retrospective report, all 62 patients treated with this method healed their fracture and there were only 2 complications. The investigators stress the particular benefits of this technique in high-energy fractures whereby an external fixator becomes a higher risk for infection with longer use and in polytrauma patients who must rely on an injured wrist for early rehabilitation of other serious injuries.

Comparative Studies

There have been many clinical studies comparing various treatment modalities in North America

since 2005. Matschke and colleagues[44] retrospectively reviewed 266 patients treated with VLP (locking compression plate 2.4 mm or 3.5 mm) and 39 patients treated with dorsal plating in a multinational study. A lower incidence of complications was seen in the dorsal group (5%) compared with the volar group (15%), which included 8 cases of tendinitis and 4 tendon ruptures (1 of each in the dorsal group). Although a significantly better range of motion was seen at 6 months in the volar group and significantly better mean Gartland and Werley score at 6 and 12 months, these differences were not seen at 2 years.

Yu and colleagues[45] retrospectively reviewed 104 cases of dorsal (n = 57) and volar (n = 47) plating of the distal radius for fracture or malunion (n = 5 dorsal plates). The follow-up was for a minimum of 1 year (mean 44 months). There was no significant difference in the rate of tendon irritation or rupture between the 2 groups (1 FPL rupture in the volar group), but a higher rate of neuropathic complications in the volar plate group. It will be interesting to see if the greater awareness of, and potential strategies of minimizing complications that have recently been brought to light with volar plating, will aid surgeons using this new technique over the next decade.

Sammer and colleagues[46] prospectively followed 14 patients who received fragment-specific fixation and compared this group with 85 patients prospectively followed at a later date who were treated with a VLP for distal radius fractures. Radiologically, volar tilt was worse in the fragment-specific group (-10° vs 10°), and the majority in this group demonstrated a loss of radial length. The complication rate was also higher in the fragment-specific group. Although the investigators favor the use of VLP in their conclusion, it should be noted that the fragment-specific group contained a higher proportion of AO type C injuries than the volar group. The investigators also note that the subsequent generation of the fragment-specific system now includes a VLP.

A randomized controlled trial (n = 45) by Rozental and colleagues[47] comparing VLP with k-wire fixation (± external fixation) demonstrated significantly lower DASH scores in the volar plate group during the first 3 months postoperatively. However, there were no significant long-term differences in any measured outcome at 1 year.

Four randomized prospective trials comparing external fixation (with or without supplementary k-wire fixation) with open reduction internal fixation (ORIF) have recently been performed in North America. Grewal and colleagues[48] randomized patients with displaced intraarticular distal radius fractures who were younger than 70 years to either dorsal pi plate fixation or external fixation with percutaneous or mini open k-wire fixation. Enrollment in the trial was stopped at midterm analysis because the dorsal plate group had a significantly higher complication rate. Comparison of the 62 enrolled patients also showed significantly higher pain levels and weaker grip strength in the same group, and so treatment with dorsal pi plating was not recommended as an option for treating displaced intraarticular distal radius fractures by the investigators. Wei and colleagues[49] randomized 46 patients to external fixation (22 patients), a locked volar plate (12 patients), or a locked radial column plate (12 patients). At 3 months, the patients who had locked volar plate treatment had significantly better DASH scores than the other 2 groups. At 12 months, the DASH scores were significantly better in the volar plate group (mean score 4) than the radial column group (mean score 18) but not the external fixation group (mean score 18). Egol and colleagues[50] randomized 88 patients to VLP or external fixation with supplementary k-wire fixation. Eleven patients were excluded in the final analysis for a variety of reasons. Fifty-eight percent of the patients in the external fixator group were AO type C compared with 38% in the volar plate group. The range of motion was better early on in the volar plate group, but at 1 year, radiological outcomes, DASH scores, and complication rates were similar between the 2 groups. A recent trial by Grewal and colleagues[51] randomized patients to external fixation (26 patients) or ORIF (27 patients). The method of ORIF changed from dorsal second-generation pi plating early on in the trial to VLP later in enrollment. A more-severe initial injury was suggested by preoperative PRWE scores in the external fixation group, although fracture classification and displacement were reported to be well matched between the 2 groups. The PRWE detected higher pain and disability at 3 months in the external fixation group. A subgroup analysis showed a significant advantage in PRWE scores in patients treated with volar plating compared with dorsal plating or external fixation at all times, including the final review at 1 year.

TREATMENT IN THE ELDERLY POPULATION

The frequency of distal radius fractures in the elderly and the role of treatment is an area of great interest in many parts of the world. In the United States, the rate of internal fixation of distal radius fractures in the elderly covered by Medicare increased from 3% in 1996 to 16% in 2005.[1] Medicare data show that patients older than 85 years were more likely to be treated nonsurgically[1] and a large variation in the treatment method according to geographic region has also been found.[52] Medicare patients treated by surgeons who were members of the American Society for Surgery of the Hand received internal fixation at a significantly higher rate than those treated by surgeons who were not members.[53] Multiple investigators have concluded that the lack of strong evidence regarding the optimal management of distal radius fractures in the elderly was a major reason for such variability.[52,53]

Shauver and Chung and colleagues[54] analyzed Medicare data from 2007 relating to distal radius fractures to accurately quantify the cost of treatment. In the United States, $170 million was spent at an average of $1983 per patient. Internal fixation was the most expensive form of treatment (average $3832 per patient) followed by external fixation ($2890), percutaneous pinning ($2791), and closed treatment ($1459). The investigators project a large increase in cost if internal fixation continues to become a more-frequent treatment method. Shauver and Chung and colleagues[55] performed a separate economic analysis of outcomes and complications in elderly patients with distal radius fractures. In their analysis, patients most preferred ORIF, followed by casting, wire fixation, and external fixation. However, the incremental preference between these 4 modalities was minimal. The incremental cost-utility ratio for ORIF over casting was $15330 per quality-adjusted life years.

Makhni and colleagues[56] compared the radiographic outcomes of distal radius fractures in 3 age groups (18–44, 45–64, and older than 65 years) treated with either cast alone or closed reduction and casting. At the time of union, they found an overall rate of further radiographic displacement in 42% of patients who had cast alone compared with 78% in patients who had reduction and casting. Of the patients who had a reduction and casting, increasing age significantly increased the risk of further displacement. Although the investigators advised close monitoring of expected fracture collapse and the consideration of surgical treatment, there are conflicting results from both current and past studies regarding the correlation between radiographic results and patient outcomes[5,14,17] in elderly patients with distal radius fractures.

Osteoporosis

Within the last 2 years, both the National Osteoporosis Foundation and the National Institutes for Health estimated osteoporosis or fragility fracture to be a major public health threat to more than 40 million Americans.[57] Osteoporosis-related fracture costs to the US health care system are estimated to increase from $19 billion per year in 2005 to more than $25 billion by 2025.[57] In 2007, Barret-Conner and colleagues[58] reported on prospective data from the National Osteoporosis Risk Assessment study showing that a previous wrist fracture increases the relative risk of any future fracture to more than 2 compared with American women who had not had a prior wrist fracture. The National Osteoporosis Foundation 2010 *Clinician's Guide to Prevention and Treatment of Osteoporosis*, which is endorsed by the American Orthopedic Association, recommends a bone mineral density scan in any adult older than 50 years who has a fracture.[57] Similarly, the Scientific Advisory Council of Osteoporosis Canada made a strong recommendation in 2010 that any man or woman older than 50 years who suffers a fragility fracture (any fall from a standing height or less that results in a fracture) should be assessed for osteoporosis.[59]

Despite 91% of patients sustaining a fragility fracture of the distal radius, meeting the World Health Organization's criteria for osteoporosis or osteopenia, a retrospective review of one North American medical hospital showed only 20% of such patients went on to have a dual-energy x-ray absorptiometry (DEXA) scan.[60] The investigators of this 2006 review concluded that orthopedic surgeons missed opportunities to initiate diagnostic and therapeutic interventions for patients presenting with fragility fractures. This worrying trend has continued in North America throughout the years. In 2008, Rozental and colleagues[61] published a rate of referral for a DEXA scan of 21.3% among 240 patients seen with a fragility fracture in their organization. Importantly, they also found in their review that the osteoporosis treatment rate for those patients who did get a DEXA scan was 2.5-fold higher than in those who did not. The investigators followed up on this data with a prospective randomization of 50 patients with fragility fractures to receive either a DEXA scan, ordered by the orthopedic surgeon but to be followed up by the primary care physician, or a letter from the orthopedic surgeon to the primary care physician outlining guidelines for osteoporosis screening. At 6 months, the patients randomized to have the orthopedic surgeon–initiated DEXA scan were almost threefold more likely to have had a discussion of osteoporosis with their primary care physician (89% vs 35%) and initiation of treatment (74% vs 26%).

For those patients already on treatment of osteoporosis, Rozental and colleagues[62] found in a separate article that bisphosphonate use was associated with an increased time to radiographic union but that this time was small (<1 week) and clinically not relevant. The treatment of fragility-related distal radius fractures represents an area of both significant importance and potential for improvement for surgeons in North America and is highly relevant as the population continues to age.

POSTOPERATIVE TREATMENT

Two articles from Massachusetts General Hospital looked at the timing and instruction of mobilization of the wrist after volar plate fixation of distal radius fractures. In the first study, 60 patients were randomized to either early motion within 2 weeks or late motion at 6 weeks after distal radius fracture ORIF with volar plate.[63] The null hypothesis that there was no difference in flexion-extension arc at 3 and 6 months after surgery between the 2 groups was proven. Additionally, there was no significant difference in grip strength, pain, or outcome scores between the early and late motion groups. The AAOS currently has a moderate strength recommendation that patients do not need to begin early wrist motion routinely following stable fracture fixation.

A second randomized controlled trial enrolled 96 patients to investigate the effect of formal occupational therapy versus surgeon-directed independent instruction on wrist function and arm-specific health status 6 months after ORIF of a distal radius fracture with volar plate.[64] At 6 months, there was a significant difference favoring the surgeon-directed instruction group regarding the primary outcome measure of wrist flexion and extension (118° vs 129°). This group also did significantly better at 6 months in terms of ulnar deviation, supination, and grip strength. The investigators thought that patient education by the surgeon and independent exercise was adequate for optimal recovery after distal radius fracture ORIF with volar plating. The AAOS gave a weak recommendation in their clinical practice guidelines that a home-based program is an option for patients prescribed therapy after a distal radius fracture.[3]

SUMMARY AND PRIORITIES FOR FUTURE RESEARCH

There is support in the literature for many surgical methods of distal radius fracture treatment but no clear best practice as of yet. Future, large, multicenter, randomized controlled trials or meta-analyses may provide better evidence for decision making. In the meantime, considerations of cost-effectiveness are made all the more relevant, especially regarding locked volar plating, which has enjoyed a huge surge in popularity in North America without strong supportive level 1 evidence for long-term outcomes. A better understanding of patient functional outcome and expectations has led to a return to the question of whether displaced distal radius fractures are best treated operatively or nonoperatively, especially in the elderly population. Given the high incidence of distal radius fracture, a sufficiently powered randomized controlled trial to help answer this question is a high priority, especially when the aging population and cost to the health care system is considered.

REFERENCES

1. Chung KC, Shauver MJ, Birkmeyer JD. Trends in the United States in the treatment of distal radial fractures in the elderly. J Bone Joint Surg Am 2009; 91(8):1868–73.
2. Koval KJ, Harrast JJ, Anglen JO, et al. Fractures of the distal part of the radius: the evolution of practice over time. Where's the evidence? J Bone Joint Surg Am 2008;90(9):1855–61.
3. Lichtman DM, Bindra RR, Boyer MI, et al. Treatment of distal radius fractures. J Am Acad Orthop Surg 2010;18(3):180–9.
4. Goldfarb CA, Rudzki JR, Catalano LW, et al. Fifteen-year outcome of displaced intra-articular fractures of the distal radius. J Hand Surg Am 2006;31(4):633–9.
5. Synn AJ, Makhni EC, Makhni MC, et al. Distal radius fractures in older patients: is anatomic reduction necessary? Clin Orthop Relat Res 2009;467(6):1612–20.
6. Knirk JL, Jupiter JB. Intra-articular fractures of the distal end of the radius in young adults. J Bone Joint Surg Am 1986;68(5):647–59.
7. Haus BM, Jupiter JB. Intra-articular fractures of the distal end of the radius in young adults: reexamined as evidence-based and outcomes medicine. J Bone Joint Surg Am 2009;91(12):2984–91.
8. Porrino JA Jr, Tan V, Daluiski A. Misquotation of a commonly referenced hand surgery study. J Hand Surg Am 2008;33(1):2–7.
9. Souer JS, Lozano-Calderon SA, Ring D. Predictors of wrist function and health status after operative treatment of fractures of the distal radius. J Hand Surg Am 2008;33(2):157–63.
10. Chung KC, Kotsis SV, Kim HM. Predictors of functional outcomes after surgical treatment of distal radius fractures. J Hand Surg Am 2007;32(1):76–83.
11. Kreder HJ, Agel J, McKee MD, et al. A randomized, controlled trial of distal radius fractures with metaphyseal displacement but without joint incongruity: closed reduction and casting versus closed reduction, spanning external fixation, and optional percutaneous k-wires. J Orthop Trauma 2006;20(2): 115–21.
12. Handoll HH, Huntley JS, Madhok R. External fixation versus conservative treatment for distal radial fractures in adults. Cochrane Database Syst Rev 2007; 3:CD006194.
13. Koenig KM, Davis GC, Grove MR, et al. Is early internal fixation preferred to cast treatment for well-reduced unstable distal radial fractures? J Bone Joint Surg Am 2009;91(9):2086–93.
14. Jaremko JL, Lambert RG, Rowe BH, et al. Do radiographic indices of distal radius fracture reduction predict outcomes in older adults receiving conservative treatment? Clin Radiol 2007;62(1):65–72.
15. Grewal R, MacDermid JC. The risk of adverse outcomes in extra-articular distal radius fractures is increased with malalignment in patients of all ages but mitigated in older patients. J Hand Surg Am 2007;32(7):962–70.
16. Amorosa LF, Vitale MA, Brown S, et al. A functional outcomes survey of elderly patients who sustained distal radius fractures. Hand 2011;6:260–7.
17. Egol KA, Walsh M, Romo-Cardoso S, et al. Distal radial fractures in the elderly: operative compared with nonoperative treatment. J Bone Joint Surg Am 2010;92(9):1851–7.
18. Liporace FA, Gupta S, Jeong GK, et al. A biomechanical comparison of a dorsal 3.5-mm T-plate and a volar fixed-angle plate in a model of dorsally unstable distal radius fractures. J Orthop Trauma 2005;19(3):187–91.
19. McCall TA, Conrad B, Badman B, et al. Volar versus dorsal fixed-angle fixation of dorsally unstable extra-articular distal radius fractures: a biomechanic study. J Hand Surg Am 2007;32(6):806–12.
20. Kandemir U, Matityahu A, Desai R, et al. Does a volar locking plate provide equivalent stability as a dorsal nonlocking plate in a dorsally comminuted distal radius fracture? A biomechanical study. J Orthop Trauma 2008;22(9):605–10.
21. Gondusky JS, Carney J, Erpenbach J, et al. Biomechanical comparison of locking versus nonlocking volar and dorsal T-plates for fixation of dorsally comminuted distal radius fractures. J Orthop Trauma 2011;25(1):44–50.
22. Knox J, Ambrose H, McCallister W, et al. Percutaneous pins versus volar plates for unstable distal radius fractures: a biomechanic study using a cadaver model. J Hand Surg 2007;32(6):813–7.
23. Jupiter JB, Marent-Huber M, LCP Study Group. Operative management of distal radial fractures with 2.4-millimeter locking plates. A multicenter prospective case series. J Bone Joint Surg Am 2009;91(1):55–65.
24. Chung KC, Watt AJ, Kotsis SV, et al. Treatment of unstable distal radial fractures with the volar locking plating system. J Bone Joint Surg Am 2006;88(12): 2687–94.

25. Chung KC, Squitieri L, Kim HM. Comparative outcomes study using the volar locking plating system for distal radius fractures in both young adults and adults older than 60 years. J Hand Surg Am 2008;33(6):809–19.

26. Rozental TD, Blazar PE. Functional outcome and complications after volar plating for dorsally displaced, unstable fractures of the distal radius. J Hand Surg Am 2006;31(3):359–65.

27. Souer JS, Ring D, Matschke S, et al. Comparison of functional outcome after volar plate fixation with 2.4-mm titanium versus 3.5-mm stainless-steel plate for extra-articular fracture of distal radius. J Hand Surg Am 2010;35(3):398–405.

28. Klug RA, Press CM, Gonzalez MH. Rupture of the flexor pollicis longus tendon after volar fixed-angle plating of a distal radius fracture: a case report. J Hand Surg Am 2007;32(7):984–8.

29. Duncan SF, Weiland AJ. Delayed rupture of the flexor pollicis longus tendon after routine volar placement of a T-plate on the distal radius. Am J Orthop 2007;36(12):669–70.

30. Soong M, Earp BE, Bishop G, et al. Volar locking plate implant prominence and flexor tendon rupture. J Bone Joint Surg Am 2011;93(4):328–35.

31. Benson EC, DeCarvalho A, Mikola EA, et al. Two potential causes of EPL rupture after distal radius volar plate fixation. Clin Orthop Relat Res 2006; 451:218–22.

32. Bhattacharyya T, Wadgaonkar AD. Inadvertent retention of angled drill guides after volar locking plate fixation of distal radial fractures. A report of three cases. J Bone Joint Surg Am 2008;90(2):401–3.

33. Soong M, van Leerdam R, Guitton TG, et al. Fracture of the distal radius: risk factors for complications after locked volar plate fixation. J Hand Surg Am 2011;36(1):3–9.

34. Simic PM, Robison J, Gardner MJ, et al. Treatment of distal radius fractures with a low-profile dorsal plating system: an outcomes assessment. J Hand Surg Am 2006;31(3):382–6.

35. Kamath AF, Zurakowski D, Day CS. Low-profile dorsal plating for dorsally angulated distal radius fractures: an outcomes study. J Hand Surg Am 2006;31(7):1061–7.

36. Mirza A, Jupiter JB, Reinhart MK, et al. Fractures of the distal radius treated with cross-pin fixation and a non-bridging external fixator, the CPX system: a preliminary report. J Hand Surg Am 2009;34(4):603–16.

37. Gradl G, Jupiter JB, Gierer P, et al. Fractures of the distal radius treated with a nonbridging external fixation technique using multiplanar k-wires. J Hand Surg Am 2005;30(5):960–8.

38. Handoll HH, Huntley JS, Madhok R. Different methods of external fixation for treating distal radial fractures in adults. Cochrane Database Syst Rev 2008;1:CD006522.

39. Egol KA, Paksima N, Puopolo S, et al. Treatment of external fixation pins about the wrist: a prospective, randomized trial. J Bone Joint Surg Am 2006;88(2): 349–54.

40. Ebraheim NA, Ali SS, Gove NK. Fixation of unstable distal radius fractures with intrafocal pins and trans-styloid augmentation: a retrospective review and radiographic analysis. Am J Orthop 2006;35(8):362–8.

41. Glickel SZ, Catalano LW, Raia FJ, et al. Long-term outcomes of closed reduction and percutaneous pinning for the treatment of distal radius fractures. J Hand Surg Am 2008;33(10):1700–5.

42. Ruch DS, Ginn TA, Yang CC, et al. Use of a distraction plate for distal radial fractures with metaphyseal and diaphyseal comminution. J Bone Joint Surg Am 2005;87(5):945–54.

43. Hanel DP, Lu TS, Weil WM. Bridge plating of distal radius fractures: the Harborview method. Clin Orthop Relat Res 2006;445:91–9.

44. Matschke S, Wentzensen A, Ring D, et al. Comparison of angle stable plate fixation approaches for distal radius fractures. Injury 2011;42(4):385–92.

45. Yu YR, Makhni MC, Tabrizi S, et al. Complications of low-profile dorsal versus volar locking plates in the distal radius: a comparative study. J Hand Surg Am 2011;36(7):1135–41.

46. Sammer DM, Fuller DS, Kim HM, et al. A comparative study of fragment-specific versus volar plate fixation of distal radius fractures. Plast Reconstr Surg 2008; 122(5):1441–50.

47. Rozental TD, Blazar PE, Franko OI, et al. Functional outcomes for unstable distal radial fractures treated with open reduction and internal fixation or closed reduction and percutaneous fixation. A prospective randomized trial. J Bone Joint Surg Am 2009;91(8): 1837–46.

48. Grewal R, Perey B, Wilmink M, et al. A randomized prospective study on the treatment of intra-articular distal radius fractures: open reduction and internal fixation with dorsal plating versus mini open reduction, percutaneous fixation, and external fixation. J Hand Surg Am 2005;30(4):764–72.

49. Wei DH, Raizman NM, Bottino CJ, et al. Unstable distal radial fractures treated with external fixation, a radial column plate, or a volar plate. A prospective randomized trial. J Bone Joint Surg Am 2009;91(7): 1568–77.

50. Egol K, Walsh M, Tejwani N, et al. Bridging external fixation and supplementary Kirschner-wire fixation versus volar locked plating for unstable fractures of the distal radius: a randomized, prospective trial. J Bone Joint Surg Br 2008;90(9):1214–21.

51. Grewal R, MacDermid JC, King GJ, et al. Open reduction internal fixation versus percutaneous pinning with external fixation of distal radius fractures: a prospective, randomized clinical trial. J Hand Surg Am 2011;36:1899–906.

52. Fanuele J, Koval KJ, Lurie J, et al. Distal radial fracture treatment: what you get may depend on your age and address. J Bone Joint Surg Am 2009; 91(6):1313–9.

53. Chung KC, Shauver MJ, Yin H. The relationship between ASSH membership and the treatment of distal radius fracture in the United States Medicare population. J Hand Surg 2011;36:1288–93.

54. Shauver MJ, Yin H, Banerjee M, et al. Current and future national costs to Medicare for the treatment of distal radius fracture in the elderly. J Hand Surg 2011;36:1282–7.

55. Shauver MJ, Clapham PJ, Chung KC. An economic analysis of outcomes and complications of treating distal radius fractures in the elderly. J Hand Surg 2011;36:1912–8.

56. Makhni EC, Ewald TJ, Kelly S, et al. Effect of patient age on the radiographic outcomes of distal radius fractures subject to nonoperative treatment. J Hand Surg Am 2008;33(8):1301–8.

57. National Osteoporosis Foundation. Available at: http://www.nof.org/node/40. Accessed November 10, 2011.

58. Barrett-Conner E, Sajjan SG, Siris ES, et al. Wrist fracture as a predictor of future fractures in younger versus older postmenopausal women: results from the National Osteoporosis Risk Assessment (NORA). Osteoporos Int 2008;19:607–13.

59. Papaioannou A, Morin S, Cheung A, et al. 2010 clinical practice guidelines for the diagnosis and management of osteoporosis in Canada: summary. CMAJ 2010. Available at: http://www.cmaj.ca/content/early/2010/10/12/cmaj.100771.full.pdf+html?ijkey=edc6c6048e7d4acdc41368fe3f1e622bf5a2deac&keytype2=tf_ipsecsha. Accessed November 10, 2011.

60. Freedman BA, Potter BK, Nesti LJ, et al. Missed opportunities in patients with osteoporosis and distal radius fractures. Clin Orthop Relat Res 2007;454:202–6.

61. Rozental TD, Makhni EC, Day CS, et al. Improving evaluation and treatment for osteoporosis following distal radial fractures. A prospective randomized intervention. J Bone Joint Surg Am 2008;90(5):953–61.

62. Rozental TD, Vazquez MA, Chacko AT, et al. Comparison of radiographic fracture healing in the distal radius for patients on and off bisphosphonate therapy. J Hand Surg Am 2009;34(4):595–602.

63. Lozano-Calderón SA, Souer S, Mudgal C, et al. Wrist mobilization following volar plate fixation of fractures of the distal part of the radius. J Bone Joint Surg Am 2008;90(6):1297–304.

64. Souer JS, Buijze G, Ring D. A prospective randomized controlled trial comparing occupational therapy with independent exercises after volar plate fixation of a fracture of the distal part of the radius. J Bone Joint Surg Am 2011;93:1761–6.

Extra-Articular Fractures of the Distal Radius—A European View Point

A. Karantana, FRCS (Orth), T.R.C. Davis, FRCS*

KEYWORDS

- Extra-articular fracture • Distal radius • European

There is no unified consensus view on the management of distal radius fractures within Europe. This is partially because of the failure of clinical studies to demonstrate overall superiority of one treatment technique over the others. Cochrane reviews have identified no definite functional advantage of percutaneous pinning[1] or external fixation[2] over nonoperative treatment in a below-elbow cast. Furthermore, recent randomized comparative studies have failed to demonstrate a consistent long-term functional benefit of volar plate fixation over less-invasive fixation techniques.[3–5]

Additional factors, not directly attributable to this fracture, also contribute to the lack of consensus in the management of this injury in Europe. They include the very different systems of health care provision and disparity in the availability of resources within the constituent countries of Europe. These differences inevitably result in variations of management, which are not determined by the characteristics of the individual fracture, but the treatment resources available within particular health systems. It is naïve to deny that nonclinical factors, such as cost and operating room availability, contribute to the decision making regarding treatment of fractures of the distal radius. This is especially true because there remains uncertainty as to the criteria that need to be fulfilled to achieve a good functional result. This article therefore does not describe a unified European viewpoint, but the viewpoint of 2 Europeans working within the health care system of 1 European country.

WHAT DETERMINES OUTCOME?

Although many studies have investigated the relationship between extra-articular malunion and outcome after fractures of the distal radius, there is little consensus on the amount of malunion that can be tolerated without loss of function.[6–9] It is generally considered that extra-articular malunion is more problematic in young active people, but clinical experience demonstrates that some young active individuals tolerate malunion of distal radius fractures well, regaining near normal function. Some older, less-active patients, however, experience persistent symptoms with milder amounts of malunion. Thus, there may be factors attributable to the individual that are not necessarily closely related to the anatomic configuration of the radiocarpal and distal radio-ulnar joints after the injury, which contribute to the final outcome.[7,10] Nevertheless, most would agree that attempts should be made to achieve union of the fracture in a position that does not cause an unsightly deformity in all but the very elderly and frail.

There is no doubt that aggressive operative intervention results in fewer malunions than closed reduction and immobilization of the fractured wrist in a below-elbow plaster cast.[11] Despite this, many centers continue to treat most distal radius fractures by closed reduction and immobilization in plaster. Even though many fractures redisplace in the weeks following initial reduction, most achieve good functional outcomes and few ever require secondary reconstructive surgery,

University Department of Trauma and Orthopaedics, Queens Medical Campus, Nottingham University Hospitals, Nottingham NG7 2UH, UK
* Corresponding author.
E-mail address: tim.davis@nuh.nhs.uk

Hand Clin 28 (2012) 145–150
doi:10.1016/j.hcl.2012.03.001
0749-0712/12/$ – see front matter © 2012 Elsevier Inc. All rights reserved.

such as corrective osteotomy or surgery to the distal radio-ulnar joint. As an example, one study of dorsally displaced distal radius fractures that were treated nonoperatively by closed reduction found 87% were initially reduced into a good position, but by 5 weeks only 30% remained in satisfactory alignment, defined as less than 10° dorsal tilt and less than 5 mm of shortening. Even so, none of these patients required subsequent corrective osteotomy. At 1 year, the Patient Evaluation Measure functional outcome score (PEM)[12] correlated with radial inclination and shortening, but not dorsal tilt[13]; however, there was no correlation between function and any parameter of malunion at 5-year follow-up.[14]

The journals contain many studies investigating the relationship between functional outcome and malunion. Many fail to find significant correlations between radiographic parameters at fracture union (radial shortening, dorsal angulation, or radial inclination) and outcome measures, such as the Patient Rated Wrist Evaluation questionnaire (PRWE)[6] or the overvalued Gartland and Werley score.[15] Statements such as "despite a high level of radiographic malunion (50%), overall function, range of movement and activities of daily living were not limited" abound.[15] This suggests surprise on the part of the investigators that most likely arises from belief in the dogma that all fractures must unite in near-anatomic alignment to achieve a good result.

In addition, there is lack of consistency in the findings of those studies that do report an effect of malunion on functional outcome. Villar and colleagues[16] found range of motion was influenced by dorsal tilt and shortening, and grip strength correlated with shortening. McQueen and Caspers[17] found dorsal tilt and radial inclination affected function, activities of daily living, and grip strength. In contrast, Keating and colleagues[18] found dorsal tilt, but not loss of radial inclination or shortening, affected grip strength. Trumble and colleagues[9] found radial inclination, but neither shortening nor dorsal tilt, affected function. Gliatis and colleagues[19] found an effect of dorsal tilt, but not shortening or loss of radial inclination, on the PEM score, whereas Earnshaw and colleagues,[13] who studied a similar cohort of patients at the same center, reported loss of radial inclination and shortening, but not dorsal tilt, affected the outcome at 1 year. However, Forward and colleagues[20] found no radiographic parameter of extra-articular malunion affected outcome at a very long follow-up.

Why is there so much disparity in the conclusions of studies attempting to correlate parameters of malunion with functional outcome? The probable answer is that, despite the careful hard work of the investigators, these studies suffer from methodological failings, including some from our own institution.[19] Future studies are required to address the failings of existing work, which are summarized as follows:

- Small study size. Most studies assessing the effect of malunion contain small numbers, and poorly powered studies lead to an increased risk of spurious findings, particularly if multiple statistical analyses are performed.
- Failure to define the original population from which the cases were collected, and to report the percentage eligible for inclusion who were recruited. This omission may mask a recruitment bias (ie, patients with poorer outcomes more willing to enter the study or more likely to attend follow-up).
- Failure to distinguish between fractures in the elderly with osteoporotic bone and limited functional demands, from those in younger age groups with good bone quality and higher functional demands.
- Failure to assess the severity of malunion. Many studies allocate cases to either a "united with malunion" group or a "united with no malunion" group and compare the functional outcomes. These groups encompass great variation and such analysis can produce erroneous results. For example, if the "malunion" group contains some very severe malunions with poor outcomes, these can negatively skew the overall outcome in this group, even if most fractures united with milder degrees of malunion and achieved functional outcomes comparable with those of the "united without malunion" group. It is thus necessary to assess not only whether malunion is present, but also to quantify it when studying its effect on clinical outcome.
- Failure to perform independent outcome assessments using validated outcome tools. Assessors should not be involved in the treatment of the injuries and, in an ideal world, should be unaware of the alignment of the fracture that is often readily discerned by looking at the wrist. Patient-centered functional self-assessment questionnaires, completed by the patients without help, such as the DASH (disabilities of the arm, shoulder, and hand),[21] PRWE,[11] and PEM[12] scores, eliminate observer bias. The Gartland and Werley score,[22] which is still used in some studies, is unsuitable for evaluating

the functional outcome of these fractures because (1) it assesses cosmetic deformity, which disadvantages fractures united in malunion; (2) it places too much weight on objective assessments and too little weight on the subjective assessment by the patient; (3) it considers radiographic features of "post traumatic osteoarthritis," which may be totally asymptomatic and nonprogressive; and (4) it is not entirely clear how to score the radiographic appearance, the range of wrist motion, and the presence of complications, such as carpal tunnel syndrome.

- Failure to assess outcome at fixed time points after injury, such as 8 weeks, 6 months, and 1 year. Instead, outcomes are often reported at "an average of 16 months (range 8 weeks to 5 years)." Most would agree that the clinical outcome of fractures of the distal radius improves with time and consequently average follow-up with a large range is not particularly useful.
- Assessing outcome solely in terms of function. Cost and cost-utility are also important, especially when the person/insurer/government paying for the treatment has a fixed budget. Providers will mostly be concerned with direct costs of treatment, whereas the injured person, if not paying for the health care, will be more concerned with the indirect costs insofar as they effect his or her income. A government health provider who provides sickness benefits will be interested in both.

Trends

In many European countries, as in the United States, increasing numbers of distal radius fractures are now treated operatively.[23] This trend has coincided with the advent of volar locking plates and their increasing popularity. The literature indicates that treatment with volar locking plates may result in better radiographic parameters of reduction than treatment by closed reduction and immobilization in plaster[13] or with percutaneous fixation methods,[24–28] but this has not been uniformly confirmed by randomized studies.[4,5] In addition, although there is evidence to suggest their use leads to an earlier recovery of function, this may not necessarily correspond to an earlier return to work. Randomized controlled studies comparing treatment with locking plates and less-invasive, percutaneous methods of fixation have failed to demonstrate a long-term

benefit, with no difference in functional outcomes at 1 year.[4,5]

A further issue regarding these studies is that they tend to be run in centers with a particular interest in fractures of the distal radius, and, thus, much of the surgery is done by experts. Such studies advise on what can be achieved, but not what would be achieved by less-experienced surgeons with no specialist interest in the distal radius. It is important to recognize that although a fixation device may work well in the hands of an expert and cause few complications, it can be associated with significant complications when used by surgeons who have little experience with these devices. It is also important to note that volar locking plate fixation is not without risks.[29] Many hand surgeons would select treatment of their own fracture with a volar locking plate if it was performed by a colleague who they knew was skilled in the use of the device. If the fracture occurred in a foreign country where they had no influence, however, would they still choose treatment with a volar locking plate by a surgeon whose competence level they did not know, and what would they recommend for treatment of the local population if they had no knowledge of the local surgeons' skill?

Health provision in Europe

As is the case for all of the industrialized world, health care in Europe is facing the significant challenge of delivering equal, efficient, and high-quality health services at affordable cost, at a time when the amount of care to be delivered is starting to exceed the resource base.[30] This crisis has been brought about by the combination of an aging population, increasingly expensive health technology, and rising public expectations.

In some countries, such as in the United Kingdom, most health care is provided by the state and there is a fixed budget that may be insufficient to cover the health needs of the population, or alternatively the health needs as perceived by patients and doctors. In such a situation, rationing inevitably occurs, either openly or overtly, and some treatments that a surgeon would otherwise recommend cannot be provided because of cost constraints. Such funding limitations almost certainly reduce the rate of open operative fixation and encourage the continued use of closed reduction and immobilization in plaster of distal radius fractures in some countries. Furthermore, in many state-funded health systems, hospitals have a fixed budget and are not necessarily paid according to what treatments they perform. As a result, they do not receive supplementary funds for performing operative fixation of these fractures rather than treating them nonoperatively in plaster. In addition, surgeons are typically salaried and not paid according to the type and number of operations they perform. Thus, they have no pecuniary incentive to offer operative rather than nonoperative treatment when there is uncertainty as to whether operative treatment produces better results. Finally, operating theater availability is often restricted in state-funded health systems. In this environment, it is inevitable that a surgeon will not only consider fracture characteristics, but also the availability of theatre time and the surgical expertise available when making the complex decision as to whether a fracture should be treated nonoperatively, with a simple short operation (closed reduction and Kirschner wire fixation) or with a potentially more expensive and lengthy open operative procedure (volar locking plate fixation). It is only human that these issues contribute to decision making.

Incentives are different in privately run health systems predominantly funded by insurance that is paid for either directly by individuals or via employers rather than by the state. In such a setting, hospitals and surgeons are usually paid for "what they do" and thus may be indirectly incentivized to treat fractures of the distal radius more aggressively, as operative fixation of these fractures usually commands superior remuneration rates than nonoperative treatment.

There is no doubt that health expenditure overall is rising and countries worldwide are looking at new methods of controlling costs. These range from a push toward market-orientated incentives, to decisions about the use of particular medical therapies by government regulators and health care providers, based on an evaluation of cost. In the setting of fractures of the distal radius, we have only recently begun to consider cost and utility comparisons.[31] We may assume that one method of fixation is cheaper than another based on direct costs,[32] but without the evidence arising from well-designed and adequately powered trials with appropriate and relevant outcome measures, the truth is that we do not actually know which method is most cost-effective.

Expectations of Outcome

Patients can reasonably expect the treatment of their distal radius fracture to have a low risk of serious complications, result in union in a position that does not cause a significant cosmetic deformity, and provide a good long-term outcome with restoration of the previous level of function. They can also reasonably hope for only a short period of incapacity when they are restricted in normal day-to-day activities at home and may also be unable to work. The purchaser (government or insurance company) of the treatment may have different expectations, which are population-based rather than centered on the individual. The purchaser would wish the treatment chosen to result in most patients achieving good outcomes, with few very poor outcomes and a cost that is reasonable and within the constraints of the available budget. The purchaser may not be as concerned as the individual by the speed of recovery, as a slow recovery affects the patient's more than the purchaser's financial situation. In addition, a faster recovery may require more expensive treatment. This is also the case in state-funded systems if, as in the United Kingdom, the health service receives no reward for returning the patient to work earlier and therefore reducing benefit payments and improving work force productivity. A quicker return to work, therefore, does not affect the amount of funding provided to the health system by the government. Thus, the provider wishes an affordable treatment that will result in satisfactory outcomes for most patients.

From a different view point, if the health purchaser is a patient who is paying directly for his or her treatment, he or she will not necessarily elect to undergo the most expensive treatment, even if it is thought to provide the best chance of achieving a fast recovery of function and an excellent long-term result. This may be because he or she does not have, or does not wish to spend, the necessary financial resources and prefers alternative treatment at a lower cost, in the knowledge that it provides a good functional outcome in most cases.

SUMMARY

Fractures of the distal radius are common and their frequency will increase with our aging populations. Despite this, the optimal management of distal radius fractures remains a topic for discussion. The advent and popularity of volar locking plate fixation has refueled the debate and stimulated a number of randomized studies to compare the outcomes of different treatment modalities. The results and conclusions of these studies may or may not be what we expect. The uncertainty about the long-term relevance of varying degrees of extra-articular malunion is unlikely to be resolved in the near future. As is the case with any new and successful fixation method, our natural enthusiasm must be checked by robust evidence and logic.

A Rolls Royce car provides the most comfortable ride, but this does not mean that everyone chooses or can afford to drive one (or is given one by the state). Most would select a more affordable car that gets one to one's destination, possibly with a few more bumps than would have been experienced in the Rolls. We should remember that even the most expensive car can be involved in a serious crash, particularly if driven by an inexperienced driver or taken off-road.

REFERENCES

1. Handoll H, Vaghela MV, Madhok R. Percutaneous pinning for treating distal radial fractures in adults. Cochrane Database Syst Rev 2007;3: CD006080.

2. Handoll H, Huntley JS, Madhok R. External fixation versus conservative treatment for distal radial fractures in adults. Cochrane Database Syst Rev 2007; 3:CD006194.

3. Wei DH, Raizman NM, Bottino CJ, et al. Unstable distal radial fractures treated with external fixation, a radial column plate, or a volar plate. A prospective randomized trial. J Bone Joint Surg Am 2009;91(7): 1568–77.

4. Rozental TD, Blazar PE, Franko OI, et al. Functional outcomes for unstable distal radial fractures treated with open reduction and internal fixation or closed reduction and percutaneous fixation. A prospective randomized trial. J Bone Joint Surg Am 2009;91(8): 1837–46.

5. Egol K, Walsh M, Tejwani N, et al. Bridging external fixation and supplementary Kirschner-wire fixation versus volar locked plating for unstable fractures of the distal radius: a randomised, prospective trial. J Bone Joint Surg Br 2008;90(9):1214–21.

6. Barton T, Chambers C, Bannister G. A comparison between subjective outcome score and moderate radial shortening following a fractured distal radius in patients of mean age 69 years. J Hand Surg Eur Vol 2007;32(2):165–9.

7. Chung KC, Kotsis SV, Kim HM. Predictors of functional outcomes after surgical treatment of distal radius fractures. J Hand Surg Am 2007;32(1): 76–83.

8. Ng CY, McQueen MM. What are the radiological predictors of functional outcome following fractures of the distal radius? J Bone Joint Surg Br 2011; 93(2):145–50.

9. Trumble TE, Schmitt SR, Vedder NB. Factors affecting functional outcome of displaced intra-articular distal radius fractures. J Hand Surg Am 1994;19(2):325–40.

10. Slutsky DJ. Predicting the outcome of distal radius fractures. Hand Clin 2005;21(3):289–94.

11. MacDermid JC, Roth JH, Richards RS. Pain and disability reported in the year following a distal

radius fracture: a cohort study. BMC Musculoskelet Disord 2003;4:24.

12. Macey AC, Burke FD, Abbott K, et al. Outcomes of hand surgery. British Society for Surgery of the Hand. J Hand Surg Br 1995;20(6):841–55.

13. Earnshaw SA, Aladin A, Surendran S, et al. Closed reduction of colles fractures: comparison of manual manipulation and finger-trap traction: a prospective, randomized study. J Bone Joint Surg Am 2002; 84(3):354–8.

14. Farmer JE, Aladin A, Earnshaw SA, et al. Patient outcome five years following colles' fracture. Boston: Orthopaedic Trauma Association; 2007.

15. Young CF, Nanu AM, Checketts RG. Seven-year outcome following Colles' type distal radial fracture. A comparison of two treatment methods. J Hand Surg Br 2003;28(5):422–6.

16. Villar RN, Marsh D, Rushton N, et al. Three years after Colles' fracture. A prospective review. J Bone Joint Surg Br 1987;69(4):635–8.

17. McQueen M, Caspers J. Colles fracture: does the anatomical result affect the final function? J Bone Joint Surg Br 1988;70(4):649–51.

18. Keating JF, Court-Brown CM, McQueen MM. Internal fixation of volar-displaced distal radial fractures. J Bone Joint Surg Br 1994;76(3):401–5.

19. Gliatis JD, Plessas SJ, Davis TR. Outcome of distal radial fractures in young adults. J Hand Surg Br 2000;25(6):535–43.

20. Forward DP, Davis TR, Sithole JS. Do young patients with malunited fractures of the distal radius inevitably develop symptomatic post-traumatic osteoarthritis? J Bone Joint Surg Br 2008;90(5):629–37.

21. Hudak PL, Amadio PC, Bombardier C. Development of an upper extremity outcome measure: the DASH (disabilities of the arm, shoulder and hand) [corrected]. The Upper Extremity Collaborative Group (UECG). Am J Ind Med 1996;29(6):602–8.

22. Gartland JJ Jr, Werley CW. Evaluation of healed Colles' fractures. J Bone Joint Surg Am 1951;33(4): 895–907.

23. Chung KC, Shauver MJ, Birkmeyer JD. Trends in the United States in the treatment of distal radial fractures in the elderly. J Bone Joint Surg Am 2009; 91(8):1868–73.

24. Marcheix PS, Dotzis A, Benko PE, et al. Extension fractures of the distal radius in patients older than 50: a prospective randomized study comparing fixation using mixed pins or a palmar fixed-angle plate. J Hand Surg Eur Vol 2010;35(8):646–51.

25. Wright TW, Horodyski M, Smith DW. Functional outcome of unstable distal radius fractures: ORIF with a volar fixed-angle tine plate versus external fixation. J Hand Surg Am 2005;30(2):289–99.

26. Oshige T, Sakai A, Zenke Y, et al. A comparative study of clinical and radiological outcomes of dorsally angulated, unstable distal radius fractures

in elderly patients: intrafocal pinning versus volar locking plating. J Hand Surg Am 2007;32(9):1385–92.

27. Jubel A. Functional outcome following fixed-angle volar plating of intra-focal K-wire fixation for extraarticular fractures of the distal part of the radius. Eur J Trauma 2005;31:44–50.

28. McFadyen I, Field J, McCann P, et al. Should unstable extra-articular distal radial fractures be treated with fixed-angle volar-locked plates or percutaneous Kirschner wires? A prospective randomised controlled trial. Injury 2011;42(2):162–6.

29. Diaz-Garcia RJ, Oda T, Shauver MJ, et al. A systematic review of outcomes and complications of treating unstable distal radius fractures in the elderly. J Hand Surg Am 2011;36(5):824–835.e2.

30. Jakubowski E. Health care systems in the EU. A comparative study. Edited by Research, D. G. f. L-2929 Luxembourg: European Parliament; 1998.

31. Shauver MJ, Clapham PJ, Chung KC. An economic analysis of outcomes and complications of treating distal radius fractures in the elderly. J Hand Surg Am 2011;36(12):1912–8 e1–3.

32. Shyamalan G, Theokli C, Pearse Y, et al. Volar locking plates versus Kirschner wires for distal radial fractures—a cost analysis study. Injury 2009;40(12):1279–81.

An Asian Perspective on the Management of Distal Radius Fractures

Sandeep J. Sebastin, MCh (Plastic)[a],*,
Kevin C. Chung, MD, MS[b]

KEYWORDS

• Asia • Distal radius fracture • Epidemiology • Wrist fracture

One of the earliest descriptions of the management of patients with distal radius and other fractures is found in *Xian Shou Li Shang Xu Duan Mi Fang* (Secrets of treating wounds and rejoining fractures handed down by a fairy), written by a Taoist priest Master Lin of the Tang dynasty (841–846) in China. It describes position, fixation, exercise, and medication as the major methods in the treatment of patients with fractures as well as depicts the method of external local immobilization with small splints and the idea of integrating immobilization and exercise. Another early description of the treatment of distal radius fractures is in a book titled *Shi Yi De Xiao Fang* (Effective Formulas from Generations of Physicians) written in 1343 by Wei Yilin from Nanfeng in Jiangxi province of China.[1] Heo Jun (**Fig. 1**) (1546–1615), a royal physician in Korea compiled a book known as the *Dong Eui Bo Gam* (Mirror of eastern medicine). He clearly defines early treatment and support after reduction in the management of distal radius fractures: "if the bone is broken or joint dislocated, reduction should be applied under the application of an anesthetic drug… immobilization with wood boards and intermittent joint motion should be started, if not

motional deficit will remain."[2] Despite these early contributions to the management of patients with distal radius fractures from Asia, the vast majority of publications dealing with distal radius fractures are from the Western countries.

The authors had the benefit of a multicultural upbringing and training, that gives them an unique perspective about the differences in the management of patients with distal radius fractures within Asia and how it compares with current treatments in the Western countries. This article discusses these differences from a surgeon and patient perspective. With increasing globalization, the cultural diversity in local populations is only bound to increase. Understanding differences in sociocultural perspectives allows one to understand and treat his/her patients better.

DEFINING ASIA

Asia is a vast continent with an amazing diversity of cultures and varying levels of economic prosperity. For the purpose of this study, the authors included only the Southeast Asian countries excluding Russia, former republics of the Soviet

Disclosure: None of the authors has a financial interest to declare in relation to the content of this article. Supported in part by grants from the National Institute on Aging and National Institute of Arthritis and Musculoskeletal and Skin Diseases (R01 AR062066) and from the National Institute of Arthritis and Musculoskeletal and Skin Diseases (2R01 AR047328-06) and a Midcareer Investigator Award in Patient-Oriented Research (K24 AR053120) (to Dr Kevin C. Chung).

[a] Department of Hand and Reconstructive Microsurgery, National University Hospital, Level 11, NUHS Tower Block, 1E Kent Ridge Road, Singapore 19228
[b] Section of Plastic Surgery, Department of Surgery, The University of Michigan Health System, 1500 E Medical Center Dr., Ann Arbor, MI 48109, USA
* Corresponding author.
E-mail address: sandeepsebastin@gmail.com

Hand Clin 28 (2012) 151–156
doi:10.1016/j.hcl.2012.03.007

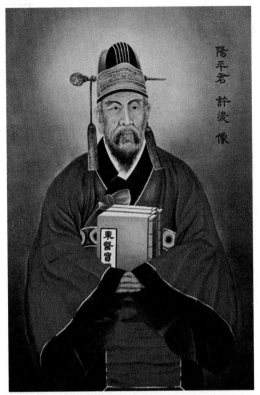

Fig. 1. Heo Jun (1537/1539–1615) was a court physician of the Yangcheon Heo clan during the reign of King Seonjo of the Joseon Dynasty in Korea.

Union, and the Middle Eastern countries. The Southeast Asian countries can be divided into advanced economies and emerging economies based on the level of economic prosperity. The countries with advanced economies include Japan and the 4 Asian Tigers namely Hong Kong (now part of China), Singapore, South Korea, and Taiwan, whereas all the remaining countries in Southeast Asia are countries with emerging economies.[3] Among the countries with emerging economies, China, India, Malaysia, Philippines, and Thailand are considered as newly industrialized (as of 2011).[3] Data regarding distal radius fractures from any of the emerging economies in Asia are limited. A search on pubmed using the term *Distal Radius Fracture* brings up 4200 articles of which approximately 100 articles are from centers in Asia. More than 70% of these articles are from Japan and the remainder from the other advanced economies.

EPIDEMIOLOGY

The epidemiologic features of distal radius fractures vary among populations and are associated with race, socioeconomic status, culture, and degree of urbanization. There have been several population-based studies in Scandinavian countries, United Kingdom, and North America that have presented the epidemiologic characteristics of distal radius fractures.[4–7] These studies demonstrated a bimodal age distribution of these fractures, with peaks of incidence occurring in the youth and in the elderly. Although the overall gender rates were similar, the fractures in men tend to occur in the younger group, whereas there is a preponderance of women in the elderly group because of osteoporosis. Only a few epidemiologic studies on distal radius fractures have been done in Asia.

Taiwan

A population-based study using claims data obtained from the National Health Insurance in Taiwan from 2000 to 2007 revealed a 42.2% overall increase in the incidence of distal radius fractures over the 8-year period (10.2–14.5 per 10,000). Women were at greater risk than men with average incidence rates of 15.1 per 10,000 persons in women and 9.5 per 10,000 persons in men. The incidence rates were lower than those in Northern Europe and America, however, the increasing incidence in the perimenopausal women was similar to that seen in Scandinavia. The authors attribute this to an increase in the prevalence of osteoporosis caused by the changes in lifestyle. The risk of fracture was higher in June and July, and the authors postulated that this was due to typhoons, which commonly occur in the summer months and may increase the risk of fractures associated with fall and slip.[8]

Japan

A study by Hagino and colleagues[9] measured the incidence of distal radius fractures in all adults older than 35 years in the Tottori prefecture of Japan from 1986 to 1987, 1992, and 1995. An increasing trend in the incidence rates of distal radius fractures, especially in women was noted. The age-adjusted incidence rates of distal radius fractures for women were 164.9 in 1986 and 211.4 in 1995, showing a significant increase with time. The investigators also noted that the highest incidence of fracture was in December (winter), although the seasonal trend was not statistically significant.[9,10] Hagino and colleagues[11] mentioned that the use of a traditional futon (as opposed to a bed) was one of the significant factors associated with reduced risk of wrist fractures among the Japanese people, and speculated that spreading futons and putting them away in a closet everyday contributes to the maintenance of muscular strength in the lower limbs, resulting in a reduced risk of falls. The investigators also conducted a similar study in patients younger than 20 years during the same time periods and concluded that the incidence of distal radius fractures in men was higher and had increased over time, peak incidence of fractures corresponded to the period of growth spurt with peaks between 12 and 13 years for men as well as between 10 and 11 years for women, and the incidences peaked in spring and autumn.[12] A similar study done in Niigata prefecture in 2004 suggested an incidence of 76.9 per 100,000 population when adjusted for the Japanese population with a male to female ratio of 1:3.2, and average age at fracture being 60.2 years.[13]

South Korea

There are 2 studies from South Korea that have data regarding the incidence of distal radius fractures obtained from the Korean Health Insurance Review Agency, which covers 97% of the population. However, both these studies deal with distal radius fractures in the elderly (>50 years) and their relationship to osteoporosis. According to these reports, the age-adjusted incidence of distal radius fractures in 2008 was 425 per 100,000 population (164/100,000 population in men and 661/100,000 population in women).

Singapore

Unpublished data from the first author's (SJS) center in Singapore based on a study done from 2008 to 2009 suggests that the incidence of distal radius fractures peaks between the ages of 50 and 60. In men, the peak incidence was between 30 and 50 years of age, whereas in women, the peak incidence was the perimenopausal age group (50–60 years). The sex ratio was 1.3:1 with slightly more distal radius fractures in men compared with women,[14] which is not consistent with that in the previous studies, because this study was not a population study and a large number of men with distal radius fractures were treated after industrial injuries and motor vehicle accidents.

Other Asian Countries

No epidemiologic data are available for any of the other Asian nations. An article on pediatric fractures from India mentions distal radius fractures as the commonest fracture pattern seen in children, accounting for 22.4% of all fractures. In this study, 112 patients with distal radius fractures were treated from a single center in Mumbai between 2004 and 2005 and the highest incidence of distal radius fractures were reported in the 13 to 16 age group followed by the 7 to 12-age group.[15] Similar data were reported from another study on

pediatric fractures from Hong Kong. In this study, 617 patients with distal radius fractures were treated from a single center in Hong Kong over a 5-year period (1986–1990). Distal radius fractures were the commonest fracture accounting for nearly 20% of all fractures, and occurred most frequently in the 8 to 11 age group followed by the 12 to 16 age group.[16]

Based on the available data, it seems that the incidence of distal radius fractures in Asia is lower than those in Europe and America, but similar to those in Australia. A higher incidence of osteoporotic fractures is seen in populations in higher latitudes (North America and Europe), and Asian populations were considered to have a low to moderate risk for osteoporotic fractures.[17] However, it seems that the incidence of osteoporosis-related distal radius fractures is increasing in Asia and similar to the rates described in the west. Epidemiologic studies have indicated that risk factors for distal forearm fractures include low bone mass, estrogen deficiency, falls, drinking alcohol, poor visual acuity, frequent walking, and walking at a brisk pace.[18] These factors combined with an increased proportion of elderly people with weakened bones who are living longer because of better medical care, especially in the advanced economies, may have contributed to this increase.[9]

Access to Health Care

There is a vast difference in the health care systems between the advanced and the emerging economies in Asia. The health care system in the advanced economies namely Hong Kong, Japan, Singapore, South Korea, and Taiwan is on par with the western countries. The people of these countries have access to quality health care that is subsidized by the respective governments. The health care system in the emerging economies faces the challenges of a predominantly rural population, low per-capita income, inadequate transportation capabilities, overcrowding, illiteracy, inadequate resources, and lack of supporting services, such as orthopedic nursing, unstructured referral practice, and a meager health insurance system. Modern orthopedic services and training are most often directed toward the urban population and a majority of the rural population receives their primary treatment from traditional bonesetters. Modern orthopedic treatment has made traditional bone setting obsolete in the advanced economies; however, this practice is prevalent in the emerging economies and is easily accessible and affordable to the poorer sections of society. The traditional bonesetter usually wraps the area with a cloth containing some herbs and applies a tight splint at the fracture site. The splints are usually made of bamboo or a wooden bar. The bonesetter also does not have a fundamental knowledge of anatomy, physiology, or radiography. This treatment often leads to complications, such as acute compartmental syndrome, complex regional pain syndrome, Volkmann contracture, chronic osteomyelitis, gangrene, amputation, tetanus, and rarely death.[19,20]

Availability of Infrastructure

In the advanced economies, the facilities are on par with those in the west. A wide variety of implants, powered drills, and intraoperative fluoroscopy machines are available in all hospitals. Although health care in the emerging economies is either free or heavily subsidized by the government, good facilities and trained manpower are often available only in the major cities. Even in the major cities, the majority of distal radius fractures are managed with some form of traction, reduction, and casting for 4 to 6 weeks. The prohibitive cost of implants makes plate fixation unavailable for most patients. In these centers, patients with complex distal radius fracture patterns who cannot be managed with closed reduction and casting usually undergo percutaneous pin fixation or external fixator application. This combination of factors, namely the patient's financial constraints, use of the cheapest technology available, and the unavailability of intraoperative fluoroscopy makes the treatment of distal radius fractures in the emerging economies suboptimal.

Surgical Training

There is no shortage of well-trained surgeons who are capable of handling varying types of distal radius fractures in the countries with advanced economies. In contrast, there is a lack of appropriate training and shortage of dedicated hand surgeons who can treat injuries of the wrist and distal radius in the countries with emerging economies. Current orthopedic or plastic surgery training in these countries does not adequately prepare the trainees to handle injuries of the wrist and distal radius. Orthopedic trainees are comfortable managing forearm fractures, whereas plastic surgery trainees are comfortable managing hand fractures. The distal radius and the wrist therefore remain a gray area that is poorly understood and treated. Another factor that improves surgical training is funding by the implant manufacturers. The manufacturers usually introduce the use of their implants to surgeons practising in advanced economies. Emerging economies are

less attractive to manufacturers because cost constraints result in the use of fewer implants.

Sociocultural Differences

The authors have noted some differences in the surgeon-patient interaction in Asia and the United States. In the United States, patients are usually more independent and prefer to decide on surgery based on the options presented to them, but in Asia (both advanced and emerging economies), the patients prefer to be guided and the surgeon usually decides what is best for the patient. The discussion regarding other options is usually limited, and the decision-making process is controlled by the surgeon. The plausible reasons for this could be a culture of implicit obedience between patient and surgeon, possible lack of patient education, and greater faith in the surgeon. With increasing westernization, this culture is gradually changing and younger patients in the countries with advanced economies are beginning to question their surgeons more often.

In Asia, patients are usually more reluctant to undergo surgery compared with their western counterparts and frequently accept some deformity to avoid surgery. Patients in Asia also seem to have more implant-related symptoms in the late postoperative period. Patients would often complain about the implant feeling cold during cold/rainy weather and request for removal of implants. Similar complaints are seldom encountered in the west. One possible reason could be that most implants manufacturers are based in Europe or North America and the implants are sized for Caucasian patients. These are usually too large, especially in the small-sized Japanese and Chinese women, and even volar plates can be easily palpated and often require removal. One peculiar question the first author (SJS) faces from patients in Singapore is whether the distal radius plate would set off the alarm in the airport. His department routinely issues a certificate to patients that they can show the airport security staff.

SCOPE FOR IMPROVEMENT
Advanced Economies

There is a large volume of good quality work being done in the 5 Asian countries with advanced economies. However, the scientific basis for treatment of distal radius fractures is still based on evidences from the west. There is an urgent need for these countries to produce better quality publications and move forward from the level 4 case series study design and technique papers. In addition, other areas of research and clinical study designs need to be considered, which include evidence-based medicine and the many options in diagnosis, prognosis, and therapeutic and economic strata. The implant manufacturers also need to consider differences between the wrists of Asians and Caucasians in designing the newer implants. The wrists of Asians are smaller and more mobile when compared with the wrists of Causcasians. This may affect the fracture pattern and the design, shape, and size of the implant. For example, the knee arthroplasty prosthesis in a Japanese population needs to flex more compared with a similar prosthesis designed for the Caucasian population because a Japanese patient needs greater flexion of the knee for his daily activities. Some progress has already been made with a few multicenter randomized-control studies from centers in Hong Kong, Singapore, and Taiwan.[21,22] A recent multimillion dollar, multicenter NIH-funded clinical trial (WRIST, Wrist and Radius Injury Study Group) led by the senior author (KCC) has included 2 centers from Singapore in addition to the 19 centers in North America to study the outcomes of surgical treatment of distal radius fractures in the elderly.[23]

Emerging Economies

The current treatment of distal radius fractures requires a technically up-to-date infrastructure and costly implants. These are usually expensive for the common man in the countries with emerging economies. A viable low-cost alternative in these countries may be to educate and train traditional bonesetters in fracture treatment both to minimize the mismanagement of fractures and to reduce the health care burden on secondary and tertiary institutions.[24] This training can include an introduction of radiographs, recognition of open and displaced fractures, guidance in the approximate duration of fracture healing, recognition of complications of fracture treatment, and the ability to decide when they should refer a patient to the hospital for management. A significant improvement in the knowledge and skills of traditional bonesetters has been seen after completion of this training.[25] Some of the traditional treatment methods have been adopted in medical education in China and India.[26]

In the urban areas of the countries with emerging economies, the emphasis should be on making the treatment of patients with distal radius fractures more affordable. Western implant manufacturers can help by making cheaper stainless steel implants available instead of titanium and allowing local firms to manufacture implants by selective transfer of technology. There is also a need for increased training and exposure of the surgeons in the developing world, which can be accomplished through training fellowships. For example, the National University of Singapore in conjunction with the Lee Foundation offers a fully funded 6-month fellowship (Tan Sri Dr Runme Shaw Fellowship in Hand and Reconstructive Microsurgery) to surgeons from countries in the Association of Southeast Asian Nations (Brunei, Cambodia, Indonesia, Laos, Malaysia, Myanmar, Philippines, Thailand, and Vietnam) to learn hand surgery in one of Singapore's tertiary hospitals. The emerging economies in Asia should contribute actively toward the current literature in distal radius fractures. Surgeons should publish in other avenues instead of the traditional "I did so many cases, and I am presenting complications and my good results." Epidemiologic studies and health services type research on distal radius fracture are needed to assess the barriers to adequate care, disparities of care, the use of costly technology, and sociocultural issues affecting choice of treatment and outcomes.

REFERENCES

1. Wang ZG, Chen P. History and development of traditional Chinese medicine. Beijing (China): IOS Press; 1999.
2. Jupiter JB. Fractures of the distal end of the radius—an historical perspective. IFFSH Ezine 2011;(1):16–7. Available at: http://www.ifssh.info/ezine.html. Accessed March 22, 2012.
3. World Economic Outlook (WEO) Tensions from the two-speed recovery: unemployment, commodities, and capital flows. Washington, DC: International Monetary Fund; 2011. p. 170–5.
4. Sanders KM, Seeman E, Ugoni AM, et al. Age- and gender-specific rate of fractures in Australia: a population-based study. Osteoporos Int 1999;10: 240–7.
5. Solgaard S, Petersen VS. Epidemiology of distal radius fractures. Acta Orthop Scand 1985;56:391–3.
6. vanStaa TP, Dennison EM, Leufkens HG. Epidemiology of fractures in England and Wales. Bone 2001;29:517–22.
7. Owen RA, Melton LJ, Johnson KA, et al. Incidence of Colles' fracture in a North American community. Am J Public Health 1982;72:605–7.
8. Muo CH, Fong YC, Lo WY, et al. A population-based study on trend in incidence of distal radial fractures in adults in Taiwan in 2000-2007. Osteoporos Int 2011;22(11):2809–15.
9. Hagino H, Yamamoto K, Ohshiro H, et al. Changing incidence of hip, distal radius, and proximal humerus fractures in Tottori Prefecture, Japan. Bone 1999; 24(3):265–70.

10. Hagino H, Yamamoto K, Teshima R, et al. The incidence of fractures of the proximal femur and the distal radius in Tottori prefecture, Japan. Arch Orthop Trauma Surg 1990;109(1):43–4.

11. Hagino H, Fujiwara S, Nakashima E, et al. Case-control study of risk factors for fractures of the distal radius and proximal humerus among the Japanese population. Osteoporos Int 2004;15:226–30.

12. Hagino H, Yamamoto K, Ohshiro H, et al. Increasing incidence of distal radius fractures in Japanese children and adolescents. J Orthop Sci 2000;5(4): 356–60.

13. Sakuma M, Endo N, Oinuma T, et al. Incidence and outcome of osteoporotic fractures in 2004 in Sado City, Niigata Prefecture, Japan. J Bone Miner Metab 2008;26(4):373–8.

14. Koo KO, Tan DM, Chong AK. Distal radius fractures: an epidemiological review. Spring meeting of British Society for Surgery of the Hand. Manchester (United Kingdom): BSSH; 2010.

15. Tandon T, Shaik M, Modi N. Paediatric trauma epidemiology in an urban scenario in India. J Orthop Surg (Hong Kong) 2007;15(1):41–5.

16. Cheng JC, Shen WY. Limb fracture pattern in different pediatric age groups: a study of 3,350 children. J Orthop Trauma 1993;7(1):15–22.

17. Kanis JA, Johnell O, Laet CD, et al. International variations in hip fracture probabilities: implications for risk assessment. J Bone Miner Res 2002;17: 1237–44.

18. Hagino H. Features of limb fractures: a review of epidemiology from a Japanese perspective. J Bone Miner Metab 2007;25(5):261–5.

19. Agarwal A, Agarwal R. The practice and tradition of bonesetting. Educ Health 2010;23(1):1–8.

20. Memon FA, Saeed G, Fazal B, et al. Complications of fracture treatment by traditional bone setters at Hyderabad. Pak J Orthop 2009;21(2):58–64.

21. Leung F, Tu YK, Chew WY, et al. Comparison of external and percutaneous pin fixation with plate fixation for intra-articular distal radial fractures. A randomized study. J Bone Joint Surg 2008;90(1):16–22.

22. Xu GG, Chan SP, Puhaindran ME, et al. Prospective randomised study of intra-articular fractures of the distal radius: comparison between external fixation and plate fixation. Ann Acad Med Singap 2009; 38(7):600–6.

23. Chung KC, Song JW, WRIST Study Group. A guide to organizing a multicenter clinical trial. Plast Reconstr Surg 2010;126(2):515–23.

24. Omololu B, Ogunlade SO, Alonge TO. The complications seen from the treatment by traditional bonesetters. West Afr J Med 2002;21:335–7.

25. Shah RK, Thapa VK, Jones DH, et al. Improving primary orthopaedic and trauma care in Nepal. Educ Health 2003;16:348–56.

26. Shang TY, Gu YW, Dong FH. Treatment of forearm bone fractures by an integrated method of traditional Chinese and Western medicine. Clin Orthop Relat Res 1987;215:56–64.

Anatomy and Biomechanics of the Distal Radioulnar Joint

Jerry I. Huang, MD*, Douglas P. Hanel, MD

KEYWORDS

- Biomechanics • Distal radioulnar joint • Instability

The distal radioulnar joint (DRUJ) is a complex diarthrodial articulation between the ulnar head and sigmoid notch of the distal radius that allows forearm pronation and supination. The longitudinal axis of forearm rotation is along a line that passes between the center of the radial head at the elbow joint and the foveal sulcus at the base of the ulnar styloid distally at the wrist. Forearm rotation involves rotation of the radiocarpal unit around a fixed and stable ulna. There is variation between individual forearm pronation and supination, ranging in total arc of motion from 150 to 180° at the distal radioulnar joint, with up to 30° of rotation through the radiocarpal and midcarpal joints. Because the joint is incongruous, with an ulnar head that is much smaller in circumference than the corresponding arc of the sigmoid notch, the bony articulation only contributes to 20% of the stability of the DRUJ.[1] The soft tissue structures responsible for maintaining stability through forearm rotation are the static constraints and the dynamic muscle stabilizers. The static constraints include the triangular fibrocartilage complex (TFCC), the dorsal radioulnar ligament (DRUL) and volar radioulnar ligament, the ulnar collateral ligament, and the joint capsule. The dynamic muscle stabilizers include the extensor carpi ulnaris tendon and the pronator quadratus muscle.

BONY ANATOMY

The ulnar head has 2 articular surfaces: the seat and the pole, which is commonly referred to as the dome. The ulnar seat articulates with the sigmoid notch of the distal radius, whereas the dome forms the gliding undersurface of the fibrocartilaginous disk of the TFCC. Approximately 220° of the ulnar head is covered in articular cartilage, with 130° of cartilage over the ulnar seat (**Fig. 1**).[2]

The seat of the ulnar head serves as the articular surface for the sigmoid notch around which the distal radius rotates. The sigmoid notch is a shallow concave articular surface with a radius of curvature between 15 and 19 mm, which is nearly twice that of the ulnar head (8–10 mm) (**Fig. 2**A).[2,3] The arc of the sigmoid notch subtends 60°, compared with 100° for the ulnar head (see **Fig. 2**B).[3] The difference in curvature leads to joint incongruity that allows both rotational and translational motion within the DRUJ. In fact, in extremes of forearm rotation, less than 10% of the ulnar head is in contact with the sigmoid notch.[2] In forearm pronation, the distal ulna translates 2.8 mm dorsally, whereas in supination the ulna translates 5.4 mm volarly.[4] In a recent cadaver study using pressure sensors, Ishii and colleagues[5] demonstrated that in neutral forearm rotation with 89 N axial load, 12.5% of the sigmoid notch was in contact with the ulnar head. Pressure is concentrated over the dorsal lip of the distal radius with forearm pronation, and pressure is concentrated volarly with forearm supination.

There is considerable variation in the anatomy of the DRUJ in both the coronal and transverse planes among individuals. In a review of

Department of Orthopaedics and Sports Medicine, University of Washington Medical Center, 4245 Roosevelt Way Northeast, Box 354740, Seattle, WA 98105, USA
* Corresponding author.
E-mail address: jihuang@uw.edu

Hand Clin 28 (2012) 157–163
doi:10.1016/j.hcl.2012.03.002

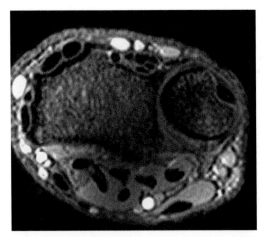

Fig. 1. T2-weighted magnetic resonance image of the DRUJ illustrating the presence of 220° arc of articular cartilage in the ulnar head.

In the transverse plane, there are 4 different types of sigmoid notch morphology. The concavity of the notch can be flat (42%), ski slope (14%), C type (30%), or S type (14%).[3] An extra-articular palmar osteocartilaginous lip that forms a stable buttress to palmar dislocation of the ulna has been found to occur in approximately 80% of wrist specimens (**Fig. 3**).[3] The buttress effect of the palmar lip must be recognized in fractures of the lunate facet in the distal radius. The volar ulnar corner is thought to be the keystone of the distal radius, and the anatomic reduction of this fragment is critical to restoring stability to the radiocarpal joint and DRUJ.

The ulnar seat articular surface represents 44% of the total ulna articular surface area, ranging from 28% to 66%.[3] During resection of areas adjacent to the ulnar seat articular surface, care must be taken to avoid complications that may affect the integrity of the DRUJ. Feldon resection with removal of the ulnar pole may eliminate a significant portion of the ulnar seat, resulting in subsequent instability, which may be especially true in the case of a type III reverse oblique sigmoid notch. Even minimal wafer resection may compromise the stability of the DRUJ.

The distal articular surface, referred to as the dome or pole, can vary from a hemispherical surface to a nearly flat contour. The ulnar styloid is a continuation of the subcutaneous ridge of the ulna on its dorsomedial aspect that varies from 2 to 6 mm in length. The ulnar styloid serves as the origin of the ulnar collateral ligament and the ulnocarpal ligaments, as well as the superficial fibers of the radioulnar ligaments. At the base of the ulnar styloid is a shallow concavity called the fovea, which is devoid of cartilage but abundant with vascular foramina. The fovea represents the geometric center of rotation for the DRUJ. The fovea is also the primary attachment of the

80 radiographs of the wrist, Tolat and colleagues[6] noted 3 basic configurations of the DRUJ in the coronal plane, type I vertical (38%), type II oblique (50%), or type III reverse obliquity (12%). Sagerman and colleagues[7] demonstrated that the inclination of the sigmoid notch and the inclination of the ulnar seat are not parallel in 98% of cases, with a mean difference of 13.3°. The sigmoid notch inclination angle ranged from −24.3 to 26.8 with a mean of 7.7, and the ulnar seat inclination angle ranged from −13.8 to 40.5 with a mean of 21.0. The presence of a reverse obliquity sigmoid notch has significant implications in the treatment of ulnocarpal impaction. Alteration in the relationship of the radius and ulna in an ulnar shortening osteotomy may lead to an increased articular pressure at the proximal edge of the sigmoid notch or cause DRUJ impingement. In the Sagerman series, 8 out of 9 cases with a reverse oblique sigmoid notch had positive ulnar variance.

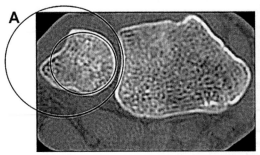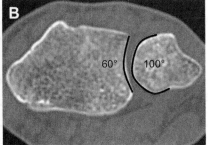

Fig. 2. Axial images of CT scans of the DRUJ demonstrating the articular incongruity between the ulnar head and sigmoid notch that allows for translation in addition to rotation at the articulation. The radius of curvature of the sigmoid notch is nearly 2 times the radius of curvature of the ulnar seat (*A*). The arc of the sigmoid notch subtends 60° compared with 100° of articulation on the ulnar head (*B*).

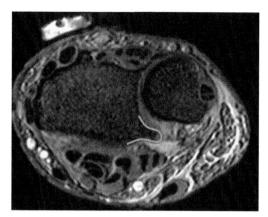

Fig. 3. T2-weighted magnetic resonance image of the DRUJ demonstrating the presence of a palmar osteochondral lip in the sigmoid notch that confers further stability as a buttress.

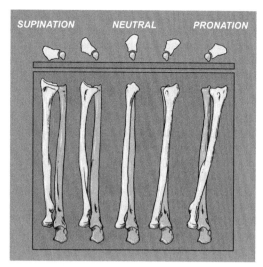

Fig. 4. As the radiocarpal unit rotates around a fixed ulna from supination to pronation, there is proximal migration of the radius, leading to ulnar positive variance in the pronated position. (*Reproduced from* Kleinman WB. Stability of the distal radioulnar joint: biomechanics, pathophysiology, physical diagnosis, and restoration of function what we have learned in 25 years. J Hand Surg Am 2007;32:1086–106; with permission from Elsevier.)

radioulnar and ulnocarpal ligaments. Dorsoradial to the ulnar styloid is a groove that houses the extensor carpi ulnaris tendon.

Ulnar variance is the index of relationship between the radius and ulna at the level of the wrist. Although there is no consensus regarding how best to measure ulnar variance, there is consensus regarding the impact or implication of variance on the mechanics of the DRUJ. Ulnar positive and ulnar minus variance describes the ulna as longer or shorter, respectively, than the radius. In the general population, the mean ulnar variance is slightly negative. However, ulnar variance differs significantly between populations, ranging from 0.7 mm in a volunteer population of black subjects to −0.9 mm in normal white subjects, with no gender differences.[8–11] Most subjects have good symmetry between right and left, with differences in ulnar variance of less than 1 mm.[8] In neutral ulnar variance, 82% of the compressive load in the wrist is transmitted through the radiocarpal joint with 18% being transmitted through the ulnocarpal articulation.[12] With an ulnar positive variance of 2.5 mm, the ulnocarpal load increases to 42%, whereas with 2.5 mm ulnar negative variance, the load is 4.3%.

Under loading conditions and grip, dynamic ulnar variance is an average of 0.9 mm greater than static ulnar variance.[8,13] During forearm pronation, the ulna migrates dorsally and distally relative to the radius, whereas in forearm supination, the ulna migrates volarly and proximally (**Fig. 4**). From full forearm pronation to full forearm supination, the mean decrease in ulnar variance is 1.0 mm.[14] Maximum ulnar variance occurs with gripping in pronation with a dynamic increase of 1.34 mm, compared with ulnar variance with the forearm relaxed in pronation.[15]

SOFT TISSUE INTRINSIC STABILIZERS

The radius and ulna are constrained from proximal to distal by the annular ligament, the interosseous ligament, and the TFCC. The TFCC is a soft tissue complex that includes the ligament complex, which stabilizes the DRUJ during normal forearm rotation, and the fibrocartilage component, which transmits load across the ulnocarpal joint. The TFCC includes the DRUL and palmar radioulnar ligament (PRUL), the articular disk, the ulnocarpal ligaments, the extensor carpi ulnaris tendon subsheath, and the meniscus homolog. Histologic studies have shown a clear distinction between the DRUL and PRUL with longitudinally oriented fibers that extend toward their ulnar insertion and the central articular disc with sheets of collagen fibers arranged in layers at various oblique angles.[16] The articular disk of the TFCC complex extends from the distal rim of the sigmoid notch, along the ulnar edge of the lunate facet, and blends peripherally with the DRUL and PRUL. During forearm rotation, the articular disk undergoes significant deformation with a nonuniform distribution of strain and change in total area.[17] Partial excisions of the articular disk, which do not violate the peripheral 2 mm and that are less than two-thirds of the total disk, have no significant effect on kinematics of the DRUJ or stability of DRUJ.[18]

Blood supply to the TFCC originates from the radiocarpal branches of the ulnar artery and the dorsal and palmar branches of the anterior interosseous artery.[19,20] The DRUL and PRUL are well vascularized, as is the peripheral 15% to 40% of the articular disk.[19–21] The inner central portion of the articular disk is completely avascular, with no vessels crossing its radial attachment. Lesions of the TFCC in the central portion (Palmer 1A and Palmer 2) and avulsions from the radial attachment (Palmer 1D) have little potential for healing. Similarly, the central portion of the TFCC is not innervated. The volar and ulnar portions of the TFCC receive innervation from the ulnar nerve, and the dorsal portion receives sensory branches from the posterior interosseous nerve.[22] A transverse branch from the dorsal ulnar sensory nerve innervates the DRUJ and the overlying skin.[23] Free nerve endings are present in the ulnar aspect of the articular disc, the ulnar collateral ligament, and the meniscal homolog.[24]

The radioulnar ligaments are the primary stabilizers of the DRUJ, which are formed by longitudinal parallel collagen fiber bundles that extend from the dorsal and palmar aspects of the sigmoid notch of the distal radius and converge in a triangular configuration onto the ulna. As each ligament extends ulnarly, it divides into a deep limb attaching to the fovea and a superficial limb attaching to the base of the ulnar styloid. The area between the insertions of the 2 limbs is a highly vascularized connective tissue called the ligamentum subcruentum. Over time, the term ligamentum subcruentum has evolved to represent the deep fibers of the DRUL and PRUL. Fractures at the base of the ulnar styloid involve injury to the superficial limb of the radioulnar ligaments, but may not lead to a significant instability of DRUJ if the deep fibers are intact.

The role of the radioulnar ligaments in the stability of dorsal and palmar DRUJ remains controversial. In 1985, af Ekestam and Hagert[2] performed excision of the central articular disc and sectioning of the DRUL or PRUL. PRUL was found to be important in preventing dorsal subluxation of the ulnar head during forearm pronation, whereas the DRUL was noted to be significant in preventing palmar subluxation of the ulnar head during forearm supination. A subsequent study by Schuind and colleagues[25] in 1991 suggested a contradicting theory on the role of the dorsal and palmar ligaments. By using a stereophotogrammetric method, ligament lengths were measured through full forearm pronation and supination. Color points placed on the superficial aspect of the ligaments were used to determine changes in ligament length and to ascertain

ligament tension. The PRUL was taut with forearm supination, as the ulna translates palmarly; the DRUL was taut with forearm pronation as the ulna translates dorsally. The findings of Schuind and colleagues were supported by Kihara and colleagues[26] in a study analyzing the roles of the DRUL and PRUL as well as the interosseous membrane (IOM) in DRUJ stability during pronation and supination. After complete sectioning of the IOM, the DRUL was found to be more important than the PRUL in stabilizing the DRUJ in pronation, whereas the PRUL was more important in preventing palmar subluxation of the distal ulna in supination. In another cadaveric study using a displacement transducer, Acosta and colleagues[27] demonstrated increased displacement of the dorsal ligament with passive forearm supination and increased displacement of the palmar ligament with supination. Based on the clinical experience and findings of the cadaveric study, the investigators concluded that the dorsal ligaments require repair or reconstruction in patients with dorsal instability of the DRUJ, and those with palmar dislocation require restoration of the PRUL.

In a biomechanical study of 11 cadaveric specimens, Ward and colleagues[28] analyzed the ligament tension of the DRUL and PRUL during forearm rotation as well as the contributions of the IOM, joint capsule, articular disk, and radioulnar ligaments, to translational stability and rotational restraint. A progressive increase in ligament tension was observed in the DRUL with forearm pronation, and increases in tension in the PRUL were observed with forearm supination. Sectioning of the DRUL led to a significant dorsal instability in pronation, whereas sectioning of the PRUL led to instability in supination. This was corroborated in a study by Adams and Holley,[17] analyzing the surface strains of the radial, central, and ulnar, portions of the articular disk. Strains along the radioulnar axis of the articular disk were found to be greatest over the radial portion of the disk. This is consistent with the arthroscopic findings of traumatic TFCC tears occurring most commonly 2 to 3 mm ulnar to its radial insertion on the sigmoid notch.[29,30] Decrease in strain was observed in all 3 regions with forearm supination. Strains along the dorsal margin of the disk increased during pronation, whereas the reverse occurred during supination.

Although the conclusions of af Ekenstam and Hagert[2] seem to be in conflict with those of Schuind and colleagues and others, the role of the superficial and deep fibers of the TFCC complex are clearly defined through careful analysis of the existing literature on biomechanical studies. In 1994, Hagert[31] reconciled the conflicting data from his earlier study and the findings of Schuind and colleagues and Acosta and colleagues in a landmark paper. Hagert's earlier study, with excision of the articular disc, dealt with only the deep components of the radioulnar ligaments inserting on the fovea, whereas Schuind and colleagues only measured tension in the superficial fibers with his phosphorescent markers. Hagert concluded that tightening of the dorsal superficial fibers and the deep palmar fibers of the ligamentum subcruentum is critical for dorsal stability in forearm pronation (**Fig. 5**). The deep fibers of the ligamentum subcruentum, as studied by af Ekenstam, provide intrinsic stability to the DRUJ. During forearm pronation, the superficial DRUL tightens and displaces the ulnar dorsally. With progressive dorsal translation of the distal ulna, the deep PRUL tightens and provides a checkrein for the distal ulna. In addition, through tensioning, the deep fibers of the PRUL pull the distal ulna into the dorsal bony buttress of the sigmoid notch. In contrast, during forearm supination the superficial PRUL fibers pull the distal ulna palmarly. The deep DRUL acts as a checkrein to

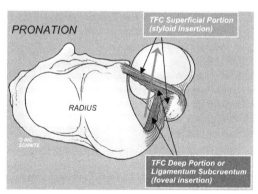

Fig. 5. An illustration showing the changes in the deep and superficial radioulnar ligaments as the distal ulna translates dorsally during forearm pronation. The deep fibers of the ligamentum subcruentum insert on the ulnar fovea whereas the superficial radioulnar ligaments insert on the base of the ulnar styloid. The deep ligaments form a more obtuse angle of attachment compared with the narrow angle of the superficial ligaments. There is tightening of both the dorsal deep fibers of the ligamentum subcruentum and the palmar superficial radioulnar ligament to prevent pathologic dorsal subluxation of the distal ulna. With progressive translation, the ulnar head herniates outside the restraining cover of the superficial fibers (*red arrow*). (*Reproduced from* Kleinman WB. Stability of the distal radioulnar joint: biomechanics, pathophysiology, physical diagnosis, and restoration of function what we have learned in 25 years. J Hand Surg Am 2007;32:1086–106; with permission from Elsevier.)

prevent further palmar translation and pulls the distal ulna into the palmar buttress of the sigmoid notch. Kleinman describes 2 critical anatomic factors supporting the deep ligamentum subcruentum as the more significant structure in DRUJ stability.[32] With full forearm pronation, the distal ulna herniates against the DRUJ capsule, outside the cover of the dorsal superficial radioulnar fibers. Thus, the deep radioulnar ligament is responsible for preventing supraphysiologic translation. Moreover, the more obtuse angle of attack of the deep radioulnar ligament allows the ligament subcruentum to have a biomechanical advantage over the narrow angle of the superficial ligaments in controlling DRUJ stability.

Kleinman and Graham[33] performed cadaveric dissections of the DRUJ capsule to characterize the anatomy of the structure as well as its contribution to forearm rotation and DRUJ stability. They described the DRUJ capsule as a continuous structure that is separate from the TFCC complex, blending seamlessly with the radioulnar ligaments dorsally and palmarly. The inferior portion of the DRUJ capsule is stout, with minimal redundancy, unlike the volar and dorsal fibers more distally, which are more patulous. The volar tissue ranges from 0.5 to 2.0 mm inferiorly, tapering distally to a fraction of a millimeter in its mid-portion, whereas the dorsal tissue is more uniform in thickness, ranging from 0.75 mm to 1.5 mm. In patients treated with limited forearm pronation and supination, the dorsal and volar joint capsules, respectively, were thickened to an average of 2 to 4 mm. Significant improvement in forearm rotation was achieved in all 9 patients with capsulectomy of the pathologic fibrosed tissue from a dorsal or volar approach. Watanabe and colleagues[34] recently showed the importance of the DRUJ capsule as a stabilizer of the DRUJ. Sectioning of the dorsal joint capsule resulted in significant dorsal instability, whereas sectioning of the volar joint capsule led to volar instability.

SOFT TISSUE EXTRINSIC STABILIZERS

The IOM functions to transfer load from the radius to the ulna as well as to provide longitudinal stability. With radial head excision, the central band of the IOM provides 71% of the soft tissue contribution to longitudinal stability to resist proximal migration of the radius.[35] However, the IOM is also important in DRUJ instability, especially in the setting of injury to the distal radioulnar ligament complex. Kihara and colleagues[26] demonstrated that with an intact IOM, sectioning of both the DRUL and PRUL did not lead to significant dorsal or palmar instability. Pfaeffle and colleagues[36] measured the magnitude and direction of force vectors in the IOM with compressive forces applied to the hand and identified the presence of transverse force vectors that act to resist distraction of the distal radius and distal ulna. Watanabe and colleagues[37] sectioned the IOM and tested for DRUJ laxity in neutral rotation, 60° pronation, and 60° supination. The distal IOM constrained volar and dorsal laxity of the DRUJ in all forearm rotation positions. The investigators also determined that the distal oblique bundle, when present, is an important stabilizer of the DRUJ. In a cadaveric study, Kitamura and colleagues[38] demonstrated the presence of the distal IOM in 40% of the specimens. In a neutral position, the specimens with a distal IOM had significantly greater DRUJ stability.

The extensor carpi ulnaris is unique in that it has its own fibro-osseous tunnel that stabilizes the tendon at the level of the distal ulna. The fibro-osseous tunnel is 1.5 to 2.0 cm in length and lies deep to and separate from the extensor retinaculum. In cadaveric dissections, if the ECU tendon is maintained in its compartment over the dorsum of the ulna, complete instability of the DRUJ does not occur even with sectioning of all the other ligaments of the TFCC.[39] The ECU tendon acts as a dynamic stabilizer by elevating the ulnar carpus dorsally while depressing the ulnar head palmarly during forearm pronation.

Several anatomic studies have demonstrated the presence of 2 heads of the pronator quadratus muscle.[40,41] The superficial head originates from the ulna and passes transversely to insert on the radius, and acts as the primary pronator of the forearm. The deep head fibers start more proximally on the ulna and are oriented obliquely as they insert distally on the radius. The deep head functions to coapt the distal ulna into the sigmoid notch during active pronation and passive supination to further stabilize the DRUJ. In a biomechanical study, sectioning of the pronator quadratus led to increased palmar subluxation of the DRUJ during forearm pronation.[42] Analysis of electromyographic activity in 14 healthy volunteers during forearm pronation and supination confirmed the importance of the deep head of the pronator quadratus as a dynamic stabilizer of the DRUJ during both forearm pronation and supination.[43]

SUMMARY

The DRUJ is a complex articulation allowing significant rotational and translational motion. Stability of the DRUJ depends on bony contact, intrinsic stabilizers of the TFCC complex, and extrinsic stabilizers of the distal forearm. Understanding the anatomy of this articulation is paramount in clinical decision making for the treatment of disorders involving the DRUJ.

REFERENCES

1. Stuart PR, Berger RA, Linscheid RL, et al. The dorsopalmar stability of the distal radioulnar joint. J Hand Surg Am 2000;25:689–99.
2. af Ekenstam F, Hagert CG. Anatomical studies on the geometry and stability of the distal radio ulnar joint. Scand J Plast Reconstr Surg 1985;19:17–25.
3. Tolat AR, Stanley JK, Trail IA. A cadaveric study of the anatomy and stability of the distal radioulnar joint in the coronal and transverse planes. J Hand Surg Br 1996;21:587–94.
4. Pirela-Cruz MA, Goll SR, Klug M, et al. Stress computed tomography analysis of the distal radioulnar joint: a diagnostic tool for determining translational motion. J Hand Surg Am 1991;16:75–82.
5. Ishii S, Palmer AK, Werner FW, et al. Pressure distribution in the distal radioulnar joint. J Hand Surg Am 1998;23:909–13.
6. Tolat AR, Sanderson PL, De Smet L, et al. The gymnast's wrist: acquired positive ulnar variance following chronic epiphyseal injury. J Hand Surg Br 1992;17:678–81.
7. Sagerman SD, Zogby RG, Palmer AK, et al. Relative articular inclination of the distal radioulnar joint: a radiographic study. J Hand Surg Am 1995;20:597–601.
8. Freedman DM, Edwards GS Jr, Willems MJ, et al. Right versus left symmetry of ulnar variance. A radiographic assessment. Clin Orthop Relat Res 1998;(354):153–8.
9. Gelberman RH, Salamon PB, Jurist JM, et al. Ulnar variance in Kienböck's disease. J Bone Joint Surg Am 1975;57:674–6.
10. Schuurman AH, Maas M, Dijkstra PF, et al. Assessment of ulnar variance: a radiological investigation in a Dutch population. Skeletal Radiol 2001;30:633–8.
11. Schuind FA, Linscheid RL, An KN, et al. A normal data base of posteroanterior roentgenographic measurements of the wrist. J Bone Joint Surg Am 1992;74:1418–29.
12. Palmer AK, Werner FW. The triangular fibrocartilage complex of the wrist–anatomy and function. J Hand Surg Am 1981;6:153–62.
13. Friedman SL, Palmer AK, Short WH, et al. The change in ulnar variance with grip. J Hand Surg Am 1993;18:713–6.
14. Yeh GL, Beredjiklian PK, Katz MA, et al. Effects of forearm rotation on the clinical evaluation of ulnar variance. J Hand Surg Am 2001;26:1042–6.
15. Jung JM, Baek GH, Kim JH, et al. Changes in ulnar variance in relation to forearm rotation and grip. J Bone Joint Surg Br 2001;83:1029–33.

16. Chidgey LK, Dell PC, Bittar ES, et al. Histologic anatomy of the triangular fibrocartilage. J Hand Surg Am 1991;16:1084–100.

17. Adams BD, Holley KA. Strains in the articular disk of the triangular fibrocartilage complex: a biomechanical study. J Hand Surg Am 1993;18:919–25.

18. Adams BD. Partial excision of the triangular fibrocartilage complex articular disk: a biomechanical study. J Hand Surg Am 1993;18:334–40.

19. Thiru RG, Ferlic DC, Clayton ML, et al. Arterial anatomy of the triangular fibrocartilage of the wrist and its surgical significance. J Hand Surg Am 1986;11:258–63.

20. Mikic Z. The blood supply of the human distal radioulnar joint and the microvasculature of its articular disk. Clin Orthop Relat Res 1992;(275):19–28.

21. Bednar MS, Arnoczky SP, Weiland AJ. The microvasculature of the triangular fibrocartilage complex: its clinical significance. J Hand Surg Am 1991;16:1101–5.

22. Gupta R, Nelson SD, Baker J, et al. The innervation of the triangular fibrocartilage complex: nitric acid maceration rediscovered. Plast Reconstr Surg 2001;107:135–9.

23. Lourie GM, King J, Kleinman WB. The transverse radioulnar branch from the dorsal sensory ulnar nerve: its clinical and anatomical significance further defined. J Hand Surg Am 1994;19:241–5.

24. Ohmori M, Azuma H. Morphology and distribution of nerve endings in the human triangular fibrocartilage complex. J Hand Surg Br 1998;23:522–5.

25. Schuind F, An KN, Berglund L, et al. The distal radioulnar ligaments: a biomechanical study. J Hand Surg Am 1991;16:1106–14.

26. Kihara H, Short WH, Werner FW, et al. The stabilizing mechanism of the distal radioulnar joint during pronation and supination. J Hand Surg Am 1995;20:930–6.

27. Acosta R, Hnat W, Scheker LR. Distal radio-ulnar ligament motion during supination and pronation. J Hand Surg Br 1993;18:502–5.

28. Ward LD, Ambrose CG, Masson MV, et al. The role of the distal radioulnar ligaments, interosseous membrane, and joint capsule in distal radioulnar joint stability. J Hand Surg Am 2000;25:341–51.

29. Osterman AL, Terrill RG. Arthroscopic treatment of TFCC lesions. Hand Clin 1991;7:277–81.

30. Osterman AL. Arthroscopic debridement of triangular fibrocartilage complex tears. Arthroscopy 1990;6:120–4.

31. Hagert CG. Distal radius fracture and the distal radioulnar joint–anatomical considerations. Handchir Mikrochir Plast Chir 1994;26:22–6.

32. Kleinman WB. Stability of the distal radioulnar joint: biomechanics, pathophysiology, physical diagnosis, and restoration of function what we have learned in 25 years. J Hand Surg Am 2007;32:1086–106.

33. Kleinman WB, Graham TJ. The distal radioulnar joint capsule: clinical anatomy and role in posttraumatic limitation of forearm rotation. J Hand Surg Am 1998;23:588–99.

34. Watanabe H, Berger RA, An KN, et al. Stability of the distal radioulnar joint contributed by the joint capsule. J Hand Surg Am 2004;29:1114–20.

35. Hotchkiss RN, An KN, Sowa DT, et al. An anatomic and mechanical study of the interosseous membrane of the forearm: pathomechanics of proximal migration of the radius. J Hand Surg Am 1989;14:256–61.

36. Pfaeffle HJ, Fischer KJ, Manson TT, et al. Role of the forearm interosseous ligament: is it more than just longitudinal load transfer? J Hand Surg Am 2000;25:683–8.

37. Watanabe H, Berger RA, Berglund LJ, et al. Contribution of the interosseous membrane to distal radioulnar joint constraint. J Hand Surg Am 2005;30:1164–71.

38. Kitamura T, Moritomo H, Arimitsu S, et al. The biomechanical effect of the distal interosseous membrane on distal radioulnar joint stability: a preliminary anatomic study. J Hand Surg Am 2011;36:1626–30.

39. Spinner M, Kaplan EB. Extensor carpi ulnaris. Its relationship to the stability of the distal radio-ulnar joint. Clin Orthop Relat Res 1970;68:124–9.

40. Stuart PR. Pronator quadratus revisited. J Hand Surg Br 1996;21:714–22.

41. Johnson RK, Shrewsbury MM. The pronator quadratus in motions and in stabilization of the radius and ulna at the distal radioulnar joint. J Hand Surg Am 1976;1:205–9.

42. King GJ, McMurtry RY, Rubenstein JD, et al. Computerized tomography of the distal radioulnar joint: correlation with ligamentous pathology in a cadaveric model. J Hand Surg Am 1986;11:711–7.

43. Gordon KD, Pardo RD, Johnson JA, et al. Electromyographic activity and strength during maximum isometric pronation and supination efforts in healthy adults. J Orthop Res 2004;22:208–13.

How to Measure Outcomes of Distal Radius Fracture Treatment

Andrew W. Ritting, MD, Jennifer M. Wolf, MD*

KEYWORDS

- Distal radius • Outcomes • Colles • Function • Fracture
- Volar plate • Recovery

The goal of any outcome measure in medicine is to evaluate the improvement or detriment of a given treatment of a condition, disease, or injury. In order for a measure to be useful, it must be easily understood and administered and have consistent reliability and validity over a wide array of demographic groups. Ultimately, a reliable outcome measure should aid in predicting the outcome of a given treatment of a specific population and then be able to guide further treatment for the benefit of patients.

Distal radius fractures represent one-sixth of all fractures evaluated in the emergency department, with greater than 450,000 fractures occurring every year in the United States.[1,2] These fractures can be treated conservatively or operatively for fracture stabilization until healing. The operative treatment of these fractures includes many modalities, such as external fixation, percutaneous pin fixation, dorsal internal fixation, and volar internal fixation, with open reduction and internal fixation via a volar approach being the most common method used today. In a recent demographic study of the Medicare population by Chung and colleagues,[3] distal radius fractures were more likely to be treated with open reduction internal fixation (ORIF) if treated by a hand surgeon rather than a general orthopedic

surgeon. However, most wrist fractures are still treated nonoperatively.

Multiple outcome measures have been described to measure the success of the treatment of distal radius fractures. These measures include general and anatomy-specific patient-reported subjective outcomes, objective measurements, and radiographic measurements. To date, there is no widely accepted outcome measure for wrist fractures that is considered the gold standard to accurately predict function after treatment. This review provides an overview of the currently used measures with an evidence-based evaluation of the advantages and disadvantages of each method and their practicality for use in clinical care.

GENERAL PATIENT-REPORTED SUBJECTIVE OUTCOMES
The 36-Item Short Form Health Survey

The 36-Item Short Form Health Survey (SF-36) is a widely used tool to estimate the general health of a population and is a commonly used outcome measure in distal radius fracture care. It was originally introduced in 1980 as a 108-question booklet for clinical practice and research, health policy evaluation, and general population surveys

Disclosures: Andrew W. Ritting has no relationship with any specific entity discussed in this article and has nothing to disclose. Jennifer M. Wolf receives salary support as a deputy editor for the *Journal of Hand Surgery* and has received research support from the Orthopedic Research and Education Foundation, the American Foundation for Surgery of the Hand, and the University of Connecticut.
Department of Orthopaedic Surgery, New England Musculoskeletal Institute, University of Connecticut Health Center, 263 Farmington Avenue, Farmington, CT 06030, USA
* Corresponding author.
E-mail address: JMWolf@uchc.edu

Important Points and Objectives for Recall

- Only reliable and valid outcome measures should be used to assess functional recovery in clinical research.
- The 36-Item Short Form Health Survey (SF-36) and European Quality of Life-5 dimensions survey (EuroquOL-5D) evaluate patients as a whole and are not specific to the extremity or injury that is being measured.
- The Disabilities of the Shoulder, Arm, and Hand (DASH) questionnaire is a validated outcome measure of the upper extremity, and although it is frequently used to assess distal radius fracture outcomes, it can be skewed by ipsilateral injury to the upper extremity and neck.
- The Patient-Rated Wrist Evaluation (PRWE) is one of the more frequently used outcome measures to assess distal radius fracture outcomes because it is more specific to wrist function.
- The Jebsen-Taylor test (JTT), Michigan Hand Outcomes Questionnaire (MHQ), and Brigham scores were developed to measure outcomes in the management of hand and finger pathologic conditions but have also been used to evaluate distal radius fracture recovery.
- The Gartland and Werley score is one of the most widely used outcome measure because it takes into consideration objective measurements to predict overall recovery; however, it has not been validated in a standard fashion to date.
- The Arthritis Impact Measurement Scale (AIMS2) is used in rheumatoid arthritis and osteoarthritis to gauge function and has been sporadically used in the measurement of distal radius fracture outcomes.
- Physical examination is one of the most important predictors of overall functional outcomes. However, the contralateral extremity may be an unreliable control. In addition, average values are highly dependent on sex, age, comorbidity, and hand dominance.
- Radiographic parameters have been created to establish normal anatomy, although they may not be predictive of functional recovery, specifically in the elderly population.
- There are few comparative trials to compare outcome measures when discussing distal radius fracture management, and there is no universally accepted gold standard to evaluate recovery.

---

as part of the Medical Outcomes Study.[4] It was thought to be too long and difficult for the average patient, so a condensed version was created to shorten the responses and improve patient compliance with completion.[5] The shortened form, the SF-36, includes 8 dimensions or scales: physical functioning, social functioning, role limitations (physical problems), role limitations (mental problems), mental health, vitality, pain, and general health perception. Brazier and colleagues[6] confirmed that the SF-36 was an acceptable measurement tool because it achieved both high reliability and constructive validity scores.

The SF-36 has been used in the outcome analysis of distal radius fracture management either using an entire score or as a specific subgroup analysis. Matschke and colleagues[7] compared volar and dorsal plate fixation of distal radius fractures and showed that the SF-36 score improved in both groups but there was no difference regarding the type of fixation method. These findings were similar to the Disabilities of the Shoulder, Arm, and Hand (DASH) questionnaire and physical examination measurements at 6 months, 1 year, and 2 years. Neidenbach and colleagues[8] compared the results of nonoperative management with a cast in patients with or without closed reduction for displaced distal radius fractures. The SF-36 was used as a primary outcome measure, and results showed that fractures treated with closed reduction lost their anatomic reduction but maintained their activities of daily living (ADL) and overall function. Lastly, Kreder and colleagues[9] used only the bodily pain subscore of the SF-36 and found a significant improvement in the 1-year outcomes when comparing percutaneous fixation with ORIF.

EuroQol Group Survey

Similar to the SF-36, the EuroquOL-5D was developed to aid research and create a reliable measure for health-related quality of life. This outcome measurement tool includes a 5-part utility index and a visual analog scale. In a study on patients with rheumatoid arthritis, Hurst and colleagues[10] found moderate to high correlations between the EQ-5D and measures of impairment and high correlations with disability measures. They concluded that the scoring system was simple to use, valid, and reliable for group comparisons.

The SF-36 and EQ-5D are to measure the impact of fractures or other events on the general health of patients. The advantage of these instruments is the ability to stratify outcomes by subscales, including pain, physical function, and emotional impact. Disadvantages include the length of the questionnaires, which are still quite detailed, and the inability to focus on extremity-specific functioning. Currently, the EQ-5D has not been evaluated as a specific measure of distal radius treatment outcomes, but Bartl and colleagues[11] plan to use it in a large prospective trial of distal radius fracture treatment as a secondary outcome measure, comparing operative fixation with nonoperative casting for intraarticular fractures.

EXTREMITY-SPECIFIC PATIENT-REPORTED SUBJECTIVE OUTCOMES
Disabilities of the Shoulder, Arm, and Hand Questionnaire

The DASH questionnaire is a patient-based survey that evaluates the upper extremity as a single functional unit. It was developed by Hudak and colleagues[12] in 1996, with the goal of having an entirely subjective way of measuring patients' upper extremity outcomes, as distinct from objective data, such as radiographic findings or physical examination findings. The final document consists of a 30-item questionnaire with 5 responses for each item. There are 2 additional optional scales to address the ability to work and to perform sports or play a musical instrument.[13]

To evaluate the clinical significance of numerical changes in the DASH questionnaire after surgical management of various upper extremity disorders, Gummesson and colleagues[14] conducted a longitudinal study to quantify the amount of score change in response to treatment. In this study, they noted that a difference of 19 points on the DASH was consistent with a change of much better or much worse, whereas a difference of 10 points was clinically significant for changes that were somewhat better or somewhat worse. The investigators concluded that a 10-point difference from preoperative and postoperative management may be considered a minimally important change. The DASH's measurement of the effectiveness of treatment was most specific for subacromial impingement and carpal tunnel syndrome.

The DASH has been widely used in the distal radius fracture literature to measure subjective patient outcomes. Hollevoet and colleagues[15] compared percutaneous K-wire fixation with volar ORIF and found no differences in DASH between study cohorts in the 3-month study follow-up. Conversely, in a prospective, randomized study comparing external fixation and volar plate ORIF for unstable extraarticular distal radius fractures, Wilcke and colleagues[16] found short-term superiority in the ORIF group in DASH scores at 3 and 6 months, with no differences by 12 months. These results were paralleled in a study comparing K-wire fixation with volar plate ORIF, with volar plate ORIF having superior DASH scores at 3 and 6 months.[17] Finally, from a postoperative perspective, Souer and colleagues[18] prospectively compared occupational therapy with independent exercise after ORIF with a volar plate and used the DASH as a primary outcome measure. Although there were short-term differences in range of motion and grip and pinch strength, arm-specific DASH scores did not differ between the 2 groups at any time.

Although the DASH is more specific than the non–anatomy-based questionnaires, it remains a regional evaluation of the limb and, therefore, is less specific for outcomes of wrist fractures. If an ipsilateral elbow or shoulder pathologic condition is present, then DASH scores could be expected to reflect this decrease in function, even if the patient has a highly functional, pain-free wrist. In a comparative analysis of the DASH with other widely used upper extremity scoring systems, Changulani and colleagues[19] found only a weak correlation of the DASH with severity of pain in the wrist joint, at 0.67, and concluded it was less valid for patients with wrist disorders. Additionally, when comparing 84 patients with an injury to the upper extremity, 73 patients with injuries to the lower extremity, and 49 control subjects, Dowrick and colleagues[20] found that DASH scores correlated with patients that had injury to the lower extremities and even found some disability in the control group. Nevertheless, in a study focused specifically on outcomes after Colles fractures, Lovgren and Hellstrom[21] found a high internal consistency and good test-retest reliability using the DASH. The investigators concluded that the DASH instrument could be reliably used to detect issues with hesitance to progress with range of motion, catastrophizing, and self-efficacy in the early and subacute treatment periods.

Patient-Rated Wrist Evaluation

The Patient-Rated Wrist Evaluation (PRWE) was developed to create a more specific means of evaluating the outcomes of patients with wrist-specific disorders and focuses on pain and functional items. The survey was designed based on a questionnaire sent to multiple physicians to determine what factors they thought were most closely related to patient recovery after wrist injury or surgery. Pain is evaluated for both intensity and frequency, and functional questions evaluate commonly performed tasks using either hand. Finally, patient-specific role-limitation questions are based on the ability to perform usual activities involved in self-care, work role, home life, and recreation. The scale was designed to be completed in 4 minutes by the average respondent. When patients with distal radius fractures (both subacute and following final treatment) or with long-term scaphoid nonunions were evaluated, the test revealed excellent reliability for the total PRWE, excellent reliability for functional subscales in all distal radius fractures, and moderate reliability for patients with chronic scaphoid nonunions. To validate the PRWE, the investigators compared results with components of the SF-36 examination and measurements of impairment (grip, range of motion, and dexterity). They found a stronger correlation between PRWE scores and SF-36 physical summary scores than for SF-36 mental summary scores. They also found moderate correlations between patient-reported pain and disability when compared with the measures of physical impairment.[22]

Based on these findings, the PRWE can be a useful tool to measure outcomes of distal radius fracture management. However, it is intended as a general tool to evaluate the wrist unit's function rather than specifically the distal radius. Additionally, some investigators have critically evaluated the results and questioned the true strength of the scores. Karnezis and Fragkiadakis[23] evaluated the recovery of 31 patients with unstable distal radius fractures and found that although grip strength was a good predictor of the PRWE score, the pronation, supination, flexion, and extension measurements were not predictive of the scores.

Michigan Hand Outcomes Questionnaire

The Michigan Hand Outcomes Questionnaire (MHQ) was developed in 1998 to evaluate overall health and function specifically in patients with hand disorders. The questionnaire was originally developed with 100 questions but was later reduced to 37 for ease of patient response and more specific content. The final questions included scoring on overall hand function, ADL, pain, work performance, aesthetics, and patient satisfaction with hand function. The final test revealed high test-retest reliability and high construct validity on each of the subscales, with the highest validity in the ADL scores. The investigators concluded that the MHQ was an excellent scale for evaluating outcomes following hand surgery.[24] In a follow-up study, the investigators asked patients with hand

disorders to repeat the MHQ with an additional question in each subcategory to evaluate their changes since the previous questionnaire. The results showed significant correlation on each scale and was, therefore, deemed responsive to patients' self-assessment of their clinical change.[25]

Chung and colleagues[26] used the MHQ as an outcome measure after 161 patients underwent ORIF of an inadequately reduced distal radius fracture with a volar locking plate system. The MHQ returned to normal at 6 months and continued to improve up to 1 year. In a similar study by Kotsis et al[27] grip strength, pinch strength, and active range of motion all improved with all subscales of the MHQ during the first 6 months following ORIF of unstable distal radius fractures, as evaluated by standardized response means (SRMs). Grip and pinch strength still had medium SRMs at 6 to 12 months, whereas active range of motion had small SRMs.[27] Sammer, Chung, and colleagues[28] used the MHQ as an outcome measure in a prospective study comparing fragment-specific fixation and fixed-angle volar plate ORIF for distal radius fractures and found that volar plate fixation was superior in most categories of the MHQ at 3 months but only in the aesthetic and work categories at 12 months.

Like many of the upper extremity and global scales, the MHQ also has weaknesses in evaluating wrist function following distal radius fracture management. The original study indicated its excellent reliability to evaluate hand function, but this is not specific to distal radius fracture and wrist function.[24] Horng and colleagues[29] found the MHQ might be more sensitive to functional changes, but the DASH correlated more closely with a patient's disability. In a study comparing outcome measures for multiple hand pathologic conditions, McMillan and Binhammer[30] identified the MHQ as being responsive to patients with carpal tunnel syndrome, wrist pain, and finger contracture, further helping to confirm its use as a hand functional outcome measure rather than a specific distal radius or wrist outcomes measure.

Gartland and Werley Score

The Gartland and Werley score was first introduced in 1951 as part of a study evaluating radiographic findings after closed reduction and splinting of distal radius fractures. The investigators used the uninjured contralateral wrist as a control and evaluated functional results in comparison with these normal values. Using a standard of 45° of dorsiflexion, 30° of palmar flexion, 15° of radial and ulnar deviation, and 50° of pronosupination, points are awarded if significant deviations from these values are found. Gartland and Werley found that a loss of dorsiflexion correlated most closely with lost function, thus resulting in greater weighting than lost palmar flexion. The sum of the points is used to classify results as excellent, good, or poor.[31] The original score was first modified by Sarmiento and colleagues[32] to include lost pronation and grip strength and then again by Lucas and Sachtjen[33] who added variables of median nerve impairment, reflex sympathetic dystrophy, and digit stiffness.

The Gartland and Werley score is commonly used throughout the distal radius literature to evaluate outcomes of management. Gereli and colleagues[34] compared 16 patients who underwent volar plate ORIF for an intraarticular, comminuted distal radius fracture with 14 who received external fixation with K-wire augmentation. They found no differences in Gartland and Werley scores at the 12-month follow-up. Moriya and colleagues[35] reviewed the results of 62 consecutive patients who underwent volar plate ORIF for both intraarticular and extraarticular distal radius fractures and used the Gartland and Werley score to conclude 35 excellent outcomes, 26 good, and 1 fair. Matschke and colleagues[7] used the Gartland and Werley score in a multicenter prospective trial of locked volar and dorsal ORIF and had good or excellent results in 89% of cases.

The Gartland and Werley score is unique in that it uses primarily objective, provider-determined measurements to create an overall score of treatment success. This score is the only true outcome measure that has a component of objective value. However, the major disadvantage to the score is that it has never been validated in the literature. Despite this fact, it continues to be used and highly regarded in the hand surgery literature.

Jebsen-Taylor Hand Function Test

The Jebsen-Taylor test (JTT) was first described in 1969 and was developed as a tool to accurately describe hand function in a variety of hand disorders based on the participant's ability to perform a battery of 7 activities. These 7 activities were created as a measure of calculating one's hand function disability.[36] Some investigators have modified the test to exclude the written component because it can be highly dependent on hand dominance and all remaining components of the test showed a strong correlation to ADLs and deformity.[37]

In examining the outcomes of distal radius fractures, Tremayne and colleagues[38] evaluated 20 nonoperatively treated patients and found a statistically significant correlation between grip strength and JTT scores but only significant correlation between 3 of the 7 tasks of the JTT and wrist

extension. In their evaluation of unstable distal radius fractures treated with ORIF using a volar locking plate, Chung and colleagues[26] used the JTT as an outcome measure and found that despite differences in physical examination parameters, the JTT on the injured side was 94.3%, 98.0%, and 96.7% of the uninjured contralateral side at 3, 6, and 12 months respectively.

The advantage of the JTT is that it is easily administered and has been previously validated.[26] The other benefit is that it can be altered to exclude the written component. Its main disadvantage is that most of the literature supporting its use is in hand and finger surgical outcomes but not specifically distal radius and wrist outcomes. Nevertheless, it can be a useful adjunct to other outcome measures in distal radius fracture management.

Arthritis Impact Measurement Scale

The Arthritis Impact Measurement Scale (AIMS2) was originally developed by Meenan and colleagues[39] to evaluate physical, emotional, and social well-being, specifically in a population of patients with rheumatoid arthritis and osteoarthritis. The original investigators further modified this scale to develop a more sensitive and comprehensive version. The new scale considered function, work, and social support and a satisfaction component. Results indicated a high reliability and validity and satisfaction had a moderate correlation with the level of function, whereas patient recognition that a specific area was a problem correlated with a poorer overall AIMS2 scale.[40]

Although the AIMS2 was designed for arthritis, it has also been used in a single study as an outcome measure for distal radius fracture management. Amadio and colleagues[41] evaluated 21 distal radius fractures treated with immobilization and then used the AIMS2 scale to evaluate improvement. They found significant improvement in the scale components of mobility, hand and finger function, arm function, self-care, satisfaction, household tasks, physical status, and affect status. Although they did find these statistically different, they cautioned against using the scale solely for distal radius fractures because 30 components of the scale did not have a significant change. They recommend that the components of the upper extremity should be used in isolation.

Brigham and Women's Hospital Carpal Tunnel Instrument

The Brigham and Women's Hospital Carpal Tunnel Instrument (Brigham) score was originally created as a specific scale to evaluate carpal tunnel syndrome and recovery after carpal tunnel release.

The parameters included a graded scale to evaluate a combination of pain, paresthesia, numbness, weakness, nocturnal symptoms, and overall functional status. Its investigators concluded that it had a high reproducibility and internal consistency and modestly or weakly positive correlation with 2-point discrimination and Semmes-Weinstein testing.[42] In Changulani and colleagues'[19] review, they found that symptom severity and functional scores correlated well with grip and pinch strength and patient satisfaction correlated with overall improvement in scores. The study was also found to be highly reproducible.

Despite being created as a scoring system to evaluate the results of carpal tunnel syndrome, the Brigham score has also been used in distal radius fracture outcome analysis because many of the components of the questionnaire are also symptoms and disabilities that are found in distal radius fractures. However, Amadio and colleagues[41] found only an improvement on the functional scale and no true correlation with clinical status that they attributed to several sensory outcomes being included in the scale, which are not usually complaints of patients with distal radius fracture. Lyngcoln and colleagues[43] used this measure to evaluate short-term outcomes after distal radius fracture in patients from initial cast removal to final follow-up at 6 months and their level of compliance with hand therapy. They noted that patients who were compliant with hand therapy demonstrated an average of 50% improvement in the Brigham outcome scores compared with those who did not follow a specific hand therapy program.

PHYSICAL EXAMINATION MEASURES OF OUTCOME

Examination of the wrist includes range of motion in the arc of flexion and extension as well as pronation and supination. Grip, key, and pinch testing are also commonly performed and reported using a dynamometer and pinch meter. Measurements are made and compared as a percentage of the values from the contralateral side. It can be difficult, however, to gain a completely accurate value for recovery because concurrent upper extremity or cervical spine pathologic conditions and hand dominance can skew these results. Additionally, within a population, gender and age can also change the definition of a normal value. Overall baseline population range of motion has been measured as a flexion of 74°, extension of 64° (flexion-extension arc of 138°), supination of 90°, and pronation of 90° (pronation-supination arc of 180°).[44] Women tend to have approximately 4°

more pronation and 5° more supination than men.[45] Normal average values of grip strength are highly dependent on gender, age, fatigue, and the instruments used for measuring and can vary anywhere from 5 kg (women aged more than 75 years, nondominant hand) to 73 kg (men, aged 24–34 years, dominant hand).[46]

Walker and colleagues[47] attempted to further define some of the population variations and found that although range of motion was similar between men and women, men had 40% stronger pinch strength and twice as much grip strength as women. Mathiowetz and colleagues[48] found that grip strengths were the highest between the ages of 25 and 39 years and then declined, whereas tip, key, and palmar pinch strength were stable from 20 to 59 years of age and then declined. Similarly, with a wide range of normal values for wrist range of motion, Brumfield and Champoux helped to identify a functional range of wrist motion by evaluating ADL in 19 normal adults. They found that a normal, functional arc was from 10° of flexion to 35° of extension.[49]

Chung and Haas[50] reviewed a prospective cohort of 125 patients with distal radius fractures who underwent surgery for definitive management. At 3 months, the adjusted range of motion compared with the uninjured hand was 79.8%, the adjusted mean grip strength was 58.2%, and the mean key grip strength was 81.8%. They found that satisfaction directly correlated with these findings and that cutoff points for satisfaction following surgery were recovery of 65% for grip strength, 87% of key grip strength, and 95% of wrist arc range of motion.[50] Another recent study evaluated 26 patients with distal radius fractures for pronosupination and grip strength 14 months after volar plate ORIF. The investigators found that patients recovered 91% of grip strength, 88% of pronation strength, and 85% of supination strength.[51] Dillingham and colleagues[52] examined 27 patients who underwent reduction and volar plate fixation for an unstable distal radius fracture and noted that all range of motion (flexion, extension, supination, and pronation) improved most rapidly within the first 3 months, with supination and pronation recovery being the fastest at 92% of the uninjured side by 3 months. All range of motion continued to improve until 12 months after injury, and grip strength improved to 94% by 12 months.

RADIOGRAPHIC MEASUREMENTS OF OUTCOMES OF DISTAL RADIUS FRACTURES

Serial radiographs are frequently used as a means of evaluating the outcome of conservative or operative treatment of distal radial fractures, with the goal of reestablishing normal anatomy. Solgaard and others[53] have defined normal radiographic landmarks at the wrist as a volar tilt of 12°, radial inclination of 23°, and length of the radial styloid (radial height) of 12 mm.[53] Using posteroanterior, lateral, and oblique radiographs, Medoff[54] reviewed normal findings of anatomic landmarks and defined normal as a radial inclination of 23.6 ± 2.5°, radial height of 11.6 ± 1.6 mm, ulnar variance of -0.6 ± 0.9 mm, and radiocarpal interval of 1.9 ± 0.2 mm. In addition, it is recommended that intraarticular step-off of 1[55,56] or 2 mm[55,57,58] be reduced and fixed to obtain a successful radiographic outcome. Chung and colleagues[59] used a regression model on 66 distal radius fractures to identify predictors of a poor outcome and found that at 3 months, radiographic incongruity with both a step-off and gap at the articular surface was the only significant predictor of poor functional outcome. However, at the 1-year follow-up, only increased age and decreased income were associated with a decreased functional result.

To date, there are many studies that have validated the correlation between radiographic restoration and functional outcomes following operative and nonoperative management of a distal radius fracture. McQueen and Caspers[60] reviewed 30 patients with a mean age of 69 years (range 56–86 years) at a minimum 4-year follow-up after manipulation with nonoperative management of an extraarticular distal radius fracture. In the group with a radiographically defined malunion (dorsal angulation between 12° and 34° and more than 2 mm of radial shift), patients had statistically poorer grip strength, less range of motion, increased pain, increased cosmetic deficit, and more difficulties performing everyday tasks compared with those with more anatomic healing on the radiographic evaluation. In addition, Porter and Stockley[61] noted that dorsal angulation greater than 20° or radial inclination of less than 10° was correlated with a reduction in grip strength of 33% at 6 months and 30% at 2 years. In this study, comminution and intraarticular involvement were associated with a decreased overall range of motion at the wrist. Finally, Batra and Gupta[62] studied 69 patients with distal radius fractures that underwent various operative and nonoperative treatments and found that at the 1-year radiographic evaluation, radial length was the most important predictor of functional recovery, followed by volar tilt.[62]

However, there is evidence that the relationship between alignment and outcome may not be reflected in self-reported function, particularly in the elderly. Grewal and MacDermid[63] noted that radiographic and clinical outcomes were not strongly correlated, particularly in the older population. In their study of 216 patients with extraarticular distal radius fractures, radiographic malalignment had a higher relative risk of poorer outcomes throughout all age ranges, but patient pain and disability reported through the DASH and PRWE scores revealed that malalignment was not associated with poor outcomes when compared with acceptable alignment in patients aged 65 years or older. In this analysis, they identified that 8 patients (when scored by the DASH) or 9 patients (when scored by the PRWE) would need correction in the older population to prevent one poor outcome when compared with 2 (DASH) or 3 (PRWE) in younger patients.[63]

Arora and colleagues[64] evaluated 73 patients aged 65 years or older and compared nonoperative treatment and locked volar plating for wrist fractures. At 3, 6, and 12 months postoperatively, their final results showed that dorsal radial tilt, radial inclination, and radial shortening were significantly better in the operatively treated group, whereas the nonoperative group had a 100% malunion rate (defined as greater than 10° dorsal tilt, greater than 2 mm of radial shortening, and greater than 1 mm of articular incongruity). Despite these findings, the operative group had lower DASH and PRWE scores only at 3 months but not at any other time; only grip strength remained better in the operative group at the final follow-up. They concluded that achieving anatomic reduction did not convey improvement in range of motion or the ability to perform ADLs. In a meta-analysis conducted by Diaz-Garcia, Chung, and colleagues,[65] 21 studies evaluated cast immobilization versus operative management for unstable distal radius fractures in the elderly and similarly concluded that although radiographic parameters were far inferior in the cast immobilization groups, this did not translate into improved clinical outcomes.

In a recent economic analysis of the cost and benefit of ORIF versus casting of distal radius fractures in elderly patients greater than 65 years old, Shauver, Chung, and colleagues[66] found that the incremental cost-utility ratio of ORIF compared with casting was $15,330 per quality-adjusted life years. They concluded that because this value was less than $50,000, ORIF was a worthwhile alternative to casting in elderly patients.

In a younger population, Goldfarb and colleagues[67] reviewed a cohort of 16 patients at 15 years after ORIF of an intraarticular distal radius fracture and found that strength and range of motion remained equal to the original 7-year data, despite the evidence of radiocarpal arthrosis in 13 of the 16 patients, which had progressed

67% from previously reported outcomes. They concluded that the presence or absence of radiographic arthrosis did not correlate with upper extremity function.

EVIDENCE-BASED COMPARISONS OF OUTCOME MEASURES

The advantages and disadvantages of each method of evaluation have been described in the previous sections. Some measures correlate well with a patient's functional outcome but may not necessarily correlate with their global outcome, whereas other measures reflect overall satisfaction or global function but are not specific to the distal radius. In addition, there is a wide array of reliability and variability, depending on the outcome measure used. Finally, the ease at which patients can complete the instrument is also a factor that must be taken into consideration.

MacDermid and colleagues[68] performed a comparative study of multiple outcome instruments and evaluated 59 patients who sustained a distal radius fracture and were treated nonoperatively. The patients completed the PRWE, DASH, and SF-36 forms at their initial visit and then again at 3 and 6 months. Using grip strength, range of motion, and dexterity, responsiveness was correlated from SRMs, which is calculated from the average change in score divided by the standard deviation of the scores, and has a good level of responsiveness that is not influenced by sample size.[69,70] The findings showed that the PRWE (SRM = 2.27) and DASH (SRM = 2.01) were more responsive than the SF-36 (SRM = 0.92). The investigators noted that during the first 3 months, when physical outcomes could not be reliably obtained because of the treatment variation, the outcome questionnaires could provide reliable information regarding patient recovery.[68]

Sears and Chung[71] conducted a prospective cohort study to compare the validity and responsiveness of the JTT with the MHQ in a group of patients with carpal tunnel syndrome, rheumatoid arthritis, osteoarthritis, and distal radius fractures. They evaluated the 2 instruments in this cohort for correlation during the preoperative period to 9 to 12 months postoperatively. Results showed a poor correlation because patients with high MHQ scores performed well on the JTT but patients with good JTT scores did not necessarily have high MHQ scores, and a change in JTT score had no true correlation with MHQ scores. A direct comparison using effect size and SRMs showed a better responsiveness of the MHQ.

Segments of the various outcome measures have also been used in the literature to create more specific tests that can reflect the distal radius rather than the function of the extremity. Gabl and colleagues[72] reviewed the consistency of the PRWE with only the wrist-specific items of the DASH. In this study, they identified a high correlation between both of these scores and found that all of the questions that were used were specific for wrist function and subjective comfort after a distal radius fracture when compared with a pathologic condition without wrist involvement. Of the 25 questions, however, only 14 of these correlated well with radiographic features of malunion, which one could consider to be a high determinant of overall functional outcome.

In their analysis of outcome measures, Changulani and colleagues[19] analyzed multiple methods of evaluating wrist outcome measures. They concluded that the Brigham score was best for patients with carpal tunnel syndrome, whereas in patients with multiple disorders involving more than one upper limb joint, the DASH was the best outcome measure. The Gartland and Werley score provided an objective measurement of wrist function but has not truly been validated. Finally, for patients with distal radius fractures, they found the PRWE to be the most reliable tool.[22] An independent review reached similar conclusions, stating that the DASH was useful in wrist and hand injuries, the MHQ was more specific for hand injuries, the Brigham score was best for carpal tunnel syndrome (although the DASH and MHQ are also responsive), and the PRWE was only slightly better than the DASH to assess patients with wrist injuries.[73]

SUMMARY

There are several different methods of evaluating patient recovery after distal radius fracture, including strictly subjective measures, objective examination measurements, or a combination of both, and radiographic outcomes. To date, there are few studies that directly compare outcome measures in a single population to identify the best outcome measures to evaluate the management of distal radius fractures. The optimal outcome instrument is easy for patients to use, provides comprehensive information about general well-being and extremity-specific function, and is responsive to change. Often, a combination of the current instruments is required to meet these goals.

REFERENCES

1. Geissler WB. Arthroscopic reduction and fixation of distal radius and ulnar styloid fractures. Operative techniques in orthopaedic surgery, vol. 3. Philadelphia: Lippincott William & Wilkins; 2011. p. 2171–82.

2. Koval KJ, Zuckerman JD. Distal radius. Handbook of fractures. 3rd edition. Philadelphia: Lippincott Williams & Wilkins; 2006. p. 226–36.

3. Chung KC, Shauver MJ, Yin H, et al. Variations in the use of internal fixation for distal radius fracture in the United States Medicare population. J Bone Joint Surg Am 2011;93(23):2154–62.

4. Ware JE, Brook RH, Williams KN, et al. Model of health and methodology. Conceptualism and measurement of health for adults in the health insurance study, vol. I. Santa Monica (CA): Rand Corporation; 1980.

5. Ware JE Jr, Sherbourne CD. The MOS 36-item short-form health survey (SF-36). I. Conceptual framework and item selection. Med Care 1992;30(6):473–83.

6. Brazier JE, Harper R, Jones NM, et al. Validating the SF-36 health survey questionnaire: new outcome measure for primary care. BMJ 1992;305(6846): 160–4.

7. Matschke S, Wentzensen A, Ring D, et al. Comparison of angle stable plate fixation approaches for distal radius fractures. Injury 2011;42(4):385–92.

8. Neidenbach P, Audige L, Wilhelmi-Mock M, et al. The efficacy of closed reduction in displaced distal radius fractures. Injury 2010;41(6):592–8.

9. Kreder HJ, Hanel DP, Agel J, et al. Indirect reduction and percutaneous fixation versus open reduction and internal fixation for displaced intra-articular fractures of the distal radius: a randomised, controlled trial. J Bone Joint Surg Br 2005;87(6):829–36.

10. Hurst NP, Kind P, Ruta D, et al. Measuring health-related quality of life in rheumatoid arthritis: validity, responsiveness and reliability of EuroQOL (EQ-5D). Br J Rheumatol 1997;36:551–9.

11. Bartl C, Stengel D, Bruckner T, et al. Open reduction and internal fixation versus casting for highly comminuted and intra-articular fractures of the distal radius (ORCHID): a protocol for a randomized clinical multi-center trial. Trials 2011;12:84.

12. Hudak PL, Amadio PC, Bombardier C. Development of an upper extremity outcome measure, the DASH. Am J Ind Med 1996;29:602–8.

13. Atroshi I, Gummesson C, Andersson B, et al. The Disability of the Arm, Shoulder and Hand (DASH) outcome questionnaire. Acta Orthop Scand 2000; 71:613–8.

14. Gummesson C, Atroshi I, Ekdahl C. The Disabilities of the Arm, Shoulder and Hand (DASH) outcome questionnaire: longitudinal construct validity and measuring self-related health change after surgery. BMC Musculoskelet Disord 2003;4:11.

15. Hollevoet N, Vanhoutie T, Vanhove W, et al. Percutaneous K-wire fixation versus palmar plating with locking screws for Colles' fracture. Acta Orthop Belg 2011;77(2):180–7.

16. Wilcke MK, Abbaszadegan H, Adolphson PY. Wrist function recovers more rapidly after volar locked plating than after external fixation but the outcomes are similar after 1 year. Acta Orthop 2011;82(1): 76–81.

17. McFayden I, Field J, McCann P, et al. Should unstable extra-articular distal radius fractures be treated with fixed-angle volar-locked plates or percutaneous Kirschner wires? A prospective randomised controlled trial. Injury 2011;42(2):162–6.

18. Souer JS, Buijze G, Ring D. A prospective randomized controlled trial comparing occupational therapy with independent exercises after volar plate fixation of a fracture of the distal part of the radius. J Bone Joint Surg Am 2011;93(19):1761–6.

19. Changulani M, Ugochuku O, Keswani T, et al. Outcome evaluation measures for wrist and hand–which one to choose? Int Orthop 2008;32:1–6.

20. Dowrick AS, Gabbe BJ, Williamson OD, et al. Does the disability of the Arm, Shoulder and Hand (DASH) scoring system only measure disability due to injuries to the upper limb? J Bone Joint Surg Br 2006;88(4):524–7.

21. Lovgren A, Hellstrom K. Reliability and validity of measurement and associations between disability and behavioural factors in patients with Colles' fracture. Physiother Theory Pract 2012;28(3):188–97.

22. MacDermid JC, Turgeon T, Richards RS, et al. Patient rating of wrist pain and disability: a reliable and valid measurement tool. J Orthop Trauma 1998; 12(8):577–86.

23. Karnezis IA, Fragkiadakis EG. Association between objective clinical variables and patient-related disability of the wrist. J Bone Joint Surg Br 2002;84:966–70.

24. Chung KC, Pillsbury MS, Walters MR, et al. Reliability and validity testing of the Michigan Hand Outcomes Questionnaire. J Hand Surg Am 1998; 23(4):575–87.

25. Chung KC, Hamill JB, Walters MR, et al. The Michigan Hand Outcomes Questionnaire (MHQ): assessment of responsiveness to clinical change. Ann Plast Surg 1999;42(6):619–22.

26. Chung KC, Watt AJ, Kotsis SV, et al. Treatment of unstable distal radius fractures with the volar locking plate system. J Bone Joint Surg Am 2006;88(12): 2687–94.

27. Kotsis SV, Lau FH, Chung KC. Responsiveness of the Michigan Hand Outcomes Questionnaire and physical measurements in outcome studies of distal radius fracture management. J Hand Surg Am 2007; 32(1):84–90.

28. Sammer DM, Fuller DS, Kim HM, et al. A comparative study of fragment-specific versus volar plate fixation of distal radius fractures. Plast Reconstr Surg 2008; 122(5):1441–50.

29. Horng YS, Lin MC, Feng CT, et al. Responsiveness of the Michigan Hand Outcomes Questionnaire and the Disabilities of the Arm, Shoulder, and Hand questionnaire in patients with hand injury. J Hand Surg Am 2010;35(3):430–6.

30. McMillan CR, Binhammer PA. Which outcome measure is the best? Evaluating responsiveness of the Disabilities of the Arm, Shoulder, and Hand questionnaire, the Michigan Hand Questionnaire and the Patient-Specific Functional Scale following hand and wrist surgery. Hand (N Y) 2009;4(3):311–8.

31. Gartland JJ Jr, Werley CW. Evaluation of healed Colles' fractures. J Bone Joint Surg Am 1951;33(4): 895–907.

32. Sarmiento A, Pratt GW, Berry NC, et al. Colles' fracture: functional bracing in supination. J Bone Joint Surg Am 1975;57:311–7.

33. Lucas GL, Sachtjen KM. An analysis of hand function in patients with Colles' fracture treated by rush rod fixation. Clin Orthop Relat Res 1981;155:172–9.

34. Gereli A, Nalbantoglu U, Kocaoglu B, et al. Comparison of palmar locking plate and K-wire augmented external fixation for intra-articular and comminuted distal radius fractures. Acta Orthop Traumatol Turc 2010;44(3):212–9.

35. Moriya K, Saito H, Takahashi Y, et al. Locking palmar plate fixation for dorsally displaced fractures of the distal radius: a preliminary report. Hand Surg 2011;16(3):263–9.

36. Jebsen RG, Taylor N, Trieschmann RB, et al. An objective and standardized test of hand function. Arch Phys Med Rehabil 1969;50(6):311–9.

37. Sharma S, Schumacher HR Jr, McLellan AT. Evaluation of the Jebsen hand function test for use in patients with rheumatoid arthritis. Arthritis Care Res 1994;1:16–9.

38. Tremayne A, Taylor N, McBurney H, et al. Correlation of impairment and activity limitation after wrist fracture. Physiother Res Int 2002;7(2):90–9.

39. Meenan RF, Gertman PM, Mason JH. Measuring health status in arthritis. The Arthritis Impact Measurement Scales. Arthritis Rheum 1980;23(2):146–52.

40. Meenan RF, Mason JH, Anderson JJ, et al. AIMST2: the content and properties of a revised and expanded Arthritis Impact Measurement Scales health status questionnaire. Arthritis Rheum 1992;35:1–10.

41. Amadio PC, Silverstein MD, Ilstrup DM, et al. Outcomes after Colles fracture: the relative responsiveness of three questionnaires and physical examination measures. J Hand Surg Am 1996;21(5):781–7.

42. Levine DW, Simmons BP, Koris MJ, et al. A self-administered questionnaire for the assessment of severity of symptoms and functional status in carpal tunnel syndrome. J Bone Joint Surg Am 1993;75: 1585–92.

43. Lyngcoln A, Taylor N, Pizzari T, et al. The relationship between adherence to hand therapy and short-term outcome after distal radius fracture. J Hand Ther 2005;18(1):2–8.

44. Franko OI, Zurakowski D, Day CS. Functional disability of the wrist: direct correlation with decreased wrist motion. J Hand Surg Am 2008;33(4):485–92.

45. Soucie JM, Wang C, Forsyth A, et al. Hemophilia Treatment Center Network. Range of motion measurements: reference values and a database for comparison studies. Haemophilia 2011;17(3):500–7.

46. Massy-Westrop N, Rankin W, Ahern M, et al. Measuring grip strength in normal adults: reference ranges and a comparison of electronic and hydraulic instruments. J Hand Surg Am 2004;29(3):514–9.

47. Walker PS, Davidson W, Erkman MJ. An apparatus to assess function of the hand. J Hand Surg Am 1978;3(2):189–93.

48. Mathiowetz V, Kashman N, Volland G, et al. Grip and pinch strength: normative data for adults. Arch Phys Med Rehabil 1985;66(2):69–74.

49. Brumfield RH, Champoux A. A biomechanical study of normal wrist motion. Clin Orthop Relat Res 1984; 187:23–5.

50. Chung KC, Haas A. Relationship between patient satisfaction and objective functional outcome after surgical treatment for distal radius fractures. J Hand Ther 2009;22(4):302–7.

51. Solgaard S. Angle of inclination of the articular surface of the distal radius. Radiologe 1984;24(7): 346–8.

52. Dillingham C, Horodyski M, Struk AM, et al. Rate of improvement following volar plate open reduction and internal fixation of distal radius fractures. Adv Orthop 2011;2011:565642.

53. Solgaard S. Classification of distal radius fractures. Acta Orthop Scand 1985;56(3):249–52.

54. Medoff RJ. Essential radiographic evaluation for distal radius fractures. Hand Clin 2005;21:279–88.

55. Fernandez DL, Geissler WB. Treatment of displaced articular fractures of the radius. J Hand Surg Am 1991;16(3):255–64.

56. Trumble TE, Schmitt SR, Vedder NB. Factors affecting functional outcome of displaced intra-articular distal radius fractures. J Hand Surg Am 1994;19(2):325–40.

57. Bradway JK, Amadio PC, Cooney WP. Open reduction and internal fixation of displaced, comminuted intra-articular fractures of the distal end of the radius. J Bone Joint Surg Am 1989;71(g):839–47.

58. Knirk JL, Jupiter JB. Intra-articular fractures of the distal end of the radius in young adults. J Bone Joint Surg Am 1986;68(5):647–59.

59. Chung KC, Kotsis SV, Kim HM. Predictors of functional outcomes after surgical treatment of distal radius fractures. J Hand Surg Am 2007;32(1): 76–83.

60. McQueen M, Caspers J. Colles fracture: does the anatomical result affect the final function? J Bone Joint Surg Br 1988;70:649–51.

61. Porter M, Stockley I. Fractures of the distal radius: intermediate and end results in relation to radiographic parameters. Clin Orthop Relat Res 1987;220:241–52.

62. Batra S, Gupta A. The effect of fracture-related factors on the functional outcome at 1 year in distal radius fractures. Injury 2002;33(6):499–502.

63. Grewal R, MacDermid JC. The risk of adverse outcomes in extra-articular distal radius fractures is increased with malalignment in patients of all ages but mitigated in older patients. J Hand Surg Am 2007;32(7):962–70.

64. Arora R, Lutz M, Deml C, et al. A prospective randomized trial comparing nonoperative treatment with volar locked plate fixation for displaced and unstable distal radius fractures in patients sixty-five years of age and older. J Bone Joint Surg Am 2011;93(23):2146–53.

65. Diaz-Garcia RJ, Oda T, Shauver MJ, et al. A systematic review of outcomes and complications of treating unstable distal radius fractures in the elderly. J Hand Surg Am 2011;36(5):824–35.

66. Shauver MJ, Clapham PK, Chung KC. An economic analysis of outcomes and complications of treating distal radius fractures in the elderly. J Hand Surg Am 2011;36(12):1912–8.

67. Goldfarb CA, Rudzki JR, Catalano LW, et al. Fifteen-year outcome of displaced intra-articular fractures of the distal radius. J Hand Surg Am 2006;31(4):633–9.

68. MacDermid JC, Richards RS, Donner A, et al. Responsiveness of the Short Form-36, Disability of the Arm, Shoulder, and Hand questionnaire, Patient-Rated Wrist Evaluation, and physical impairment measurements evaluating recovery after a distal radius fracture. J Hand Surg Am 2000;25:330–40.

69. Stratford PW, Binkley JM, Riddle DL. Health status measures: strategies and analytic methods for assessing change scores. Phys Ther 1996;76:1109–23.

70. Liang MH, Fossel AH, Larson MG. Comparisons of five health status instruments for orthopedic evaluation. Med Care 1990;28:632–42.

71. Sears DE, Chung KC. Validity and responsiveness of the Jebsen-Taylor Hand Function Test. J Hand Surg Am 2010;35(1):30–7.

72. Gabl M, Krappinger D, Arora R, et al. Acceptance of patient-related evaluation of wrist function following distal radius fracture (DRF). Handchir Mikrochir Plast Chir 2007;39(1):68–72.

73. Hoang-Kim A, Pegreffi F, Moroni A, et al. Measuring wrist and hand function: common scales and checklists. Injury 2011;42(3):253–8.

Treatment Strategies of Distal Radius Fractures

Joshua G. Bales, MD*, Peter J. Stern, MD

KEYWORDS

- Treatment strategies • Distal radius fractures
- Closed reduction • Fixation

Key Points

- Evaluate the fracture based on mechanism, associated injuries, and the overall health of the patients.
- Review different treatment modalities for distal radius fractures, including casting, closed reduction, percutaneous pinning, external fixation, and various methods of internal fixation.
- Discuss treatment options with patients and review patients' expectations before devising a treatment plan.

In recent years, there has been a surge in the operative management of distal radius fractures. A review of the Medicare database from 1997 to 2005 found that more than 85,000 beneficiaries sustain distal radius fractures annually, only second to hip fractures.[1] Overall, the lifetime risk of sustaining a distal radius fracture is 15% for women and 2% for men.[2] In the past, many of these fractures were managed nonoperatively; however, advances in internal fixation have spawned an increase in operative management. In 1997, 83% of distal radius fractures sustained by Medicare beneficiaries were treated nonoperatively, this number declined to 70% in 2005.[1] Over this period, no new level 1 evidence has been published to support the increased use of internal fixation. In 2007 alone, Medicare paid $170 million for the treatment of distal radius fractures.[3] With an aging population in the United States, this number will undoubtedly increase in the coming years. Along similar lines, in 2008, Koval and colleagues[4] reviewed the case lists from orthopedic surgeons taking part II (oral) of the American Board of Orthopedic Surgery examination and found a "striking shift" toward operative management among younger surgeons. Another striking article from Mattila and colleagues[5] in Finland found a shift during an 11-year period from external fixation to internal fixation despite evidence-based medicine not supporting this change. The investigators also found the incidence and number of surgeries doubled for distal radius fractures in this time period for unknown reasons.

Along with the increased use of internal fixation for distal radius fractures, there has been an increase in surgical implant options. A myriad of dorsal, volar, and fragment specific plates have evolved in the past decade, each claiming acceptable outcomes. Despite the increase in distal radius publications, the Cochrane Collaboration concludes that there is not enough evidence to decide best practices regarding conservative interventions, surgical interventions, anesthesia for these surgeries, rehabilitation, and closed reduction techniques.[6–10] Thus, the question for the surgeon is: What factors are important in determining the optimal treatment of distal radius fractures?

Hand Surgery Specialists, Inc, 538 Oak Street, Cincinnati, OH 45219, USA
* Corresponding author.
E-mail address: jbales@handsurg.com

Hand Clin 28 (2012) 177–184
doi:10.1016/j.hcl.2012.02.003
0749-0712/12/$ – see front matter © 2012 Elsevier Inc. All rights reserved.

The mechanism of injury is an important factor in clinical decision making because it allows the clinician to determine the amount of energy involved in the creation of the fracture and reveals vital information regarding the quality of the bone and the injury to associated ligaments and soft tissue. For example, a kinetic low-energy injury, such as a fall from a standing height, should alert the clinician to rule out osteoporosis or other metabolic diseases affecting bone quality. High-energy distal radius fractures more frequently occur in active, young adults and usually require operative intervention for bony stabilization and management of damage to the soft tissue envelope. In addition to the distal radius fracture, the surgeon should always evaluate the status of the carpus, elbow, shoulder, and neck for associated injuries.

The next step in the decision-making process should be to review the timing of definitive treatment. Fractures more than 14 days old are difficult to reduce by closed means, secondary to callus formation. On the contrary, acute treatment of a distal radius fracture, within the first few days, may not allow sufficient time for the acute swelling to subside. Unfortunately, the exact timing of when to fix these fractures is not so exact and based more on surgeon experience than a high level of evidence. In the authors' practice, when internal surgical management is indicated, the fracture is either fixed the day of the injury or the initial swelling is allowed to subside, and the operation occurs 7 to 14 days later.

Another important concept involves shared decision making with patients.[11] The authors attempt to provide patients with the risks and benefits of conservative care versus surgery based on the patients' expectations, lifestyle, and associated injuries. Lurie and Weinstein[12] have championed this idea of shared decision making in orthopedics as a method that allows patient preferences and values to determine the correct rate of health care use.

TREATMENT STRATEGIES FOR DISTAL RADIUS FRACTURES
Closed Reduction

A well-executed closed reduction is nearly always indicated. By recreating the fracture mechanism, disengaging the fragments, reducing the fracture, and placing a 3-point mold, many distal radius fractures may be treated closed. In the authors' practice, nearly all extraarticular fractures and most intraarticular fractures, excluding unstable shear fractures, warrant a closed reduction.

Following closed reduction, repeat radiographic assessment of fracture alignment is mandatory. Many fracture reductions are acceptable yet fall out of alignment at follow-up. The question remains, will these patients develop posttraumatic osteoarthritis? Forward and colleagues[13] reviewed 106 adults with malunited distal radius fractures sustained in patients younger than 40 years of age and found that at a mean follow-up of 38 years, no patient required a salvage procedure and the Disabilities of the Arm, Shoulder, Hand (DASH) scores did not differ from the population norms. The investigators concluded that imperfect reduction may not correlate with late symptomatic arthritis.

Recent literature has shown that many distal radius fractures in the elderly may be treated non-operatively, even after a loss of initial closed reduction.[14] Arora and colleagues[14] randomized patients who failed an initial closed reduction, aged 65 years and older, to either open reduction internal fixation (ORIF) with a volar locked plate or nonoperative treatment. They found that range of motion, pain, and subjective outcomes did not differ between the 2 groups at the 12-month follow-up examination. No significant difference existed in DASH or patient related wrist evaluation scores at 6 and 12 months. Grip strength, however, was significantly better at all time points. Although the radiographic parameters of dorsal tilt, inclination, and shortening of the radius were all better in the operative treatment group, this did not correspond to subjective outcomes.

In a similar study, Egol and colleagues[15] examined elderly patients, older than 65 years of age, who failed initial closed reduction and either received surgery or continued cast immobilization. The investigators found no statistically significant functional differences. Grip strength and radiographic outcomes were significantly better in the operative group at 1 year; however, these parameters did not correlate with subjective outcomes. Both of these studies suggest that minor limitations in objective parameters, such as grip strength, do not seem to limit functional recovery. The limitation of these 2 studies is that follow-up is limited to only 1 year.

Closed reduction outcomes have also been compared with external fixation. Aktekin and colleagues[16] retrospectively reviewed patients aged 65 years and older who received external fixation or closed reduction and casting for dorsally displaced AO/ASIF type A or C fractures. The investigators followed the patients for roughly 2 years and found no significant differences in DASH scores. Wrist extension and ulnar deviation, clinically, were the only significantly improved parameters with external fixation.

Despite the historic impetus to always attempt closed reduction initially, Neidenbach and colleagues[17] prospectively reviewed patients with a mean age of 62 years whose wrists were treated conservatively with or without closed reduction before casting. The investigators found that all patients attained a "successful level of activities in their daily life" regardless of treatment. There was no difference in DASH or 36-Item Short Form Health Survey scores and no difference in radiological parameters for these 2 groups of patients. The conclusions of this article echo what was found by Arora and colleagues[14] and Egol and colleagues[15]: perhaps closed reduction is not necessary in every patient older than 65 years of age. However, more evidence-based, long-term data are needed before definitively arriving at this conclusion.

External Fixation or Percutaneous Fixation

Over the past 50 years, external fixation devices have evolved with new configurations and modifications, but the principles of external fixation remain the same. Most external fixation devices rely on ligamentotaxis to provide stability and reduction. The ligamentotaxis, in the form of traction, is transmitted through the radioscaphocapitate and long radiolunate ligaments.[18]

Biomechanically, external fixation provides relative stability compared with the absolute stability of a plate construct. Despite external fixation being a nonrigid construct, it must resist loads of up to 245 N, which is the intraarticular pressure within the wrist in radial deviation and the forearm in supination.[19] To achieve this strength, the surgeon needs to use the proper configuration and size of fixator rods, clamps, and bars. To increase the rigidity of the construct, use more than one parallel spanning rod, place the rod as close to the skin as possible, and consider large diameter rods. In addition, underdrilling the pin hole by 0.1 mm provides better pin fixation and less risk of pin loosening or pullout. When planning the placement of the pins for optimal stability, one pin should be close to the fracture site and the other as far away as possible.[20]

Despite a well-placed external fixator, unacceptable intraarticular displacement may be present. In such instances, the authors do not hesitate to augment the fixation with percutaneous pins. These pins can stabilize a radial styloid fragment or buttress a sheared component of the fracture. Dunning and colleagues[21] found that combining an external fixator with 1.6-mm K pins closely approximates the strength of a 3.5-mm dorsal AO plate (Synthes, Paoli, Pennsylvania). In these

instances, the external fixator is more of a neutralization force than a distraction force. Kreder and colleagues[22] reviewed the results of ORIF versus external fixation augmented with pinning and found that there was no statistically significant difference in the radiological alignment or range of motion at 2 years. The investigators also found that external fixation and pinning provided a more rapid return of function and better functional outcome than ORIF in cases whereby intraarticular step-off and gap were minimal.

Bindra lists the following indications for both temporary and definitive external fixation: temporizing polytrauma patients, transferring patients to a higher level of care, and initial treatment of severe open fractures with extensive soft tissue loss.[23] The authors would also consider external fixation for an extremely unstable fracture to supplement suboptimal internal fixation. In the extraarticular distal radius fractures that are candidates for external fixation, nonbridging (fixation does not span radiocarpal joint) external fixation allows early range of motion of the wrist with some promising results.[24,25] Slutsky also describes arthroscopic assisted reduction with nonbridging external fixation for more than 2-mm articular displacement in isolated radial styloid fractures and simple 3-part distal radius fractures to allow for early range of motion.[18] However, difficulty exists in the reproduction of complex wrist kinematics while maintaining ligamentotaxis.[26] Fracture stability is not sacrificed for early range of motion. In fact, Lozano-Calderon and colleagues[27] have found that early mobilization, 2 weeks versus 6 weeks, after operative fixation of a distal radius fracture does not affect outcomes. Contraindications to external fixation include volar or dorsal shear fractures, fractures with disruption of volar radiocarpal ligaments, and ulnar translocation secondary to an unstable distal radioulnar joint (DRUJ).

Complications are a common problem with external fixation. Up to 30% of patients will develop pin track infections necessitating oral or intravenous antibiotics and possible early removal of the pin. The pins may loosen, cause tendon irritation or attritional rupture, or irritate the superficial branch of the radial nerve. The poor outcomes with external fixation are largely derived from overdistraction of the carpus. This distraction leads to intrinsic tightness, finger stiffness, increased carpal tunnel pressures, and a higher incidence of complex regional pain syndrome.[18,28] Early motion at the metacarpophalangeal (MCP) joint combined with MCP dynamic splinting may partially prevent some of these complications.

Results are mixed when comparing external fixation with internal fixation. A meta-analysis by

Margaliot, Chung and colleagues[28] did not detect a significant difference in grip strength, wrist range of motion, radiographic alignment, pain, and physician-rated outcomes between external or internal fixation of distal radius fractures. However, external fixation was associated with higher rates of infection, hardware failure, and nerve irritation than internal fixation. More recently, Richard and colleagues[29] reviewed 59 patients treated with external fixation and 56 with volar plates for comminuted intraarticular distal radius fractures and found that volar plate fixation had an overall decreased incidence of complications and better wrist motion than external fixation. The investigators also found that patients with volar plates had less pain and better functional outcomes at 1 year.

Percutaneous Pinning

Many distal radius fractures may also benefit from percutaneous K-wire fixation alone. In a 2007 Cochrane database review, Handoll and colleagues[30] found "some evidence" to support the use of percutaneous pinning, both across-fracture and Kapandji (interfocal) pinning. However, the reviewers found higher rates of complications with Kapandji pinning and biodegradable pins, thus cautioning their use. Hollevoet and colleagues[31] recently performed a prospective randomized study comparing percutaneous K-wire fixation with volar plates in patients older than 50 years of age. They found at greater than 1-year follow-up, no significant differences in clinical outcomes or DASH scores between the 2 groups. Volar plates were only statistically superior to K wires in restoring radiographic ulnar variance. Rozental and colleagues[32] specifically randomized patients with displaced, unstable extraarticular or simple intraarticular fractures of the distal radius to either pin fixation or volar plating. These patients were then assessed at 6, 9, and 12 weeks after surgery then again at 1 year. The investigators found better functional results in the early postoperative period with volar plating. However, at 1 year, there was no significant difference in the DASH scores between the groups. From a cost-analysis perspective, Shyamalan and colleagues[33] compared volar locked plating with k-wire fixation and found that locked volar plating increases costs more than threefold. In the authors' practice, percutaneous pinning is considered in patients with unstable extraarticular or simple intraarticular fractures particularly if bone stock is satisfactory. In the shared-decision-making approach, these patients are also offered volar plating for these fractures based on age, lifestyle, work, and preferences.

INTERNAL FIXATION
Volar Plates

Since the early 1990s, there has been an exponential growth in volar plate fixation for the treatment of distal radius fractures.[34–36] Chung and colleagues[37,38] noted that American Society for Surgery of the Hand members perform internal fixation in the Medicare population at a statistically significantly higher rate than their surgical colleagues. Whatever the reason for the popularity of volar plates for distal radius fractures, we still need rigorous scientific trials to validate their utility in these fractures.

When comparing dorsal with volar plating, many surgeons prefer the volar approach because it is less disruptive to the extrinsic tendons.[39] In addition, the volar cortical surface is not routinely comminuted, and precontoured plates can be applied to facilitate accurate and anatomic reduction. The volar plate may also be covered with the pronator quadratus, minimizing tendon irritation. Many investigators have also shown volar plate effectiveness in the treatment of dorsally displaced, unstable fractures of the distal radius.[40–42] Volar plating also preserves the vascular supply to dorsal metaphyseal fragments. Finally, most surgeons do not routinely remove volar plates as opposed to those placed dorsally.

The disadvantages of volar plating include the lack of direct visualization of articular fragments, screw penetration irritating extensor tendons, prominent plating causing flexor tendon attritional rupture, and joint penetration of the screws. Soong and colleagues[43] reviewed patients who underwent volar locked plating and found that plates that extend volarly past a line drawn tangentially to the most volar extent of the rim of the distal radius were at an increased risk of flexor tendon rupture. Tanaka and colleagues[44] performed an excellent cadaveric study showing that plates placed volarly, distal to the watershed line, impinge on the flexor pollicis longus tendon risking attritional rupture, even in cases of anatomic fracture healing. In intraarticular fractures, arthroscopy can be of assistance with reduction and assessing ligamentous injury but this increases surgical costs, time, and may be subject to the same attritional rupture as nonsurgically treated fractures.[45]

In the authors' practice, volar plating is the preferred treatment of unstable fractures in younger patients, volar shear fractures, articular impaction (die-punch) fractures, and intraarticular step off and gap formation (>2 mm) that cannot be controlled with closed reduction. Koenig and colleagues[46] created an analytic model to compare internal fixation with a volar plate to nonoperative management of a displaced, distal radius fracture. They found that the plate proved a higher probability of painless union based on the current literature. They qualify this conclusion with the caveat that older patients, who have more tolerance for malunion, may be candidates for nonoperative treatment.

Dorsal Plates

Surgeons may elect dorsal plating when there is considerable dorsal comminution or dorsal displacement. Dorsal plating initially fell out of favor because of the first-generation plates irritating and, in some cases, causing attritional rupture of the extensor tendons.[47] As technology advanced, newer, low-profile plates have been designed to avoid this complication. In one of the first comparative articles of volar versus dorsal plating, Ruch and colleagues[11] found that both methods had similar DASH scores, yet Gartland and Werley scores were significantly better in those treated with volar plating. The investigators also reported higher rates of volar collapse and late complications in dorsal plating.

On the contrary, Yu and colleagues[48] reviewed purely low-profile dorsal plates versus volar locking plates and found no significant difference in tendon irritation or rupture. In fact, Yu and colleagues found that volar plating was associated with a higher rate of neuropathic complications. The authors favor dorsal plating in those fractures with considerable intraarticular dorsal comminution or dorsal displacement that cannot be controlled with volar plates. Fragment-specific fixation or special T- or L-plates are also used to stabilize a dorsal, displaced die-punch fracture. Dorsal plates are routinely removed because of concerns of tendon irritation and rupture. The authors also remove volar plates (6 months after internal fixation) when the distal lip of the plate is anterior to the watershed line of the volar cortex.

Fragment-Specific Fixation

Because of the somewhat bulky profile of volar and dorsal plates and the impetus to avoid tendon irritation, low-profile fragment-specific plates were subsequently developed. Despite small size, these plates were designed to withstand forces associated with immediate wrist motion. In a small series, Konrath and colleagues[49] reported good initial results with fragment-specific fixation but with a high rate of complications: 29% radial sensory nerve paresthesias (secondary to application of a precontoured radial column plate) and reoperation in 18%. Benson and colleagues[50] retrospectively reviewed a larger series of 81 patients with

intraarticular fractures using this system and found that all patients had excellent or good results with an average DASH score of 9. Ten patients in Benson's series had radial sensory numbness, and hardware was removed in 5 of the patients. The authors rarely use fragment-specific fixation because of concerns of radial sensory neuropathy and the length of time required to apply such plates. Many of these fragment-specific fractures may be effectively treated with percutaneous pinning or dorsal or volar plating with supplemental percutaneous pinning as needed. Sammer and colleagues[51] prospectively evaluated fragment-specific fixation versus volar plating and found better subjective and objectives outcomes and fewer complications with volar plates.

Special Considerations for ORIF

Open fractures of the distal radius pose an additional controversy in fracture management. Traditionally, it was recommended that all open fractures have a surgical debridement within 6 hours, and it was considered inappropriate to incorporate any internal fixation in these types of fractures. More recent literature by Kurylo and colleagues[52] suggests that open grade I and grade II distal radius fractures do not require early (<6 hours) debridement. In addition to these findings, Kurylo and colleagues[52] found that temporary external fixation with staged conversion to plating actually increases the risk of complications. Severe or grade III open fractures of the distal radius do experience a considerable number of initial complications with poorer long-term clinical outcomes regardless of operative treatment.[53]

Another consideration is the presence of an ulnar styloid fracture because it relates to the stability of the distal radioulnar joint. Kim and colleagues[53] reviewed a prospective cohort of 138 patients who underwent volar plating for distal radius fractures associated with ulnar styloid fractures. The investigators then separated the patients into those without an ulnar styloid fracture, those with a base fracture, and those with a nonbase fracture. There was a 59% nonunion rate regardless of location of the styloid fracture. They also found no measurable differences in motion, strength, or functional scores at a mean follow-up of 23 months in patients with or without an ulnar styloid fracture. In a similar study, Sammer, Chung, and colleagues[54] found a nonunion rate of 68% of ulnar styloid fractures associated with distal radius fractures. The presence of a nonunion had no correlation with functional scores and none of the patients had DRUJ instability. On the other hand, when managing distal radius fractures nonoperatively, Oskarsson and colleagues[55] reviewed 158 fractures and found that an ulnar styloid fracture was a greater predictor of fracture instability than intraarticular involvement of the fracture on the distal radius. This study, however, reviewed a nonoperative group of patients, making it impossible to extrapolate to fractures treated surgically. May and colleagues[56] reviewed 130 distal radius fractures and assessed for DRUJ stability, dividing the patients to those with and without ulnar styloid fractures. The investigators are unclear on the type of fixation and stated that 49% were treated with open or percutaneous fixation. Nonetheless, they report a higher incidence of DRUJ instability with ulnar styloid base fractures and styloid fractures displaced greater than 2 mm.

Souer and colleagues[57] matched 2 cohorts of patients, those with fractures of the ulnar styloid and those without. They found that an unrepaired fracture of the base of the ulnar styloid did not seem to influence function or outcome of a distal radial fracture with plate and screw fixation. It should be noted that anatomic reduction of the distal radius fracture yielded stability of the DRUJ in these fractures.

In an evidence-based review of ulnar styloid fractures associated with distal radius fractures, Wysocki and Ruch[58] state that only in the uncommon case of DRUJ instability after volar plate fixation of the distal radius would they consider fixing a concomitant ulnar styloid fracture. Based on existing current literature, most ulnar styloid fractures do not require operative treatment. The authors would fix the ulnar styloid only if there were obvious instability of the DRUJ or radiographic evidence of ulnar head subluxation or dislocation.

An additional consideration of distal radius fractures is a review of concurrent injuries, such as scaphoid or elbow fractures. Routine radiographs of the elbow should be obtained in patients with distal radius fractures, especially in those fractures secondary to high-energy trauma. In combined elbow and distal radius fractures, anatomic reduction of the distal radius fracture with internal fixation is most always necessary, in addition to appropriate treatment of the concomitant elbow injury. In the authors' practice, the combination of scaphoid/distal radius fractures is usually treated with ORIF of both fractures. Rutgers and colleagues[59] reviewed this combination of fractures and found no consensus in the literature regarding fixation. However, the investigators stated that from their retrospective review, combined fractures of the distal radius and scaphoid were usually the result of high-energy trauma and best treated with internal fixation of both fractures.

In certain instances, bridge plating, as popularized by Hanel and colleagues,[60] may be an excellent solution to severely comminuted distal radius fractures. Bridge plating high-energy distal radius fractures, especially those fractures that extend into the diaphysis, allows early weight bearing in trauma patients. Hanel and colleagues[60] reviewed 62 patients with bridge plating and found excellent maintenance of reduction with few reported complications.

Compartment syndrome may occur in both low- and high-energy distal radius fractures.[61] Compartment syndrome may also develop after surgical treatment, which can require a second surgery for decompression fasciotomies. Pain out of proportion in the wrist and hand during the physical examination should alert the surgeon to the possibility of compartment syndrome. In addition, signs and symptoms of carpal tunnel syndrome (CTS) should be appropriately evaluated in all patients with distal radius fractures. In patients with worsening CTS after a distal radius fracture, urgent treatment of the fracture and carpal tunnel release should be strongly considered.

SUMMARY

When counseling patients with distal radius fractures, especially low-energy fragility fractures, the caregiver should discuss both operative and nonoperative options because the literature is inconclusive regarding the superiority of one treatment option over the other. The surgeon should also remember to discuss important health concerns, such as osteoporosis, and appropriate referrals to either a primary care physician or an endocrinologist for follow-up if needed. In addition, recent guidelines from the American Academy of Orthopaedic Surgeons have encouraged the surgeon to offer vitamin C to avoid complications of complex regional pain syndrome.

Closed reduction, external fixation, and ORIF each have advantages and disadvantages. The purpose of this review is not to provide the clinician with an algorithm for the treatment of distal radius fractures. These fractures span an extensive spectrum of severity across age groups and demographics. Fortunately, the surgeon holds a vast array of options to provide care for patients with distal radius fractures. The choice of fixation or conservative care resides in the personality of the fracture and the needs of the patients.

REFERENCES

1. Chung KC, Shauver MJ, Birkmeyer JD. Trends in the United States in the treatment of distal radial

fractures in the elderly. J Bone Joint Surg 2009;91: 1868–73.

2. Ruch DS. Fractures of the distal radius and ulna. In: Bucholz RW, Heckman JD, Court-Brown C, editors. Rockwood and green's fractures in adults, vol. 1, 6th edition. Philadelphia: Lippincott Williams and Wilkins; 2006. p. 909–88.

3. Shauver MJ, Yin H, Banerjee M, et al. Current and future national costs to Medicare for the treatment of distal radius fracture in the elderly. J Hand Surg 2011;36:1282–7.

4. Koval KJ, Harrast JJ, Anglen JO, et al. Fractures of the distal part of the radius, the evolution of practice over time. Where's the evidence. J Bone Joint Surg 2008;90:1855–61.

5. Mattila VM, Huttunen TT, Sillanpaa P, et al. Significant change in the surgical treatment of distal radius fractures: a nationwide study between 1998 and 2008 in Finland. J Trauma 2011;71(4):939–42.

6. Handoll HH, Madhok R. Closed reduction methods for treating distal radial fractures in adults. Cochrane Database Syst Rev 2003;1:CD003763.

7. Handoll HH, Madhok R. Surgical interventions for treating distal radial fractures in adults. Cochrane Database Syst Rev 2003;3:CD003209.

8. Handoll HH, Madhok R. Conservative interventions for treating distal radial fractures in adults. Cochrane Database Syst Rev 2003;2:CD000314.

9. Handoll HH, Madhok R, Dodds C. Anaesthesia for treating distal radial fracture in adults. Cochrane Database Syst Rev 2002;3:CD003320.

10. Handoll HH, Madhok R, Howe TE. Rehabilitation for distal radial fractures in adults. Cochrane Database Syst Rev 2006;3:CD003324.

11. Ruch DS, Papadonikolakis A. Volar versus dorsal plating in the management of intra-articular distal radius fractures. J Hand Surg 2006;31:9–16.

12. Lurie JD, Weinstein JN. Shared decision-making and the orthopaedic workforce. Clin Orthop Relat Res 2001;(385):68–75.

13. Forward DP, Davis TR, Sithole JS. Do young patients with malunited fractures of the distal radius inevitably develop symptomatic post-traumatic osteoarthritis. J Bone Joint Surg Br 2008;90(5):629–37.

14. Arora R, Lutz M, Deml C, et al. A prospective randomized trial comparing nonoperative treatment with volar locking plate fixation for displaced and unstable distal radial fractures in patients sixty-five years of age and older. J Bone Joint Surg Am 2011;93:2146–53.

15. Egol KA, Walsh M, Romo-Cardoso S, et al. Distal radial fractures in the elderly: operative compared with nonoperative treatment. J Bone Joint Surg Am 2010;92(9):1851–7.

16. Aktekin CN, Altay M, Gursoy Z, et al. Comparison between external fixation and cast treatment in the management of distal radius fractures in patients aged 65 years and older. J Hand Surg Am 2010; 35(5):736–42.

17. Neidenbach P, Audige L, Wilhelmi-Mock M, et al. The efficacy of closed reduction in displaced distal radius fractures. Injury 2010;41(6):592–8.

18. Slutsky DJ. External fixation of distal radius fractures. J Hand Surg 2007;32:1624–37.

19. Rikli DA, Honigmann P, Babst R, et al. Intra-articular pressure measurement in the radioulnocarpal joint using a novel sensor: in vitro and in vivo results. J Hand Surg 2007;32:67–75.

20. Behrens F, Johnson WD, Koch TW, et al. Bending stiffness of unilateral and bilateral fixator frames. Clin Orthop Relat Res 1983;178:103–10.

21. Dunning CE, Lindsay CS, Bicknell RT, et al. Supplemental pinning improves the stability of external fixation in distal radius fractures during simulated finger and forearm motion. J Hand Surg 1999;24: 992–1000.

22. Kreder HJ, Hanel DP, Agel J, et al. Indirect reduction and percutaneous fixation versus open reduction and internal fixation for displaced intra-articular fractures of the distal radius: a randomised, controlled trial. J Bone Joint Surg 2005;87:829–36.

23. Bindra RR. Biomechanics and biology of external fixation of distal radius fractures. Hand Clin 2005; 21:363–73.

24. McQueen MM. Redisplaced unstable fractures of the distal radius. A randomised, prospective study of bridging versus non-bridging external fixation. J Bone Joint Surg 1998;80:665–9.

25. McQueen MM. Metaphyseal external fixation of the distal radius. Bull Hosp Jt Dis 1999;58:9–14.

26. Sommerkamp TG, Seeman M, Silliman J, et al. Dynamic external fixation of unstable fractures of the distal part of the radius. A prospective, randomized comparison with static external fixation. J Bone Joint Surg 1994;76:1149–61.

27. Lozano-Calderon SA, Souer S, Mudgal C, et al. Wrist mobilization following volar plate fixation of fractures of the distal part of the radius. J Bone Joint Surg Am 2008;90(6):1297–304.

28. Margaliot Z, Haase SC, Kotsis SV, et al. A meta-analysis of outcomes of external fixation versus plate osteosynthesis for unstable distal radius fractures. J Hand Surg 2005;30:1185–99.

29. Richard MJ, Wartinbee DA, Riboh J, et al. Analysis of the complications of palmar plating versus external fixation for fractures of the distal radius. J Hand Surg 2011;36:1614–20.

30. Handoll HH, Vaghela MV, Madhok R. Percutaneous pinning for treating distal radius fractures in adults. Cochrane Database Syst Rev 2007;3:CD006080.

31. Hollevoet N, Vanhoutie T, Vanhove W, et al. Percutaneous K-wire fixation versus palmar plating with locking screws for Colles' fractures. Acta Orthop Belg 2011;77(2):180–7.

32. Rozental TD, Blazar PE, Franko OI, et al. Functional outcomes for unstable distal radial fractures treated with open reduction and internal fixation or closed reduction and percutaneous fixation. A prospective randomized trial. J Bone Joint Surg Am 2009;91(8): 1837–46.

33. Shyamalan G, Theokli C, Pearse Y, et al. Volar locking plates versus Kirschner wires for distal radial fractures a cost analysis study. Injury 2009;40(12): 1279–81.

34. Jupiter JB. Fractures of the distal end of the radius. J Bone Joint Surg 1991;73:461–9.

35. Leibovic SJ, Geissler WB. Treatment of complex intra-articular distal radius fractures. Orthop Clin North Am 1994;25:685–706.

36. Jakob M, Rikli DA, Regazzoni P. Fractures of the distal radius treated by internal fixation and early function. A prospective study of 73 consecutive patients. J Bone Joint Surg 2000;82B:340–4.

37. Chung KC, Shauver MJ, Yin H. The relationship between ASSH membership and the treatment of distal radius fracture in the United States Medicare population. J Hand Surg 2011;36:1288–93.

38. Chung KC, Shauver MJ, Yin H, et al. Variations in the use of internal fixation for distal radial fracture in the United States Medicare population. J Bone Joint Surg Am 2011;93:2154–62.

39. Orbay JL, Touhami A. Current concepts in volar fixed-angle fixation of unstable distal radius fractures. Clin Orthop Relat Res 2006;445:58–67.

40. Osada D, Kamei S, Masuzaki K, et al. Prospective study of distal radius fractures treated with a volar locking plate system. J Hand Surg 2008;33:691–700.

41. Carter PR, Frederick HA, Laseter GF. Open reduction and internal fixation of unstable distal radius fractures with a low-profile plate: a multicenter study of 73 fractures. J Hand Surg 1998;23:300–7.

42. Fitoussi F, Ip WY, Chow SP. Treatment of displaced intra-articular fractures of the distal end of the radius with plates. J Bone Joint Surg 1997;79:1303–12.

43. Soong M, Earp BE, Bishop G, et al. Volar locking plate implant prominence and flexor tendon rupture. J Bone Joint Surg Am 2011;93(4):328–35.

44. Tanaka Y, Aoki M, Izumi T, et al. Effect of distal radius volar plate position on contact pressure between the flexor pollicis longus tendon and the distal plate edge. J Hand Surg 2011;36:1790–7.

45. Herzberg G. Intra-articular fracture of the distal radius: arthroscopic-assisted reduction. J Hand Surg Am 2010;35(9):1517–9.

46. Koenig KM, Davis GC, Grove MR, et al. Is early internal fixation preferred to cast treatment for well-reduced unstable distal radial fractures? J Bone Joint Surg Am 2009;91(9):2086–93.

47. Nana AD, Joshi A, Lichtman DM. Plating of the distal radius. J Am Acad Orthop Surg 2005;13(3):159–71.

48. Yu YR, Makhni MC, Tabrizi S, et al. Complications of low-profile dorsal versus volar locking plates in the distal radius: a comparative study. J Hand Surg 2011;36:1135–41.

49. Konrath GA, Bahler S. Open reduction and internal fixation of unstable distal radius fractures: results using the trimed fixation system. J Orthop Trauma 2002;16:578–85.

50. Benson LS, Minihane KP, Stern LD, et al. The outcome of intra-articular distal radius fractures treated with fragment specific fixation. J Hand Surg Am 2006;31(8):1333–9.

51. Sammer DM, Fuller DS, Kim HM, et al. A comparative study of fragment-specific versus volar plate fixation of distal radius fractures. Plast Reconstr Surg 2008;122(5):1441–50.

52. Kurylo JC, Axelrad TW, Tornetta P 3rd, et al. Open fractures of the distal radius: the effects of delayed debridement and immediate internal fixation on infection rates and the need for secondary procedures. J Hand Surg Am 2011;36(7):1131–4. [Epub 2011 Jun 2].

53. Kim JK, Koh YD, Do NH. Should an ulnar styloid fracture be fixed following volar plate fixation of a distal radial fracture? J Bone Joint Surg 2010; 92A:1–6.

54. Sammer DM, Shah HM, Shauver MJ, et al. The effect of ulnar styloid fractures on patient-rated outcomes after volar locking plating of distal radius fractures. J Hand Surg 2009;34:1595–602.

55. Oskarsson GV, Aaser P, Hjall A. Do we underestimate the predictive value of the ulnar styloid affection in Colles fractures? Arch Orthop Trauma Surg 1997;116:341–4.

56. May MM, Lawton JN, Blazar PE. Ulnar styloid fractures associated with distal radius fractures: incidence and implications for distal radioulnar joint instability. J Hand Surg 2002;27:965–71.

57. Souer JS, Ring D, Matschke S, et al. Effect of an unrepaired fracture of the ulnar styloid base on outcome after plate and screw fixation of a distal radial fracture. J Bone Joint Surg Am 2009;91(4): 830–8.

58. Wysocki RW, Ruch DS. Ulnar styloid fracture with distal radius fracture. J Hand Surg Am 2011 Oct 21. [Epub ahead of print].

59. Rutgers M, Mudgal CS, Shin R. Combined fractures of the distal radius and scaphoid. J Hand Surg Eur Vol 2008;33(4):478–83.

60. Hanel DP, Lut TS, Weil WM. Bridge plating of distal radius fractures: the Harborview method. Clin Orthop Relat Res 2006;445:91–9.

61. Kupersmith LM, Weinfeld SB. Acute volar and dorsal compartment syndrome after a distal radius fracture: a case report. J Orthop Trauma 2003;17(5): 382–6.

Avoiding and Treating Perioperative Complications of Distal Radius Fractures

Peter C. Rhee, DO[a], David G. Dennison, MD[b],
Sanjeev Kakar, MD, MRCS[b],*

KEYWORDS

- Distal radius • Fracture • Perioperative complication
- Treatment

Numerous methods of treatment are available for the management of distal radius fractures, with modern trends favoring volar fixed-angle distal radius plates. Whatever the method of fixation, recognition, management, and prevention of the known associated complications are essential to achieve a good outcome. This article reviews the common preventable complications that are associated with operative treatment of distal radius fractures, including tendon injuries, inadequate reduction, subsidence or collapse, intra-articular placement of pegs or screws, nerve injuries, complex regional pain syndrome, carpal tunnel syndrome, and compartment syndrome.

TENDON INJURY

Flexor and extensor tendon problems after surgical fixation of distal radius fractures may range from simple irritation, adhesion formation, tenosynovitis, to laceration or attritional rupture. McKay and colleagues[1] noted 85 physician-reported complications in their series of 250 distal radius fractures treated operatively and nonoperatively, including tendon adhesions (n = 6), tendon rupture (n = 4), and tenosynovitis (n = 12). The cause can be attributed to mechanical or vascular insult to the tendons from the fracture itself, the surgical procedure, or prominent hardware.[2] Yu and colleagues[3] examined the complication rates between a low-profile dorsal plate and volar locking plate fixation in 104 distal radius fractures (n = 57 and n = 47, respectively). The use of a volar locking plate resulted in 1 rupture of the flexor pollicis longus (FPL) (n = 1) and 6 cases of tendon irritation. Conversely, low-profile dorsal plate fixation resulted in no tendon ruptures and 7 cases of tendon irritation.

Extensor Tendon

Extensor tendon dysfunction can arise from either dorsal or volar fixation of distal radius fractures. Ring and colleagues[4] reported on 5 cases of extensor tendon irritation in 22 distal radius fractures treated with dorsal plate fixation (π-plate, Synthes Ltd, Paoli, PA). Hardware removal was required in 4 patients with resolution of symptoms. Rozental and colleagues[5] noted 7 cases of extensor tendon irritation and 1 rupture of the extensor digitorum communis (EDC) to the ring finger out of 19 patients treated with the Synthes π-plate. The investigators reported complete

[a] Department of Orthopedic Surgery, Mayo Clinic, 200 First Street Southwest, Rochester, MN 55905, USA
[b] Division of Hand and Microvascular Surgery, Department of Orthopedic Surgery, Mayo Clinic, 200 First Street Southwest, Rochester, MN 55905, USA
* Corresponding author.
E-mail address: kakar.sanjeev@mayo.edu

Hand Clin 28 (2012) 185–198
doi:10.1016/j.hcl.2012.03.004
0749-0712/12/$ – see front matter © 2012 Elsevier Inc. All rights reserved.

resolution of tendon irritation after hardware removal and functional recovery of the affected digit after tendon reconstruction.

To minimize the risk of tendon irritation, several local tissue interposition flaps have been proposed to serve as a protective interface between a dorsal plate and the overlying tendons. Chiang and colleagues[6] described splitting the extensor retinacular flap in half to produce ulnar-based and radial-based flaps that can be used to cover the floor of the fourth extensor compartment over the dorsal plate. However, 12 of 20 patients continued to have symptoms of dorsal wrist pain. Althausen and Szabo advocated elevating the dorsal distal radius periosteum with the third and fourth extensor compartments and subsequent reapproximation of the periosteum over the dorsal plate.[7] If the thickness of the dorsal plate would not allow full periosteal coverage of the hardware, the investigators used an acellular dermal matrix patch to reapproximate the 2 ends of the periosteum (AlloDerm, Lifecell Corp., Branchburg, NJ). They reported no cases of tenosynovitis, tendon adhesions, or tendon ruptures with this technique.

The incidence of extensor tendon injury after volar plate fixation has been reported to be 3% to 5%,[8,9] with the extensor pollicis longus (EPL) known to be the most commonly affected extensor tendon. It may be secondary to drill-bit penetration,[10] a prominent edge of the dorsal cortex, or the sharp turn distal to the Lister's tubercle.[11] Benson and colleagues[11] noted that prominent screws were also a predominant cause. The investigators advocated placing the screws directed into the third extensor compartment short, or not placing them because of the difficulty in assessing prominent hardware at the dorsal surface. The EPL tendon adjacent to the Lister tubercle may also be susceptible to vascular insufficiency because it is devoid of intrinsic vascular supply and thus is at risk of rupture in minimally displaced distal radius fractures.[2]

Traditional anteroposterior and lateral radiographs may not allow accurate assessment of screw length along the dorsal rim of the distal radius. This problem was highlighted by Thomas and Greenberg[12] who showed a low sensitivity (56%) of standard lateral and oblique radiographs for detecting screw tip penetration through the dorsal cortex. Many investigators have described a technique of using fluoroscopic imaging with the beam aimed along the dorsal longitudinal axis of the radius with the wrist in hyperflexion to obtain a better view of the appropriate screw length along the dorsal cortex (skyline view[13] or the dorsal horizon view[14]). Riddick and colleagues[15] demonstrated improved accuracy in correctly detecting long screws with the skyline view in 83% of cases compared with the lateral (77%, $P = .05$) and pronated oblique (50%, $P<.01$) views.[15] Using these imaging techniques, Joseph and colleagues[14] detected 3 cases of dorsal cortex screw penetration (out of 15 wrists) that were not apparent on standard radiographic views. Maschke and colleagues[16] advocated obtaining a lateral radiograph of the distal radius with varying degrees of pronation and supination to evaluate the ulnar and radial dorsal surfaces relative to the Lister tubercle to confirm appropriate screw length. Technically, the placement of screws of appropriate length is a combination of accurate drilling with a calibrated drill guide, accurate depth measurement, and selection of a screw with a length 2 mm less than the shortest measurement from either drilling with a calibrated drill guide or with the depth gauge.

In cases of EPL rupture, transfer of the extensor indicis proprius (EIP) or free tendon graft (FTG) reconstruction can restore thumb function. Noorda and Hage[17] reported on the transfer of the EIP to the EPL in 22 patients at a mean follow-up of 7 years. Based on the Geldmacher criteria (radial abduction, deficit in thumb extension, opposition deficit, and finger flexion-extension deficit), there were 5 excellent (23%), 4 good (18%), 12 satisfactory (55%), and 1 poor (4%) outcome with 8% loss of pinch strength compared with the uninjured side. Lemmen and colleagues[18] noted similar Geldmacher scores (7 excellent, 4 good, 5 satisfactory, and 1 poor) in 17 patients with EIP to EPL transfer. A recent study by Schaller and colleagues[19] compared EPL reconstruction with EIP transfer (n = 28) or palmaris longus FTG reconstruction (n = 17). The investigators noted very good to good Geldmacher scores in 86% and 77% of patients at a mean of 4.3 years, respectively. There were no significant differences in thumb abduction (51° ± 11° vs 52° ± 9°, $P = .64$) and thumb lift-off (1.0 ± 0.3 cm vs 1.1 ± 0.3 cm, $P = .94$) for the EIP transfer compared with palmaris longus FTG reconstruction groups.

Recommendations to Avoid and Treat Extensor Tendon Injuries

- Prominent dorsal plates can result in extensor tendon irritation and attritional rupture.
- Coverage of the dorsal hardware with extensor retinaculum or other biomaterials may decrease the occurrence of extensor tendon dysfunction.
- Removal of symptomatic dorsal plates or volar screws after fracture healing can resolve symptoms.

- The skyline or dorsal horizon may help to identify prominent screw tips dorsally, particularly adjacent to the Lister tubercle.
- Multiple oblique fluoroscopic views are recommended in every case.
- Drilling should be performed carefully with volar plate fixation to prevent iatrogenic injury to the extensor tendons. Care should be taken to ensure that the drill does not pass through the cortex into the adjacent tendons.
- With the use of volar locking plates, shorter, unicortical screws or smooth pegs should be used.
- If EPL rupture does occur, EIP to EPL transfer or palmaris longus FTG EPL reconstruction can restore thumb function.

Flexor Tendon

Injury to the flexor tendons after volar plate fixation for distal radius fractures is thought to be secondary to hardware irritation. Although several causes have been proposed,[9,10,20–24] a cadaveric study noted increased contact pressure within the FPL at 30° to 60° of wrist extension when a volar plate was placed distal to the so-called watershed line.[25] The watershed line was described by Orbay and Touhami[26] as a transverse ridge proximal to the articular surface (2 mm from the lunate facet and 10–15 mm from the scaphoid facet) that is devoid of pronator quadratus coverage. As such, volar distal radius plates that are placed distal to this line can act as a mechanical irritant to overlying flexor tendons, resulting in tenosynovitis and possible rupture.[10,26] Soong and colleagues[27] reported 3 cases of flexor tendon ruptures in 73 distal radius fractures at a mean of 20 months after surgery. In 2 of these patients, the volar locking plate was prominent on or distal to the watershed line. Rozental and colleagues[5] removed 2 plates in 41 patients for flexor carpi radialis (FCR) irritation and FPL subluxation over the plate. Similarly, Arora and colleagues[9] observed flexor tenosynovitis in 9 of 141 patients who required volar hardware removal. Tada and colleagues[28] removed volar plates in 9 of 12 patients who complained of FPL tendon irritation; 3 of the 9 patients with FPL irritation had evidence of FPL injury. The investigators concluded that volar plate removal in patients with symptomatic FPL irritation may prevent FPL rupture. Because attritional ruptures tend to occur more than 1 year after surgery, patients should be educated about this potential late complication so that they may return for evaluation if needed.

Coverage of the volar plate with adequate pronator quadratus coverage has been theorized to provide protection to the flexor tendons.[29]

Brown and Lifchez[30] reported a case of FPL erosion through an anatomically repaired pronator quadratus (confirmed at the time of reoperation) causing tendon irritation and partial-thickness laceration at 2.5 years after the initial operation.

In cases of refractory pain or tendon irritation, volar locking plates can be removed. Gyuricza and colleagues[31] reported on the complications associated with volar locking plate removal in 28 wrists with symptoms pertaining to retained hardware. There were 2 intraoperative complications, a cross-threaded screw into the plate, and a stripped screw head, but all hardware was removed in all patients without morbidity. Hardware removal may also be complicated by broken pegs or screws. If a broken screw remains within the bone and is not prominent along the dorsal cortex, it may be safer to leave the screw in this position versus further bone destruction associated with removal. If a broken screw is prominent dorsally, it can be retrieved through a small dorsal incision. If the locking screw head is stripped, all remaining screws may be removed and the plate may then be used as a handle to remove the stripped locking screw.

In cases of symptomatic attritional FPL rupture, the tendon is usually not suitable for direct repair. In such cases, flexor digitorum superficialis (FDS) transfer to the FPL can result in recovery of thumb flexion.[32,33] Posner[32] reported on 23 patients who underwent transfer of the ring finger FDS to the FPL through a single-stage (n = 18) or 2-stage reconstruction (n = 5), with initial silicone-rod insertion if significant scarring was present. The mean recovery of thumb interphalangeal (IP) joint flexion was 53.5° (range 25–70°) after surgery with preservation of ring finger mobility.[32] Klug and colleagues[34] used an interposition palmaris longus autograft for FPL reconstruction in 1 patient with recovery of grade 4 pinch strength and restoration of IP and metacarpophalangeal joint motion at 1 year after surgery. In patients with thumb IP joint degenerative arthritis, or inability to comply with a flexor tendon reconstruction therapy program, an IP joint arthrodesis is an excellent alternative to restore pinch.

Recommendations to Avoid and Treat Flexor Tendon Injuries

- Flexor tendon injuries are less common with dorsal plate fixation
- Volar plates should be placed proximal to the watershed line to prevent attritional rupture to the flexor tendons
- Pronator quadratus closure over a volar plate may decrease irritation to the flexor tendons

- With symptomatic tendonitis or tendon rupture that requires operative intervention, removal of the volar plate and screws (or any offending hardware) is recommended
- FPL rupture may be reconstructed with direct repair, interposition grafting, tendon transfer, or thumb IP joint arthrodesis

INADEQUATE INITIAL OR PROGRESSIVE LOSS OF REDUCTION

Nonanatomic reduction may result from a failure to achieve an initial reduction during surgery or can develop from a loss of reduction after surgery. Radiographic goals for operative fixation of distal radius fractures include (1) less than 5 mm of radial shortening, (2) radial inclination greater than 15°, (3) sagittal plane alignment between neutral and 20° volar tilt, (4) less than 2 mm of intra-articular gap or step-off at the radiocarpal joint, and (5) less than 2 mm of intra-articular incongruity at the sigmoid notch.[35] Reduction of the volar cortex can serve as a buttress or hinge to aid in the restoration of volar tilt and radial length. Because of the precontoured nature of volar locking plates and the fixed-angle screw positions, near-normal anatomy is necessary to allow proper screw positioning within the subchondral bone of the articular surface and to avoid intra-articular placement of screws or pegs.

Obtaining adequate initial reduction requires an understanding of the fracture anatomy and appropriate surgical approach. The reduction can be facilitated by adequate surgical exposure and knowledge of the common fracture fragments associated with a distal radius fracture: radial styloid, ulnar corner (volar and dorsal), dorsal wall, and the volar rim.[36] In general, the FCR-based approach to the volar distal radius, in conjunction with release of the brachioradialis insertion, allows visualization of the fracture, including the dorsal surface.[29] However, the surgical approach (radial column, volar-ulnar, and dorsal) should be dictated by the major fracture fragments to allow adequate exposure and fixation.[36] Nonetheless, progressive loss of reduction after initial anatomic reduction usually occurs as a result of dorsal collapse, loss of radial length, or loss of reduction at the lunate facet.[10] Arthrotomy or arthroscopy should be used to evaluate the reduction when there is any question of significant articular incongruity, especially in young, active patients. Fracture stability after fixation should be confirmed during surgery by physical examination in addition to fluoroscopic evaluation. The sequelae of inadequate initial reduction or stability of fracture fragments, or progressive loss of reduction, may include malunion, nonunion, or posttraumatic arthritis.

Dorsal Collapse

Despite the advent of volar fixed-angle plates, progressive dorsal collapse can occur and result in loss of reduction. In a series by Rozental and colleagues,[5] dorsal collapse was noted at final radiographic follow-up in 2 of 41 patients treated with a volar locking plate. Similarly, Drobetz and Kutscha-Lissberg[23] reported angular malalignment in 4 of 50 distal radius fractures operatively stabilized with a volar fixed-angle plate. The sequelae with dorsal collapse include persistent wrist pain, increased risk for flexor tendon injury, and loss of wrist flexion, often requiring surgical revision.[5,26] Many clinical studies have emphasized the importance of placing the distal screws/pegs into subchondral bone to prevent dorsal collapse.[23,37,38] A biomechanical study by Mehling and colleagues[39] found that a volar fixed-angle plate with screws inserted in all available distal and proximal row screw holes provided the most stable construct to stabilize an extra-articular distal radius fracture. This finding was compared with using the distal row only, proximal row only, or alternating screw holes in both the distal and proximal rows. Weninger and colleagues[40] also produced a more stable construct when a locking protection screw was placed distal to a compression screw within the proximal fragment with a specific volar plate (Aptus Radius 2.5, Medartis, Switzerland).

Loss of Radial Length

Radial shortening may be avoided by proper screw and plate positioning. Orbay and Fernandez[37] reported 2 cases of fracture settling with resultant radial shortening in 31 patients treated with volar fixed-angle plates, both of which had distal pegs more than 3 mm proximal to the subchondral bone. A biomechanical study by Drobetz and colleagues[41] confirmed that distal fixation (screw or peg) more than 4 mm proximal to the subchondral bone resulted in 50% loss of radial height and 50% reduction in construct load to failure. Although bone grafting has been advocated to prevent radial shortening in the presence of metaphyseal bone defects,[42,43] a Cochrane Database Review and a recent prospective randomized trial found no additional benefit with the use of bone scaffolding materials (bone grafts or substitutes).[44,45] Some investigators have recommended the use of volar fixed-angle plates that allow for 2 rows of distal interlocking screws or pegs to improve fracture stability, particularly when extensive dorsal cortex comminution or bone loss exists.[29,46] Other investigators have recommended the use of combined external and internal fixation to initially aid reduction, maintain precise reduction, and prevent radial shortening.[47] In cases of significant metaphyseal-diaphyseal comminution, distraction plate fixation that can bridge the region of bone loss is another treatment option. Ruch and colleagues[48] reported fracture union in all 22 patients treated with distraction plate fixation at a mean of 110 days, with a mean loss of radial length of 2 mm, and final mean wrist range of motion consisting of flexion to 57°, extension to 65°, pronation to 77°, and supination to 76° after plate removal (mean 124 days).

Lunate Facet Malreduction

Incomplete reduction of the lunate facet can occur at the time of operative fixation or progress after surgery. Obtaining reduction of the lunate facet can be challenging because of the difficulty in visualizing the articular surface. The tilted or tangential lateral radiograph, 15° to 23° from the horizontal, can be helpful to evaluate the congruency of the lunate facet, especially when combined with standard imaging.[49–51] In addition, the tangential anteroposterior radiograph, obtained with the forearm in full pronation and tilted 10° to 15° from the plane of the operating table, allows a true profile of the articular surface at the scaphoid and lunate facet.[52] Arthroscopically assisted procedures are advocated to evaluate the articular reduction and when triangular fibrocartilage or other associated ligamentous injuries are suspected.[53] An open dorsal arthrotomy can provide direct visualization when there is a question of an acceptable reduction. The arthroscope may also be used in a dry manner when an open arthrotomy is already present to improve the ability to see the reduction.

Loss of reduction can occur with volar and dorsal rim fractures.[54,55] Harness and colleagues[54] reported on 7 patients with postoperative loss of volar rim reduction at the lunate facet. The investigators recommended an ulnarly based approach to improve visualization and reduction of the volar-ulnar fragment, or alternative fixation other than volar plating, such as a tension-band technique,[56] scaffolding K-wires, radiolunate K-wire, or an external fixator in this scenario.[54,57] In fractures with an intra-articular split between the scaphoid and lunate facet (3-part, arbeitsgemeinschaft für osteosynthesefragen [AO] 23-C), a combination of volar fixed-angle and fragment-specific radial column plates has been shown in a cadaveric biomechanical study to have less fracture displacement compared with a volar locking plate alone.[58] The use of fragment-specific

fixation, including a volar or dorsal wire form, may be indicated for certain fractures with ulnar column or radial styloid fragments.[36]

Recommendations to Avoid Inadequate Initial or Progressive Loss of Reduction

- An understanding of the fracture anatomy is necessary to dictate the appropriate surgical approach and method of fixation
- With more complicated fractures, a computed tomography scan may provide valuable information
- Dorsal collapse may be prevented when using a volar fixed-angle plate by inserting at least 4 screws within the distal fragment, with at least 2 in the most distal row
- The distal screws of a volar locking plate should be placed within 3 mm of the subchondral bone
- If extensive dorsal comminution or metaphyseal bone loss is present, all distal row screws of a volar locking plate, external fixation alone, a hybrid volar locking plate and external fixation, or a dorsal distraction plate can be used
- Anatomic reduction of the lunate facet articular surface can be confirmed with the tilted or tangential lateral and tangential anteroposterior view, arthroscopy, or arthrotomy
- Volar rim (volar-ulnar or volar marginal fragments) fractures may require alternative methods of fixation other than volar fixed-angle plate fixation
- Addition of a radial column plate to a volar locking plate can augment fracture stability when an intra-articular splint is present between the scaphoid and lunate facet

INTRA-ARTICULAR SCREW PLACEMENT

Intra-articular screw penetration may occur because of the difficulty in obtaining adequate visualization of the radiocarpal joint during surgery. Soong and colleagues[8] reported on 8 intra-articular screws out of 594 (1.3%) distal radius fractures treated with a volar locking plate that had a complication. As described earlier, the tilted lateral image can be helpful to evaluate for any intra-articular screws during surgery.[49–51] Soong and colleagues[59] performed a cadaveric imaging study of wrists with a volar fixed-angle plate (DVR-A, Hand Innovations, Miami, FL, USA). They noted sufficient visualization of the ulnar-most screws with a low-angle (15°–23°), tilted lateral view and the styloid screw with a high-angle (30°) tilted lateral view in combination with a standard posteroanterior (PA) and tilted PA (11°) view. The investigators recommended placement of the ulnar screws first, followed by the radial styloid screw, because radial styloid screws placed first may obscure visualization of the ulnar-most screw tips. Alternatively, Smith and Henry described the 45° pronated oblique view to better visualize the scaphoid and lunate facet articular surface in 1 radiographic image.[60] Tweet and colleagues[61] noted the highest sensitivity (93%) and specificity (96%) for detecting intra-articular screws with continuous, rotational fluoroscopic imaging. In osteoporotic bone in which fracture settling may occur, smooth pegs have been advocated to avoid intra-articular injury, which may occur with threaded screws.[29,38]

Recommendations to Avoid Intra-articular Screw Placement

- Multiple fluoroscopic and radiographic views can be helpful to detect intra-articular screws during surgery (tilted lateral, lateral, PA, and tilted PA imaging)
- Ulnar-to-radial screw placement may decrease the occurrence of intra-articular screw placement
- A 45° pronated oblique image can be used to visualize both the lunate and scaphoid facet
- If intra-articular screws cannot be excluded with standard and tilted fluoroscopic imaging, consider continuous, rotational fluoroscopic imaging, arthroscopy, or arthrotomy
- If fracture settling is a concern (osteoporotic bone), consider smooth pegs in the distal row of the volar locking plate to prevent intra-articular injury

NERVE INJURY

The incidence of nerve injuries associated with distal radius fractures ranges from 2% to 8%.[62–64] Symptoms can be attributed to direct compression from the fracture, inappropriate traction, edematous tenosynovium, hematoma, scar adhesions, or iatrogenic injury from the operative procedure. McKay and colleagues[1] noted 33 physician-reported neuropathies out of 250 patients after a distal radius fracture involving the median nerve (19), the radial nerve (9), and the ulnar nerve (5).

Carpal Tunnel Syndrome and Median Neuropathy

The development of median nerve neuropathy associated with distal radius fractures can present acutely or be delayed. Patients at risk for acute carpal tunnel syndrome (CTS) may be identified before surgery. In a case-control study of 100 distal radius fractures treated with operative fixation with or without acute CTS, Dyer and colleagues[65] noted that, when concomitant hand fractures were excluded, ipsilateral upper extremity trauma ($P = .01$) (proximal humerus, olecranon, humerus, and ulna fractures) and fracture translation ($P = .01$) were significant predictors for developing acute median nerve neuropathy. The investigators also noted that women less than 48 years of age and patients with fracture translation greater than 35% were at high risk for the development of acute CTS. Henry and Stutz[66] prospectively evaluated 169 out of 374 distal radius fracture patients at risk for acute CTS based on the presence of paresthesias within the median nerve distribution, and a positive Semmes-Weinstein monofilament test (at least 4.31 g or 1 monofilament grade less than the uninjured side). Those patients who were considered at risk had either a single portal endoscopic carpal tunnel release (CTR), or division of the transverse carpal ligament (TCL) from the radial margin of the FCR sheath, along with an FCR approach to the distal radius. With this protocol, the investigators noted complete resolution of symptoms in patients who were at risk and none of the remaining patients developed signs or symptoms of CTS after surgery.[66] Patients who present with a worsening sensory examination and pain in the volar wrist after a distal radius fracture with a concern for an acute CTS should be treated with a CTR.

Prophylactic CTR without preoperative signs or symptoms of median nerve neuropathy remains controversial[10,35] and may be associated with increased postoperative median nerve dysfunction.[67,68] Odumala and colleagues[67] reviewed 69 distal radius fractures stabilized with a volar plate with (n = 24) and without (n = 45) concurrent prophylactic CTR. Carpal tunnel syndrome developed in 9 patients (36%) who underwent prophylactic CTR. In fact, prophylactic CTR was associated with a 2.7 times increase in relative odds for developing median nerve neuropathy. Similarly, Lattmann and colleagues[68] compared 2 cohorts of volar plate fixation for a distal radius fracture treated through an extended carpal tunnel approach with concurrent CTR (plane between the palmaris longus/FDS and the median nerve/FCR; n = 83) or via the distal Henry approach (n = 91) without prophylactic CTR. At 6 weeks after treatment, there was significantly less median nerve dysfunction in the distal Henry approach group without prophylactic CTR compared with the extended carpal tunnel approach group with prophylactic CTR (n = 4 vs n = 31; $P<.05$). In addition, 4 patients in the prophylactic CTR group had persistent median nerve dysfunction at 1 year after surgery, and only 2 had resolution of symptoms after revision CTR. The American Academy of Orthopedic Surgeons (AAOS) does not condone or condemn prophylactic CTR.[69]

Physicians should be aware of the delayed onset of median neuropathy in patients with distal radius fractures. Arora and colleagues[9] diagnosed CTS in 3 of 141 (2.1%) patients after volar locking plate fixation at a mean of 7 months after surgery. All patients had resolution of symptoms after CTR and hardware removal. Ho and colleagues[64] reported 24 cases of postoperative hand numbness in 282 (8.5%) distal radius fractures treated with volar plate fixation at least 2 months after surgery. Although the time from surgery to the development of median nerve dysfunction was not specified, late CTS developed in 9 patients and late median nerve neuropathy (numbness at the wrist or forearm) in 15 patients. Nonoperative treatment including splinting, vitamin supplementation, and observation resulted in the improvement of symptoms for 16 patients.[64] In the remaining 8 patients, there were 5 CTR and 3 median nerve neurolysis and hardware removals with resolution of symptoms in all but 1 patient in each operative group (CTR or median nerve neurolysis).[64] Intraoperative retraction may also produce median nerve neuropraxia. To minimize the risk of iatrogenic traction or compression injury to the median nerve during operative fixation of a distal radius fracture, retractors should be placed carefully and should be removed (or may be used intermittently) as soon as possible to limit pressure on the median nerve. Blunt retractors may also be favorable to limit injury to the median nerve and radial artery. Tourniquet time and pressures should be minimized as well.

Nourbakhsh and Tan[70] reported on a patient with progressive median nerve palsy after volar plate fixation caused by median nerve fibrosis in the forearm. Symptoms improved after plate removal and neurolysis. In addition, positioning the wrist in flexion greater than 20°, or also with ulnar deviation (the so-called Cotton-Loder position),[71] should be avoided because Gelberman and colleagues[72,73] noted increased carpal tunnel pressures with wrist positioning in neutral (mean 18 mm Hg) to 20° (mean 27 mm Hg) and 40° of flexion (mean 47 mm Hg).

Several methods of CTR with a concurrent volar approach to the distal radius have been described.[74–76] The TCL can be divided through a separate palmar incision or an extension of the volar Henry approach to the distal radius. The proposed advantage of the latter approach is that the TCL can be released through 1 incision, thus theoretically decreasing the risk of pillar pain. Weber and Sanders[77] reported resolution of symptoms in 79 of 87 (91%) patients with isolated CTS (without a distal radius fracture) by releasing the TCL from its radial attachment on the scaphoid and trapezium. In a cadaveric study, a single, extensile hybrid FCR-based approach to the distal radius, with TCL division as described by Weber and Sanders,[77] resulted in significant reduction of carpal tunnel pressure ($P<.001$) compared with controls (FCR approach without CTR) without iatrogenic tendon or nerve injury.[78] Gwathmey and colleagues[74] performed volar plate fixation and concurrent prophylactic CTR through the hybrid FCR approach in 68 distal radius fractures and noted no additional complications related to the extensile approach.

Recommendations to Avoid and Treat CTS and Median Nerve Neuropathies

- Patients with fracture translation greater than 35% and ipsilateral upper extremity injury should be monitored for CTS
- In the presence of acute CTS, release of the TCL should be performed urgently along with fracture fixation
- If a CTR is performed through an extension of the distal volar Henry incision, the palmar cutaneous branch of the median nerve must be protected
- Volar plate fixation and concurrent CTR can be performed effectively through an extensile FCR approach
- Prophylactic CTR should not be performed in all patients without clinical suspicion for concurrent acute CTS or the development of late CTS
- Late (nonacute) CTS may be managed with nonoperative methods (splinting, vitamin supplementation, and observation)
- If nonoperative measures fail, CTR, median nerve neurolysis, and hardware removal have been associated with resolution of symptoms
- Wrist and forearm immobilization should not place the wrist in excessive flexion (>20°) and ulnar deviation because this increases carpal tunnel pressure

Radial Nerve Neuropathy

Iatrogenic injury to the superficial branch of the radial nerve (SBRN) can be seen with operative fixation of distal radius fractures. Lee and colleagues[63] noted transient neuropraxia of the SBRN in 3 of 22 distal radius fractures treated with volar plate fixation. This finding was primarily attributed to traction and resolved with observation. There have been multiple reports of SBRN injury with percutaneous pin or Kirschner wire (K-wire) fixation.[79,80] One anatomic study noted that the volar radial styloid and dorsal radial styloid K-wire positions were on average 1.47 ± 1.7 mm and 0.35 ± 0.64 mm from the SBRN, respectively.[81] They recommended a small incision to facilitate protection of the SBRN with K-wire insertion. A safe zone was suggested by Steinberg and colleagues[82] located distal to the radial styloid and dorsal to the first extensor compartment that would allow safe percutaneous K-wire insertion, negating the need for a mini–open approach. Subsequently, Korcek and Wongworawat[83] observed many variations on the branching pattern and course of the SBRN about the wrist and deemed that a true safe zone does not exist for percutaneous pin insertion near the radial styloid. Therefore, a limited open technique for pin, K-wire, or external fixation insertion is recommended to avoid injury to the SBRN. Smooth pins may be inserted using an oscillation mode on the wire driver to minimize soft tissue injury during insertion. Hassan and Johnston[84] used a limited open approach (5–10 mm) for external fixation half-pin insertion in the dorsolateral plane (between the brachioradialis and the extensor carpi radialis longus) of the distal radius in 20 cadaveric specimens and noted no iatrogenic injury to the SBRN. Emami and Mjoberg[85] recommended half-pin insertion in a more dorsal location (between the extensor carpi radialis brevis and extensor digitorum) if stab incisions are used, based on their experience with this technique in 40 patients without SBRN injuries.

Recommendations to Avoid and Treat Radial Nerve Neuropathies

- No safe zone exists for placement of a percutaneous K-wire
- A mini–open approach with protection of the soft tissues is recommended for percutaneous pin fixation
- Pin insertion with oscillation rather than rotation can limit binding of soft tissue structures
- Observation is indicated for SBRN neuritis because most cases are transient
- K-wires may be used as fixed-angle support through K-wire holes in the volar plates to stabilize the distal fragment and avoid the need for additional percutaneous pins

Ulnar Nerve Neuropathy

Injury to the ulnar nerve is rare and can occur with the distal radius fracture or at the time of surgical fixation of an associated distal ulna fracture. Soong and Ring[62] noted 5 (2%) preoperative, acute, complete ulnar nerve palsies (motor and sensory) in 280 distal radius fractures treated operatively over a 2-year study period. These distal radius fractures were associated with ulna fractures (styloid n = 2, combined styloid and distal diaphysis n = 1) and triangular fibrocartilage complex avulsions (n = 1). The ulnar nerve was explored and released in 3 patients. However, resolution of symptoms occurred in all 5 patients regardless of treatment. Dennison[86] reported 2 cases of transient paresthesias in the dorsal cutaneous branch of the ulnar nerve (DCUN) out of 5 patients with a distal ulna fracture after volar locking plate fixation. Irritation to the nerve was attributed to retraction during surgery and full recovery was noted at 3 months with observation. Puna and Poon[87] performed a cadaveric study of the DCUN and noted its subcutaneous course from palmar to dorsal at a mean of 0.2 cm proximal to the tip of the ulnar styloid (range 2.5 cm distal to 2.5 cm proximal). The investigators noted palmar and radial displacement of the DCUN with full pronation at the wrist, and therefore recommend this position for initial skin incision around the distal ulna.

Recommendations to Avoid and Treat Ulnar Nerve Neuropathies

- Caution should be maintained with surgical approaches to the distal ulna, specifically within the range of 2.5 cm proximal and distal to the tip of the ulnar styloid, to avoid injury to the DCUN
- Positioning the wrist and forearm in full pronation with initial surgical approaches about the distal ulna displaces the DCUN palmarly away from the incision
- If DCUN paresthesias are present after a surgical approach to the distal ulna, observation is recommended initially because most cases are transient

COMPLEX REGIONAL PAIN SYNDROME

Complex regional pain syndrome (CRPS) can occur after nonoperative and operative treatment of distal radius fractures. Symptoms of CRPS type I (global nerve dysfunction attributed to a noxious event), as opposed to type II (related to a specific peripheral nerve), consist of allodynia, persistent soft tissue edema, skin and temperature changes, and decreased active range of motion (ROM).[88] Although CRPS may be perceived to have a psychological cause, Puchalski and Zyluk[89] did not find any differences in personality or depression scales in 9 of 50 patients (18%) diagnosed with CRPS after closed reduction and percutaneous K-wire fixation of a distal radius fracture compared with those who did not exhibit the symptoms of

CRPS. In an attempt to identify patients at risk for developing CRPS, Goris and colleagues[90] developed a regional inflammation score (based on pain and differences in skin temperature, edema, color, and active ROM compared with the uninjured extremity) that positively correlated with length of time to full recovery ($P = .01$) and predicted the development of CRPS with a regional inflammation score of more than 5 points out of 10 (sensitivity 100% and specificity 16%). However, scoring systems to predict the development of CRPS are not widely used at this time.

Although the pathophysiology of CRPS is not fully understood, Zollinger and colleagues[91] evaluated 427 distal radius fractures and observed a prevalence of 10.1% (10 of 99) for CRPS in a placebo group and 2.4% (8 of 328) in a group receiving variable daily doses of vitamin C (200 mg, 500 mg, or 1500 mg) for 50 days after operative or nonoperative management ($P = .002$). There was no additional reduction in the risk of developing CRPS in doses in excess of 500 mg daily. The investigators suggested vitamin C in 500-mg doses daily for 50 days after a wrist fracture, and stressed the importance of early diagnosis and a multidisciplinary approach toward treatment of CRPS if it does occur (psychiatric, occupational therapy, and pain management). Given these and other findings,[92] the AAOS recommends the use of vitamin C in the management of patients with distal radius fractures to decrease the development of CRPS.[69] Although adverse effects from vitamin C supplementation is dose dependent, these usually do not occur in doses of less than 1000 mg a day. However, vitamin C should be given with caution in patients with hyperoxaluria and hyperuricosuria, which may predispose them to the development of renal calculi.[93]

Recommendations to Avoid and Treat CRPS Type I

- There does not seem to be a psychological cause associated with the development of CRPS type I after a distal radius fracture
- All patients with a distal radius fracture, or those at risk for the development of CRPS type I, may benefit from vitamin C (500 mg) daily for 50 days
- Vitamin C should be cautiously administered to patients with hyperoxaluria and hyperuricosuria because of the risk of developing renal calculi
- A multidisciplinary approach (psychiatric, occupational therapy, and pain management) should be instituted if CRPS type I is diagnosed

INFECTION

Postoperative infections can occur around percutaneous K-wires or external fixation pins. The rates of infection after K-wire or external fixation have been reported to be 33% and 21%, respectively.[94,95] Hargreaves and colleagues[94] reported 12 infected K-wires out of 99 wires in 56 patients who underwent open or closed reduction, forearm cast immobilization, and pin removal at 6 weeks for treatment of a distal radius fracture. They noted pin-site infections in 10 of 29 percutaneous pins compared with 2 of 27 buried pins ($P = .02$) that required pin removal before 6 weeks in 5 and 0 patients, respectively. Based on their series of 137 patients with 422 percutaneous, unthreaded pins used for distal radius stabilization, Botte and colleagues[96] observed pin-site infections in 10 patients (7%), of whom 2 had osteomyelitis, at a mean of 10 weeks after surgery. They concluded that infection was more common if left in situ for longer than 8 weeks. Similarly, external fixator pins became infected in 65 out of 314 (21%) wrists and required oral antibiotics (in all cases) and early pin removal (in 9 wrists) without any cases of osteomyelitis being noted.[95]

To determine the best protocol for pin-site care, Egol and colleagues[97] performed a prospective randomized trial comparing (1) weekly dry dressing changes without pin-site care, (2) daily pin-site care with 1:1 normal saline and hydrogen peroxide, and (3) weekly placement of a chlorhexidine-impregnated disc around the pin after external fixation for an unstable distal radius fracture. They noted 23 pin-tract infections (19%) without significant differences between pin-site care protocols. Therefore, they recommended weekly dry dressing changes without additional wound care for the sake of simplicity and cost-efficiency.

Open distal radius fractures can also develop postoperative infections. Rozental and colleagues reported on 18 patients with open distal radius fractures (Gustilo-Anderson type I n = 9, type II n = 3, type IIIa n = 3, type IIIb n = 2, type IIIc n = 1)[98] after immediate irrigation, debridement, and initial fracture stabilization.[99] Postoperative infections occurred in 8 patients (pin-site infection n = 4, fracture-site osteomyelitis n = 3, and deep wound infection n = 1) who were treated successfully with intravenous or oral antibiotics, serial debridements, or resection arthroplasty (1 patient with osteomyelitis). They noted that wound severity was associated with an increased number of complications ($P = .015$), higher number of surgical procedures ($P = .003$), and fair or poor results at final follow-up ($P = .03$).[99] Kurylo and colleagues[100] evaluated 32 open distal radius fractures (Gustilo-Anderson type I n = 19, type II n = 11, and type IIIA n = 3) and observed no infections regardless of time to debridement (less than or more than 6 hours after hospital admission) or immediate fracture stabilization (definitive external fixation n = 20, plating n = 7, staged external fixation to plating n = 3). Glueck and colleagues[101] advocated that wound contamination is the single best predictor of developing an infection, therefore immediate fixation is feasible in non-contaminated open distal radius fractures following debridement and antibiotics.[102]

Recommendations to Avoid and Treat Infections

- Pins and K-wires should be buried under the skin if possible
- K-wires and external fixator pins should be removed before 8 weeks
- Pin-site infections may be treated with local wound care and oral or intravenous antibiotics, or local debridement in addition to pin removal
- No formal pin-site care is necessary and weekly dry dressing changes are adequate
- Wound severity and contamination are predictors of postoperative infection
- Clean, open, distal radius fractures with moderate wound severity (Gustilo-Anderson type I and II) can be treated with immediate open reduction and internal fixation
- If a superficial or deep infection (osteomyelitis) develops, treatment consisting of irrigation, debridement, and intravenous or oral antibiotics is recommended until fracture union is noted with subsequent hardware (pins or K-wires) removal

COMPARTMENT SYNDROME

Compartment syndrome most often occurs acutely after the initial injury, but it may also develop after surgery. Careful monitoring for signs and symptoms should always be part of the perioperative plan. Although more common in the volar forearm compartment, acute compartment syndrome can occur in the dorsal compartment[103] and within the pronator quadratus.[104] McQueen and colleagues[105] reported on 16 cases of compartment syndrome (15 involving the volar forearm) in 6395 patients with a distal radius fracture. Hwang and colleagues[106] noted a higher incidence of forearm compartment syndrome in patients with a combined distal radius fracture and ipsilateral elbow injury (15%, 9 of 59 patients) compared with an isolated distal radius fracture (0.3%, 3 of 869 patients). In this series, compartment syndrome evolved more than 27 hours after presentation, 3 of which

occurred after initial operative fixation of the distal radius. Postoperative compartment syndrome is uncommon, possibly because of the hematoma decompression and limited fasciotomy performed with the surgical approach. However, formal forearm fasciotomy may be needed in select cases, and a surgical approach to the distal radius does not effectively decompress all of the forearm compartments. In cases in which patients may have altered mental status, polytrauma, or other combined injuries, even greater attention must be directed toward surveillance and treatment of compartment syndrome. Regional anesthesia should be used carefully when there is any concern for compartment syndrome or CTS.

Recommendations to Avoid Compartment Syndrome

- Acute compartment syndrome is rare after operative fixation of a distal radius fracture
- Patients with an ipsilateral elbow injury, in addition to a distal radius fracture, may be at a higher risk for the development of compartment syndrome
- Patients at risk for the development of compartment syndrome should not be placed into a circumferential postoperative splint or cast
- If there is concern for a potential compartment syndrome, refrain from using regional or local anesthesia during surgery
- Balance postoperative extremity elevation with dependency because perfusion pressure will be decreased but soft tissue edema increased, respectively.[107]

SUMMARY

Operative treatment of unstable distal radius fractures are widely successful but can be fraught with postoperative complications. This article presents the most common postoperative complications that can be avoided with a heightened sense of perioperative awareness. In general, most of the presented complications can be prevented from developing after surgery with careful attention to detail during surgery and modification of surgical techniques on an individualized basis.

REFERENCES

1. McKay SD, MacDermid JC, Roth JH, et al. Assessment of complications of distal radius fractures and development of a complication checklist. J Hand Surg Am 2001;26(5):916–22.
2. Engkvist O, Lundborg G. Rupture of the extensor pollicis longus tendon after fracture of the lower

end of the radius–a clinical and microangiographic study. Hand 1979;11(1):76–86.

3. Yu YR, Makhni MC, Tabrizi S, et al. Complications of low-profile dorsal versus volar locking plates in the distal radius: a comparative study. J Hand Surg Am 2011;36(7):1135–41.

4. Ring D, Jupiter JB, Brennwald J, et al. Prospective multicenter trial of a plate for dorsal fixation of distal radius fractures. J Hand Surg Am 1997;22(5): 777–84.

5. Rozental TD, Beredjiklian PK, Bozentka DJ. Functional outcome and complications following two types of dorsal plating for unstable fractures of the distal part of the radius. J Bone Joint Surg Am 2003;85(10):1956–60.

6. Chiang PP, Roach S, Baratz ME. Failure of a retinacular flap to prevent dorsal wrist pain after titanium Pi plate fixation of distal radius fractures. J Hand Surg Am 2002;27(4):724–8.

7. Althausen PL, Szabo RM. Coverage of distal radius internal fixation and wrist fusion devices with Allo-Derm. Tech Hand Up Extrem Surg 2004;8(4):266–8.

8. Soong M, van Leerdam R, Guitton TG, et al. Fracture of the distal radius: risk factors for complications after locked volar plate fixation. J Hand Surg Am 2011;36(1):3–9.

9. Arora R, Lutz M, Hennerbichler A, et al. Complications following internal fixation of unstable distal radius fracture with a palmar locking-plate. J Orthop Trauma 2007;21(5):316–22.

10. Berglund LM, Messer TM. Complications of volar plate fixation for managing distal radius fractures. J Am Acad Orthop Surg 2009;17(6):369–77.

11. Benson EC, DeCarvalho A, Mikola EA, et al. Two potential causes of EPL rupture after distal radius volar plate fixation. Clin Orthop Relat Res 2006; 451:218–22.

12. Thomas AD, Greenberg JA. Use of fluoroscopy in determining screw overshoot in the dorsal distal radius: a cadaveric study. J Hand Surg Am 2009; 34(2):258–61.

13. Jacob J, Clay NR. Re: Pichler et al. Computer tomography aided 3D analysis of the distal dorsal radius surface and the effects on volar plate osteosynthesis. J Hand Surg Eur. 2009, 34: 598-602. J Hand Surg Eur Vol 2010;35(4):335–6.

14. Joseph SJ, Harvey JN. The dorsal horizon view: detecting screw protrusion at the distal radius. J Hand Surg Am 2011;36(10):1691–3.

15. Riddick AP, Hickey B, White SP. Accuracy of the skyline view for detecting dorsal cortical penetration during volar distal radius fixation. J Hand Surg Eur 2011. [Epub ahead of print].

16. Maschke SD, Evans PJ, Schub D, et al. Radiographic evaluation of dorsal screw penetration after volar fixed-angle plating of the distal radius: a cadaveric study. Hand (N Y) 2007;2(3):144–50.

17. Noorda RJ, Hage JJ. Extensor indicis proprius transfer for loss of extensor pollicis longus function. Arch Orthop Trauma Surg 1994;113(6):327–9.

18. Lemmen MH, Schreuders TA, Stam HJ, et al. Evaluation of restoration of extensor pollicis function by transfer of the extensor indicis. J Hand Surg Br 1999;24(1):46–9.

19. Schaller P, Baer W, Carl HD. Extensor indicistransfer compared with palmaris longus transplantation in reconstruction of extensor pollicis longus tendon: a retrospective study. Scand J Plast Reconstr Surg Hand Surg 2007;41(1):33–5.

20. Cross AW, Schmidt CC. Flexor tendon injuries following locked volar plating of distal radius fractures. J Hand Surg Am 2008;33(2):164–7.

21. Casaletto JA, Machin D, Leung R, et al. Flexor pollicis longus tendon ruptures after palmar plate fixation of fractures of the distal radius. J Hand Surg Eur Vol 2009;34(4):471–4.

22. Adham MN, Porembski M, Adham C. Flexor tendon problems after volar plate fixation of distal radius fractures. Hand (N Y) 2009;4(4):406–9.

23. Drobetz H, Kutscha-Lissberg E. Osteosynthesis of distal radial fractures with a volar locking screw plate system. Int Orthop 2003;27(1):1–6.

24. Bhattacharyya T, Wadgaonkar AD. Inadvertent retention of angled drill guides after volar locking plate fixation of distal radial fractures. A report of three cases. J Bone Joint Surg Am 2008;90(2):401–3.

25. Tanaka Y, Aoki M, Izumi T, et al. Effect of distal radius volar plate position on contact pressure between the flexor pollicis longus tendon and the distal plate edge. J Hand Surg Am 2011;36(11): 1790–7.

26. Orbay JL, Touhami A. Current concepts in volar fixed-angle fixation of unstable distal radius fractures. Clin Orthop Relat Res 2006;445:58–67.

27. Soong M, Earp BE, Bishop G, et al. Volar locking plate implant prominence and flexor tendon rupture. J Bone Joint Surg Am 2011;93(4):328–35.

28. Tada K, Ikeda K, Shigemoto K, et al. Prevention of flexor pollicis longus tendon rupture after volar plate fixation of distal radius fractures. Hand Surg 2011;16(3):271–5.

29. Orbay JL. The treatment of unstable distal radius fractures with volar fixation. Hand Surg 2000;5(2): 103–12.

30. Brown EN, Lifchez SD. Flexor pollicis longus tendon rupture after volar plating of a distal radius fracture: pronator quadratus plate coverage may not adequately protect tendons. Eplasty 2011; 11:e43.

31. Gyuricza C, Carlson MG, Weiland AJ, et al. Removal of locked volar plates after distal radius fractures. J Hand Surg Am 2011;36(6):982–5.

32. Posner MA. Flexor superficialis tendon transfers to the thumb–an alternative to the free tendon graft for

treatment of chronic injuries within the digital sheath. J Hand Surg Am 1983;8(6):876–81.

33. Schneider LH, Wiltshire D. Restoration of flexor pollicis longus function by flexor digitorum superficialis transfer. J Hand Surg Am 1983;8(1):98–101.

34. Klug RA, Press CM, Gonzalez MH. Rupture of the flexor pollicis longus tendon after volar fixed-angle plating of a distal radius fracture: a case report. J Hand Surg Am 2007;32(7):984–8.

35. Nana AD, Joshi A, Lichtman DM. Plating of the distal radius. J Am Acad Orthop Surg 2005;13(3):159–71.

36. Schumer ED, Leslie BM. Fragment-specific fixation of distal radius fractures using the Trimed device. Tech Hand Up Extrem Surg 2005;9(2):74–83.

37. Orbay JL, Fernandez DL. Volar fixation for dorsally displaced fractures of the distal radius: a preliminary report. J Hand Surg Am 2002;27(2):205–15.

38. Orbay JL, Fernandez DL. Volar fixed-angle plate fixation for unstable distal radius fractures in the elderly patient. J Hand Surg Am 2004;29(1):96–102.

39. Mehling I, Muller LP, Delinsky K, et al. Number and locations of screw fixation for volar fixed-angle plating of distal radius fractures: biomechanical study. J Hand Surg Am 2010;35(6):885–91.

40. Weninger P, Schueller M, Drobetz H, et al. Influence of an additional locking screw on fracture reduction after volar fixed-angle plating-introduction of the "protection screw" in an extra-articular distal radius fracture model. J Trauma 2009;67(4):746–51.

41. Weninger P, Dall'Ara E, Leixnering M, et al. Volar fixed-angle plating of extra-articular distal radius fractures–a biomechanical analysis comparing threaded screws and smooth pegs. J Trauma 2010;69(5):E46–55.

42. Leung KS, So WS, Chiu VD, et al. Ligamentotaxis for comminuted distal radial fractures modified by primary cancellous grafting and functional bracing: long-term results. J Orthop Trauma 1991;5(3):265–71.

43. Leung KS, Shen WY, Leung PC, et al. Ligamentotaxis and bone grafting for comminuted fractures of the distal radius. J Bone Joint Surg Br 1989;71(5):838–42.

44. Handoll HH, Watts AC. Bone grafts and bone substitutes for treating distal radial fractures in adults. Cochrane Database Syst Rev 2008;2:CD006836:

45. Jakubietz MG, Gruenert JG, Jakubietz RG. The use of beta-tricalcium phosphate bone graft substitute in dorsally plated, comminuted distal radius fractures. J Orthop Surg Res 2011;6:24.

46. Buzzell JE, Weikert DR, Watson JT, et al. Precontoured fixed-angle volar distal radius plates: a comparison of anatomic fit. J Hand Surg Am 2008;33(7):1144–52.

47. McAuliffe JA. Combined internal and external fixation of distal radius fractures. Hand Clin 2005;21(3):395–406.

48. Ruch DS, Ginn TA, Yang CC, et al. Use of a distraction plate for distal radial fractures with metaphyseal and diaphyseal comminution. J Bone Joint Surg Am 2005;87(5):945–54.

49. Lundy DW, Quisling SG, Lourie GM, et al. Tilted lateral radiographs in the evaluation of intra-articular distal radius fractures. J Hand Surg Am 1999;24(2):249–56.

50. Boyer MI, Korcek KJ, Gelberman RH, et al. Anatomic tilt x-rays of the distal radius: an ex vivo analysis of surgical fixation. J Hand Surg Am 2004;29(1):116–22.

51. Matullo KS, Dennison DG. Lateral tilt wrist radiograph using the contralateral hand to position the wrist after volar plating of distal radius fractures. J Hand Surg Am 2010;35(6):900–4.

52. Kumar D, Breakwell L, Deshmukh SC, et al. Tangential views of the articular surface of the distal radius-aid to open reduction and internal fixation of fractures. Injury 2001;32(10):783–6.

53. Wiesler ER, Chloros GD, Mahirogullari M, et al. Arthroscopic management of distal radius fractures. J Hand Surg Am 2006;31(9):1516–26.

54. Harness NG, Jupiter JB, Orbay JL, et al. Loss of fixation of the volar lunate facet fragment in fractures of the distal part of the radius. J Bone Joint Surg Am 2004;86(9):1900–8.

55. Kim JK, Cho SW. The effects of a displaced dorsal rim fracture on outcomes after volar plate fixation of a distal radius fracture. Injury 2012;43(2):143–6.

56. Chin KR, Jupiter JB. Wire-loop fixation of volar displaced osteochondral fractures of the distal radius. J Hand Surg Am 1999;24(3):525–33.

57. Smith RS, Crick JC, Alonso J, et al. Open reduction and internal fixation of volar lip fractures of the distal radius. J Orthop Trauma 1988;2(3):181–7.

58. Grindel SI, Wang M, Gerlach M, et al. Biomechanical comparison of fixed-angle volar plate versus fixed-angle volar plate plus fragment-specific fixation in a cadaveric distal radius fracture model. J Hand Surg Am 2007;32(2):194–9.

59. Soong M, Got C, Katarincic J, et al. Fluoroscopic evaluation of intra-articular screw placement during locked volar plating of the distal radius: a cadaveric study. J Hand Surg Am 2008;33(10):1720–3.

60. Smith DW, Henry MH. The 45 degrees pronated oblique view for volar fixed-angle plating of distal radius fractures. J Hand Surg Am 2004;29(4):703–6.

61. Tweet ML, Calfee RP, Stern PJ. Rotational fluoroscopy assists in detection of intra-articular screw

penetration during volar plating of the distal radius. J Hand Surg Am 2010;35(4):619–27.

62. Soong M, Ring D. Ulnar nerve palsy associated with fracture of the distal radius. J Orthop Trauma 2007;21(2):113–6.

63. Lee HC, Wong YS, Chan BK, et al. Fixation of distal radius fractures using AO titanium volar distal radius plate. Hand Surg 2003;8(1):7–15.

64. Ho AW, Ho ST, Koo SC, et al. Hand numbness and carpal tunnel syndrome after volar plating of distal radius fracture. Hand (N Y) 2011;6(1):34–8.

65. Dyer G, Lozano-Calderon S, Gannon C, et al. Predictors of acute carpal tunnel syndrome associated with fracture of the distal radius. J Hand Surg Am 2008;33(8):1309–13.

66. Henry M, Stutz C. A prospective plan to minimise median nerve related complications associated with operatively treated distal radius fractures. Hand Surg 2007;12(3):199–204.

67. Odumala O, Ayekoloye C, Packer G. Prophylactic carpal tunnel decompression during buttress plating of the distal radius–is it justified? Injury 2001;32(7):577–9.

68. Lattmann T, Dietrich M, Meier C, et al. Comparison of 2 surgical approaches for volar locking plate osteosynthesis of the distal radius. J Hand Surg Am 2008;33(7):1135–43.

69. Lichtman DM, Bindra RR, Boyer MI, et al. Treatment of distal radius fractures. J Am Acad Orthop Surg 2010;18(3):180–9.

70. Nourbakhsh A, Tan V. Median nerve fibrosis at the distal forearm after volar plate fixation of distal radius fracture. J Hand Surg Eur Vol 2010;35(9):768–9.

71. Patel VP, Paksima N. Complications of distal radius fracture fixation. Bull NYU Hosp Jt Dis 2010;68(2):112–8.

72. Turner RG, Faber KJ, Athwal GS. Complications of distal radius fractures. Hand Clin 2010;26(1):85–96.

73. Gelberman RH, Szabo RM, Mortensen WW. Carpal tunnel pressures and wrist position in patients with Colles' fractures. J Trauma 1984;24(8):747–9.

74. Gwathmey FW Jr, Brunton LM, Pensy RA, et al. Volar plate osteosynthesis of distal radius fractures with concurrent prophylactic carpal tunnel release using a hybrid flexor carpi radialis approach. J Hand Surg Am 2010;35(7):1082–1088.e4.

75. Orbay JL, Badia A, Indriago IR, et al. The extended flexor carpi radialis approach: a new perspective for the distal radius fracture. Tech Hand Up Extrem Surg 2001;5(4):204–11.

76. Szabo RM. Acute carpal tunnel syndrome. Hand Clin 1998;14(3):419–29, ix.

77. Weber RA, Sanders WE. Flexor carpi radialis approach for carpal tunnel release. J Hand Surg Am 1997;22(1):120–6.

78. Pensy RA, Brunton LM, Parks BG, et al. Single-incision extensile volar approach to the distal radius and concurrent carpal tunnel release: cadaveric study. J Hand Surg Am 2010;35(2):217–22.

79. Das AK, Sundaram N, Prasad TG, et al. Percutaneous pinning for non-comminuted extra-articular fractures of distal radius. Indian J Orthop 2011;45(5):422–6.

80. Singh S, Trikha P, Twyman R. Superficial radial nerve damage due to Kirschner wiring of the radius. Injury 2005;36(2):330–2.

81. Chia B, Catalano LW 3rd, Glickel SZ, et al. Percutaneous pinning of distal radius fractures: an anatomic study demonstrating the proximity of K-wires to structures at risk. J Hand Surg Am 2009;34(6):1014–20.

82. Steinberg BD, Plancher KD, Idler RS. Percutaneous Kirschner wire fixation through the snuff box: an anatomic study. J Hand Surg Am 1995;20(1):57–62.

83. Korcek L, Wongworawat M. Evaluation of the safe zone for percutaneous Kirschner-wire placement in the distal radius: cadaveric study. Clin Anat 2011;24(8):1005–9.

84. Hassan DM, Johnston GH. Safety of the limited open technique of bone-transfixing threaded-pin placement for external fixation of distal radial fractures: a cadaver study. Can J Surg 1999;42(5):363–5.

85. Emami A, Mjoberg B. A safer pin position for external fixation of distal radial fractures. Injury 2000;31(9):749–50.

86. Dennison DG. Open reduction and internal locked fixation of unstable distal ulna fractures with concomitant distal radius fracture. J Hand Surg Am 2007;32(6):801–5.

87. Puna R, Poon P. The anatomy of the dorsal cutaneous branch of the ulnar nerve. J Hand Surg Eur Vol 2010;35(7):583–5.

88. Field J, Warwick D, Bannister GC. Features of algodystrophy ten years after Colles' fracture. J Hand Surg Br 1992;17(3):318–20.

89. Puchalski P, Zyluk A. Complex regional pain syndrome type 1 after fractures of the distal radius: a prospective study of the role of psychological factors. J Hand Surg Br 2005;30(6):574–80.

90. Goris RJ, Leixnering M, Huber W, et al. Delayed recovery and late development of complex regional pain syndrome in patients with an isolated fracture of the distal radius: prediction of a regional inflammatory response by early signs. J Bone Joint Surg Br 2007;89(8):1069–76.

91. Zollinger PE, Tuinebreijer WE, Breederveld RS, et al. Can vitamin C prevent complex regional pain syndrome in patients with wrist fractures? A randomized, controlled, multicenter dose-response study. J Bone Joint Surg Am 2007;89(7):1424–31.

92. Amadio PC. Vitamin C reduced the incidence of reflex sympathetic dystrophy after wrist fracture. J Bone Joint Surg Am 2000;82(6):873.

93. Shah AS, Verma MK, Jebson PJ. Use of oral vitamin C after fractures of the distal radius. J Hand Surg Am 2009;34(9):1736–8.

94. Hargreaves DG, Drew SJ, Eckersley R. Kirschner wire pin tract infection rates: a randomized controlled trial between percutaneous and buried wires. J Hand Surg Br 2004;29(4):374–6.

95. Ahlborg HG, Josefsson PO. Pin-tract complications in external fixation of fractures of the distal radius. Acta Orthop Scand 1999;70(2):116–8.

96. Botte MJ, Davis JL, Rose BA, et al. Complications of smooth pin fixation of fractures and dislocations in the hand and wrist. Clin Orthop Relat Res 1992;(276):194–201.

97. Egol KA, Paksima N, Puopolo S, et al. Treatment of external fixation pins about the wrist: a prospective, randomized trial. J Bone Joint Surg Am 2006;88(2):349–54.

98. Gustilo RB, Anderson JT. Prevention of infection in the treatment of one thousand and twenty-five open fractures of long bones: retrospective and prospective analyses. J Bone Joint Surg Am 1976;58(4):453–8.

99. Rozental TD, Beredjiklian PK, Steinberg DR, et al. Open fractures of the distal radius. J Hand Surg Am 2002;27(1):77–85.

100. Kurylo JC, Axelrad TW, Tornetta P, et al. Open fractures of the distal radius: the effects of delayed debridement and immediate internal fixation on infection rates and the need for secondary procedures. J Hand Surg Am 2011;36(7):1131–4.

101. Glueck DA, Charoglu CP, Lawton JN. Factors associated with infection following open distal radius fractures. Hand (N Y) 2009;4(3):330–4.

102. Jawa A. Open fractures of the distal radius. J Hand Surg Am 2010;35(8):1348–50.

103. Kupersmith LM, Weinfeld SB. Acute volar and dorsal compartment syndrome after a distal radius fracture: a case report. J Orthop Trauma 2003;17(5):382–6.

104. Summerfield SL, Folberg CR, Weiss AP. Compartment syndrome of the pronator quadratus: a case report. J Hand Surg Am 1997;22(2):266–8.

105. McQueen MM, Gaston P, Court-Brown CM. Acute compartment syndrome. Who is at risk? J Bone Joint Surg Br 2000;82(2):200–3.

106. Hwang RW, de Witte PB, Ring D. Compartment syndrome associated with distal radial fracture and ipsilateral elbow injury. J Bone Joint Surg Am 2009;91(3):642–5.

107. Zhang Q, Styf J, Lindberg LG. Effects of limb elevation and increased intramuscular pressure on human tibialis anterior muscle blood flow. Eur J Appl Physiol 2001;85(6):567–71.

Management of the Distal Radioulnar Joint and Ulnar Styloid Fracture

Douglas M. Sammer, MD[a],*, Kevin C. Chung, MD, MS[b]

KEYWORDS

- Distal radius • Ulnar styloid • Distal radioulnar joint • DRUJ

INTRODUCTION

The ulna is the fixed unit of the forearm, around which the radius, carpus, and hand rotate. The distal radioulnar joint (DRUJ) and adjacent supporting structures form an anatomically complex unit at the distal end of the forearm, and along with the proximal radioulnar joint allow for rotation of the forearm. Motion at the DRUJ is not purely rotational, however, as axial and translational motion also occur. During forearm pronation, the radius axially shortens and translates palmarly relative to the ulna. During supination the reverse occurs with relative lengthening and dorsal translation of the radius relative to the ulna at the level of the DRUJ.[1–7]

DRUJ stability is maintained through the bony anatomy of the joint as well as by various soft tissue stabilizers. Because the radius of curvature of the sigmoid notch is greater than that of the seat of the ulnar head (**Fig. 1**), the bony geometry of the DRUJ contributes only approximately 20% of total joint stability.[8] Furthermore, because of the axial and translational motion in the joint during forearm rotation, the amount of articular contact can vary from 60% with the forearm in neutral position to as little as 10% with the forearm at extremes of rotation.[9,10] Therefore, in certain positions the joint itself has very little intrinsic stability, and relies almost completely on soft tissue constraints.

The primary stabilizer of the DRUJ is the triangular fibrocartilaginous complex (TFCC), specifically the dorsal and palmar radioulnar ligaments.[8,11,12] These ligaments arise from the dorsal and palmar margin of the sigmoid notch and converge to insert on the base of the ulnar styloid and the fovea (**Fig. 2**). Both ligaments consist of superficial and deep components (the deep component is also called the ligamentum subcruentum), each with a different role. The superficial fibers of the radioulnar ligaments insert onto the base of the ulnar styloid, and the deep fibers insert onto the fovea. In pronation, the superficial fibers of the dorsal ligament and the deep fibers of the palmar ligament become taut and constrain the joint. In supination the reverse occurs; the superficial fibers of the palmar ligament and the deep fibers of the dorsal ligament become taut and constrain the joint.[8,12–17] In addition to the radioulnar ligaments there are secondary soft tissue stabilizers of the DRUJ, such as the interosseous membrane (IOM), the extensor carpi ulnaris (ECU) and its subsheath, the joint capsule, and the pronator quadratus, which can be static or dynamic in nature.[18–20]

The function of the DRUJ can be adversely affected by the fractures of the distal radius and ulnar styloid in several ways. A distal radius fracture that is intra-articular at the DRUJ can lead to posttraumatic arthritis, particularly if the fracture heals with a step-off at the sigmoid notch. Displacement of an extra-articular distal radius fracture with shortening, dorsal angulation, or radial translation can result in DRUJ instability or loss of forearm rotation. An associated TFCC tear with injury to the radioulnar ligaments can

[a] Department of Plastic Surgery, UT Southwestern Medical Center, 1801 Inwood Road, Dallas, TX 75390, USA
[b] Section of Plastic Surgery, Department of Surgery, The University of Michigan Health System, 2130 Taubman Center, 1500 East Medical Center Drive, Ann Arbor, MI 48109, USA
* Corresponding author.
E-mail address: Douglas.Sammer@UTSouthwestern.edu

Hand Clin 28 (2012) 199–206
doi:10.1016/j.hcl.2012.03.011
0749-0712/12/$ – see front matter © 2012 Published by Elsevier Inc.

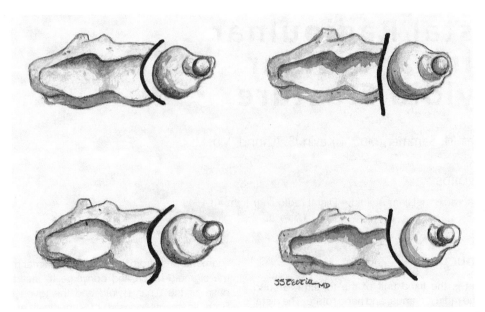

Fig. 1. Although the geometry of the DRUJ can vary, the sigmoid notch generally has a greater radius of curvature than the seat of the ulnar head. The bony geometry of the joint therefore provides limited stability.

contribute to DRUJ instability, as can some ulnar styloid base avulsion fractures.

ARTICULAR STEP-OFF AT THE SIGMOID NOTCH

Distal radius fracture lines often extend into the DRUJ and are present in 55% of dorsally angulated intra-articular fractures.[21] Axial plane fracture lines that enter the sigmoid notch are readily recognized on plain radiographs (**Fig. 3**). Coronal plane fractures that enter the sigmoid notch may be more difficult to identify on plain radiographs but are easily distinguishable on an axial computed tomography scan image (**Fig. 4**).[21] Similar to articular fractures at any location, these injuries have the potential to lead to arthrosis. Although multiple retrospective clinical and biomechanical studies have addressed the issue of radiocarpal step-offs in distal radius fractures,[21–32] less attention has been paid to the sequelae of articular step-offs at

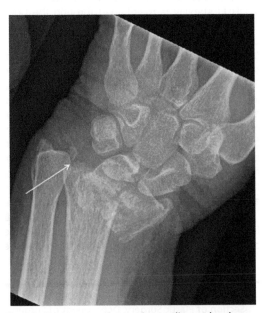

Fig. 3. Posteroanterior wrist radiograph demonstrating a comminuted intra-articular distal radius and ulnar styloid fracture. The white arrow points to the intra-articular fracture line at the DRUJ. Also, note the displacement of the ulnar styloid fragment.

Fig. 2. The radioulnar ligaments are seen to converge on the ulnar styloid and fovea. The deep and superficial components, which are confluent, have been separated for visualization. The deep fibers insert on the fovea, whereas the superficial fibers insert on the ulnar styloid base.

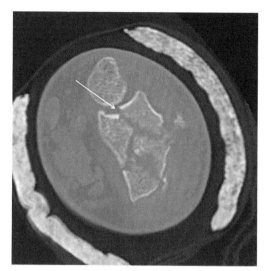

Fig. 4. Axial CT scan image demonstrating a step-off (*white arrow*) at the DRUJ of an oblique coronal plane fracture line.

the DRUJ. The conclusion of most of these studies is that an articular step-off of greater than 2 mm almost always results in radiographic arthritis, and that the incidence of arthritis is lower with improved articular reduction. Additionally, even though some patients with arthritis were symptomatic, many had very good or even excellent function despite radiographic arthritis.[22,23,26,31] Because most of these studies focus on the radiocarpal joint, it is unknown exactly what degree of step-off is acceptable at the DRUJ. The decision of whether or not to operate on a patient with a step-off at the DRUJ should be based on the evidence in the literature regarding step-offs at the radiocarpal joint as well as other fracture characteristics and patient factors.

EXTRA-ARTICULAR MALUNION

Extra-articular malunion of the distal radius can affect DRUJ mechanics, altering joint loading, contact surfaces, and congruity. Clinically, these changes may result in limited forearm rotation, DRUJ instability, pain, or arthritis.[33–37] Although the numbers vary, adverse clinical outcomes including loss of forearm rotation and DRUJ arthritis have been associated with fractures that malunite with substantial deformity (shortening ≥5 mm, radial inclination ≤12°, or dorsal angulation >20°).[26,33,38–41] In vivo biomechanical studies suggest that DRUJ symptoms, such as limited forearm rotation or pain, are not caused by a bony block or altered forearm kinematics,[42] but instead may be caused by the altered DRUJ mechanics and changes in the soft tissue constraints of the DRUJ.[43] In malunions with shortening and dorsal angulation, the radioulnar contact

area is diminished and shifted proximally. In addition, the radioulnar ligaments become stretched, and in some positions of forearm rotation the dorsal radioulnar ligament may be tented over the ulnar head.[43] These mechanical and soft tissue changes may limit forearm rotation, alter DRUJ stability, and contribute to early arthritis.

The effect of radial displacement of the distal fragment (probably better described as ulnar displacement of the proximal fragment) on DRUJ stability has not been extensively studied (**Fig. 5**). However, correcting radial displacement results in re-tensioning of the interosseous membrane, which would enhance DRUJ stability in patients with an intact interosseous membrane (**Fig. 6**), and is particularly important in patients with radioulnar ligament injury or avulsion. Substantial fracture displacement, angulation, and shortening should be corrected to preserve forearm rotation and prevent articular or ligamentous changes at the DRUJ that may lead to instability, pain, or arthrosis.

TFCC INJURY

Because the radioulnar ligaments are the primary stabilizers of the DRUJ, injury to the TFCC in patients with a distal radius fracture can contribute to DRUJ instability. Some degree of TFCC injury occurs in a large percentage of patients with unstable distal radius fractures (40%–85%),[44,45] and there is a positive correlation between the severity of initial fracture displacement and the incidence of TFCC injury.[46]

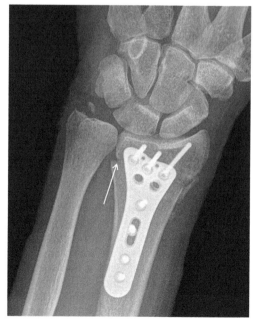

Fig. 5. Persistent radial translation of the distal fragment after ORIF is demonstrated (*white arrow*).

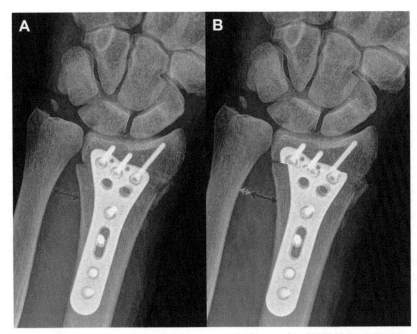

Fig. 6. (*A*) Persistent radial translation of the distal fragment is present after open reduction internal fixation (*red arrow*). (*B*) the radiograph has been digitally altered to correct the radial translation. Note the increase in the interosseous space between the radius and ulna, which would result in re-tensioning of the interosseous membrane. The red arrow indicates the original interosseous space, and the blue arrow indicates the increase in the interosseous space after achieving reduction.

Although some degree of TFCC injury is common, complete peripheral TFCC tears are less common but are strongly associated with DRUJ instability.[45,47] Patients with DRUJ instability due to TFCC injury should ideally be treated early, rather than attempting to treat patients with chronic instability later.[48,49] The degree of DRUJ instability influences management of patients. When the DRUJ is unstable only in certain positions of forearm rotation, it can be treated by long-arm cast immobilization or by radioulnar pinning in the position of stability. However, when gross instability is present in all positions of forearm rotation, closed management results in persistent instability.[50] Direct repair of the TFCC injury via arthroscopic or open approach has been associated with good clinical outcomes.[47,51]

ASSOCIATED ULNAR STYLOID FRACTURES

Ulnar styloid fractures accompany 50% or more of distal radius fractures[46,52,53] and approximately 25% of fractures fail to unite.[38,48] Despite a high incidence of nonunion, they are usually asymptomatic.[27,48] Nevertheless, they have been occasionally associated with pain at the nonunion site, stylocarpal impaction, and ECU tendonitis,[49,54,55] all of which can be treated by excision of the styloid fragment. Displaced fractures involving the ulnar styloid base or fovea are more concerning because

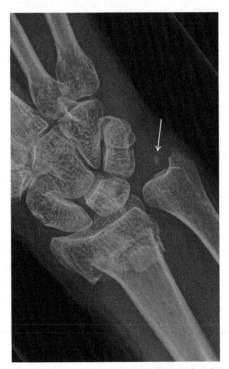

Fig. 7. Posteroanterior wrist radiograph demonstrating a small ulnar styloid tip fracture (*white arrow*) that is likely due to capsular avulsion, rather than radioulnar ligament avulsion.

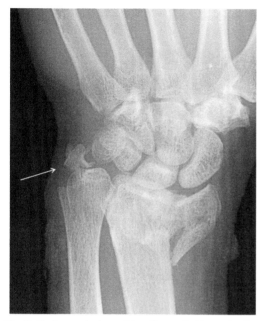

Fig. 8. Posteroanterior wrist radiograph demonstrating a large ulnar styloid base fracture (*white arrow*) that is likely attached to the radioulnar ligaments.

they have the potential to result in DRUJ instability (**Figs. 7** and **8**).[49] However, several studies suggest that regardless of styloid fracture size or degree of displacement, ulnar styloid fractures are poor predictors of DRUJ instability.[47,53,56] Recent research also supports the idea that most ulnar styloid fractures do not affect objective or subjective clinical outcomes, particularly when the distal radius is treated with open reduction internal fixation (ORIF).[53,56,57] Hence, the author treats large ulnar styloid base fractures with ORIF only if the DRUJ is unstable after anatomic ORIF of the distal radius.[53] Anatomic reduction and rigid internal fixation of the distal radius results in indirect reduction of an associated ulnar styloid base fracture,[16,56]

and ulnar styloid ORIF may be unnecessary even when the DRUJ is unstable before distal radius ORIF.[16,56] It is critical to recognize that these studies were performed in patients who underwent near anatomic reduction with rigid internal fixation. In patients with distal radius fractures that are allowed to heal with some degree of malunion, ulnar styloid base fractures are probably more clinically relevant.

TREATMENT

In the acute setting after closed reduction and splint immobilization has been performed, patients with distal radius fractures with shortening of 5 mm or more, radial inclination of up to 12°, dorsal angulation greater than 20°, and substantial radial displacement or a step-off of more than 1 mm are candidates for operative treatment, with the goal of achieving healing in near anatomic reduction. Intra-operatively after reduction and fixation of the distal radius fracture and reduction of the DRUJ, the DRUJ should be tested and compared with the preoperative examination of the contralateral DRUJ.[53,56,58] If the DRUJ is unstable, forearm rotation is limited, or there is a clunk or grind, the fracture reduction and hardware position should be reevaluated and corrected if necessary. If the DRUJ is persistently unstable in only some positions of forearm rotation but is stable in other positions (usually supination), the forearm can be immobilized in the position of stability for 6 weeks, either by long-arm cast immobilization or more reliably by radioulnar pinning (**Fig. 9**). If the DRUJ is unstable in all positions of forearm rotation, treatment depends on the presence or absence of an ulnar styloid base fracture. If ulnar styloid base fracture is present, ulnar styloid ORIF is indicated and typically results in DRUJ stability. If there is no ulnar styloid base fracture or if ORIF of the ulnar styloid fracture does not restore

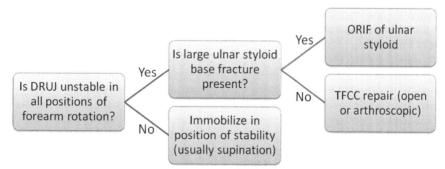

Fig. 9. An algorithm is presented to guide the management of DRUJ instability that is present after distal radius ORIF and DRUJ reduction.

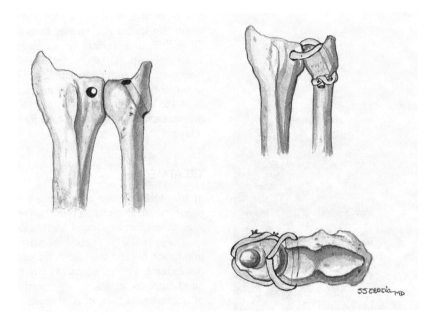

Fig. 10. Radioulnar ligament reconstruction described by Adams and Berger. On the left, the bone tunnels in the radius and ulna are demonstrated. On the right, the final reconstruction using tendon graft is demonstrated.

DRUJ stability, a complete tear of the TFCC, often located at the foveal insertion, may be present, which should be repaired with an open or arthroscopic approach. The forearm is immobilized in supination for 6 weeks followed by rehabilitation.

When DRUJ symptoms, such as instability, pain, or limited forearm rotation, are detected in the subacute or chronic setting after fracture healing has occurred, the principles of management remain the same (assuming that arthrosis is not present). The first goal is to reestablish the normal anatomy of the radius with corrective osteotomy. Often, restoration of DRUJ stability can be appreciated intra-operatively after shortening and dorsal angulation have been corrected. If the DRUJ remains unstable intra-operatively after correcting the radius malunion, an associated ulnar styloid base fracture or TFCC tear should be repaired, which may not be feasible in the chronic setting. In such situations, one should be prepared to reconstruct the radioulnar ligaments as described by Adams and Berger.[59]

SUMMARY

The anatomy, mechanics, and function of the DRUJ and associated soft tissue structures can be altered in distal radius and ulnar styloid fractures, resulting in symptoms that include reduced forearm rotation, pain, instability, and arthritis. The DRUJ can be adversely affected in several ways, including by extension of a fracture line into the sigmoid notch, extra-articular distal radius malunion, associated injury to the substance of the TFCC, avulsion fracture at the base of the ulnar styloid, and disruption of secondary stabilizers, such as the interosseous membrane. In both the acute and chronic setting, assuming that arthrosis has not developed, the principles of management are the same and include restoration of the normal anatomy of the radius, followed by the repair of associated TFCC injuries or ulnar styloid base fractures if necessary. In the chronic setting, radioulnar ligament reconstruction may be required (**Fig. 10**).

ACKNOWLEDGMENTS

The author would like to acknowledge the artistry of Dr Sumeet Teotia, and thank him for his contributions to this article.

REFERENCES

1. af Ekenstam FW, Palmer AK, Glisson RR. The load on the radius and ulna in different positions of the wrist and forearm. A cadaver study. Acta Orthop Scand 1984;55(3):363–5.
2. Drobner WS, Hausman MR. The distal radioulnar joint. Hand Clin 1992;8(4):631–44.
3. Epner RA, Bowers WH, Guilford WB. Ulnar variance–the effect of wrist positioning and roentgen filming technique. J Hand Surg Am 1982;7(3):298–305.
4. Palmer AK, Werner FW. Biomechanics of the distal radioulnar joint. Clin Orthop Relat Res 1984;(187):26–35.

5. Bruckner JD, Lichtman DM, Alexander AH. Complex dislocations of the distal radioulnar joint. Recognition and management. Clin Orthop Relat Res 1992;(275):90–103.

6. Linscheid RL. Biomechanics of the distal radioulnar joint. Clin Orthop Relat Res 1992;(275):46–55.

7. Ray RD, Johnson RJ, Jameson RM. Rotation of the forearm; an experimental study of pronation and supination. J Bone Joint Surg Am 1951;33(4):993–6.

8. Stuart PR, Berger RA, Linscheid RL, et al. The dorsopalmar stability of the distal radioulnar joint. J Hand Surg Am 2000;25(4):689–99.

9. af Ekenstam F, Hagert CG. Anatomical studies on the geometry and stability of the distal radio ulnar joint. Scand J Plast Reconstr Surg 1985;19(1):17–25.

10. Hagert CG. The distal radioulnar joint. Hand Clin 1987;3(1):41–50.

11. Palmer AK, Werner FW. The triangular fibrocartilage complex of the wrist–anatomy and function. J Hand Surg Am 1981;6(2):153–62.

12. Hagert CG. Distal radius fracture and the distal radioulnar joint–anatomical considerations. Handchir Mikrochir Plast Chir 1994;26(1):22–6.

13. Kleinman WB. Stability of the distal radioulnar joint: biomechanics, pathophysiology, physical diagnosis, and restoration of function what we have learned in 25 years. J Hand Surg Am 2007;32(7):1086–106.

14. Xu J, Tang JB. In vivo changes in lengths of the ligaments stabilizing the distal radioulnar joint. J Hand Surg Am 2009;34(1):40–5.

15. Rose-Innes AP. Anterior dislocation of the ulna at the inferior radio-ulnar joint. Case report, with a discussion of the anatomy of rotation of the forearm. J Bone Joint Surg Br 1960;42:515–21.

16. Buterbaugh GA, Palmer AK. Fractures and dislocations of the distal radioulnar joint. Hand Clin 1988;4(3):361–75.

17. Hui FC, Linscheid RL. Ulnotriquetral augmentation tenodesis: a reconstructive procedure for dorsal subluxation of the distal radioulnar joint. J Hand Surg Am 1982;7(3):230–6.

18. Kihara H, Short WH, Werner FW, et al. The stabilizing mechanism of the distal radioulnar joint during pronation and supination. J Hand Surg Am 1995;20(6):930–6.

19. Garcia-Elias M. Soft-tissue anatomy and relationships about the distal ulna. Hand Clin 1998;14(2):165–76.

20. Gordon KD, Pardo RD, Johnson JA, et al. Electromyographic activity and strength during maximum isometric pronation and supination efforts in healthy adults. J Orthop Res 2004;22(1):208–13.

21. Tanabe K, Nakajima T, Sogo E, et al. Intra-articular fractures of the distal radius evaluated by computed tomography. J Hand Surg Am 2011;36(11):1798–803.

22. Forward DP, Davis TR, Sithole JS. Do young patients with malunited fractures of the distal radius inevitably develop symptomatic post-traumatic osteoarthritis? J Bone Joint Surg Br 2008;90(5):629–37.

23. Anderson DD, Bell AL, Gaffney MB, et al. Contact stress distributions in malreduced intraarticular distal radius fractures. J Orthop Trauma 1996;10(5):331–7.

24. Baratz ME, Des Jardins J, Anderson DD, et al. Displaced intra-articular fractures of the distal radius: the effect of fracture displacement on contact stresses in a cadaver model. J Hand Surg Am 1996;21(2):183–8.

25. Bradway JK, Amadio PC, Cooney WP. Open reduction and internal fixation of displaced, comminuted intra-articular fractures of the distal end of the radius. J Bone Joint Surg Am 1989;71(6):839–47.

26. Catalano LW 3rd, Cole RJ, Gelberman RH, et al. Displaced intra-articular fractures of the distal aspect of the radius. Long-term results in young adults after open reduction and internal fixation. J Bone Joint Surg Am 1997;79(9):1290–302.

27. Fernandez DL, Geissler WB. Treatment of displaced articular fractures of the radius. J Hand Surg Am 1991;16(3):375–84.

28. Knirk JL, Jupiter JB. Intra-articular fractures of the distal end of the radius in young adults. J Bone Joint Surg Am 1986;68(5):647–59.

29. Mehta JA, Bain GI, Heptinstall RJ. Anatomical reduction of intra-articular fractures of the distal radius. An arthroscopically-assisted approach. J Bone Joint Surg Br 2000;82(1):79–86.

30. Missakian ML, Cooney WP, Amadio PC, et al. Open reduction and internal fixation for distal radius fractures. J Hand Surg Am 1992;17(4):745–55.

31. Steffen T, Eugster T, Jakob RP. Twelve years follow-up of fractures of the distal radius treated with the AO external fixator. Injury 1994;25(Suppl 4):S-D44-54.

32. Trumble T, Allan CH, Miyano J, et al. A preliminary study of joint surface changes after an intraarticular fracture: a sheep model of a tibia fracture with weight bearing after internal fixation. J Orthop Trauma 2001;15(5):326–32.

33. Fernandez DL. Correction of post-traumatic wrist deformity in adults by osteotomy, bone-grafting, and internal fixation. J Bone Joint Surg Am 1982;64(8):1164–78.

34. Adams BD. Effects of radial deformity on distal radioulnar joint mechanics. J Hand Surg Am 1993;18(3):492–8.

35. Kihara H, Palmer AK, Werner FW, et al. The effect of dorsally angulated distal radius fractures on distal radioulnar joint congruency and forearm rotation. J Hand Surg Am 1996;21(1):40–7.

36. Bronstein AJ, Trumble TE, Tencer AF. The effects of distal radius fracture malalignment on forearm rotation: a cadaveric study. J Hand Surg Am 1997;22(2):258–62.

37. Schuind F, An KN, Berglund L, et al. The distal radioulnar ligaments: a biomechanical study. J Hand Surg Am 1991;16(6):1106–14.

38. Bacorn RW, Kurtzke JF. Colles' fracture; a study of two thousand cases from the New York State Workmen's Compensation Board. J Bone Joint Surg Am 1953;35(3):643–58.

39. DePalma AF. Comminuted fractures of the distal end of the radius treated by ulnar pinning. J Bone Joint Surg Am 1952;34:651–62.

40. Porter M, Stockley I. Fractures of the distal radius. Intermediate and end results in relation to radiologic parameters. Clin Orthop Relat Res 1987;(220):241–52.

41. Hirahara H, Neale PG, Lin YT, et al. Kinematic and torque-related effects of dorsally angulated distal radius fractures and the distal radial ulnar joint. J Hand Surg Am 2003;28(4):614–21.

42. Moore DC, Hogan KA, Crisco JJ 3rd, et al. Three-dimensional in vivo kinematics of the distal radioulnar joint in malunited distal radius fractures. J Hand Surg Am 2002;27(2):233–42.

43. Crisco JJ, Moore DC, Marai GE, et al. Effects of distal radius malunion on distal radioulnar joint mechanics–an in vivo study. J Orthop Res 2007; 25(4):547–55.

44. Geissler WB, Freeland AE, Savoie FH, et al. Intracarpal soft-tissue lesions associated with an intra-articular fracture of the distal end of the radius. J Bone Joint Surg Am 1996;78(3):357–65.

45. Lindau T, Adlercreutz C, Aspenberg P. Peripheral tears of the triangular fibrocartilage complex cause distal radioulnar joint instability after distal radial fractures. J Hand Surg Am 2000;25(3):464–8.

46. Richards RS, Bennett JD, Roth JH, et al. Arthroscopic diagnosis of intra-articular soft tissue injuries associated with distal radial fractures. J Hand Surg Am 1997;22(5):772–6.

47. Fujitani R, Omokawa S, Akahane M, et al. Predictors of distal radioulnar joint instability in distal radius fractures. J Hand Surg Am 2011;36(12):1919–25.

48. Geissler WB, Fernandez DL, Lamey DM. Distal radioulnar joint injuries associated with fractures of the distal radius. Clin Orthop Relat Res 1996;(327): 135–46.

49. May MM, Lawton JN, Blazar PE. Ulnar styloid fractures associated with distal radius fractures: incidence and implications for distal radioulnar joint instability. J Hand Surg Am 2002;27(6):965–71.

50. Strehle J, Gerber C. Distal radioulnar joint function after Galeazzi fracture-dislocations treated by open reduction and internal plate fixation. Clin Orthop Relat Res 1993;(293):240–5.

51. Varitimidis SE, Basdekis GK, Dailiana ZH, et al. Treatment of intra-articular fractures of the distal radius: fluoroscopic or arthroscopic reduction? J Bone Joint Surg Br 2008;90(6):778–85.

52. Villar RN, Marsh D, Rushton N, et al. Three years after Colles' fracture. A prospective review. J Bone Joint Surg Br 1987;69(4):635–8.

53. Sammer DM, Shah HM, Shauver MJ, et al. The effect of ulnar styloid fractures on patient-rated outcomes after volar locking plating of distal radius fractures. J Hand Surg Am 2009;34(9):1595–602.

54. Hauck RM, Skahen J 3rd, Palmer AK. Classification and treatment of ulnar styloid nonunion. J Hand Surg Am 1996;21(3):418–22.

55. Cerezal L, del Pinal F, Abascal F, et al. Imaging findings in ulnar-sided wrist impaction syndromes. Radiographics 2002;22(1):105–21.

56. Kim JK, Koh YD, Do NH. Should an ulnar styloid fracture be fixed following volar plate fixation of a distal radial fracture? J Bone Joint Surg Am 2010;92(1):1–6.

57. Souer JS, Ring D, Matschke S, et al. Effect of an unrepaired fracture of the ulnar styloid base on outcome after plate-and-screw fixation of a distal radial fracture. J Bone Joint Surg Am 2009;91(4):830–8.

58. Jupiter JB. Commentary: the effect of ulnar styloid fractures on patient-rated outcomes after volar locking plating of distal radius fractures. J Hand Surg Am 2009;34(9):1603–4.

59. Adams BD, Berger RA. An anatomic reconstruction of the distal radioulnar ligaments for posttraumatic distal radioulnar joint instability. J Hand Surg Am 2002;27(2):243–51.

Management of Malunions of the Distal Radius

Steven C. Haase, MD*, Kevin C. Chung, MD, MS

KEYWORDS

- Distal radius • Fracture • Malunion • Volarly displaced
- Dorsally displaced • Intra-articular

DEFINITION AND CLASSIFICATION

A malunion occurs when a fractured bone heals with improper alignment, incorrect length, articular incongruity, or a combination of these factors. Malunions of the distal radius may be intra-articular or extra-articular, and may be asymptomatic or symptomatic. As with many conditions of the hand and wrist, the degree of radiographic abnormality does not correlate well with patient symptom severity. Nonetheless, radiographic criteria are commonly used to describe (and define) distal radius malunions.

The key radiographic parameters used to define proper reduction and/or alignment of distal radius fractures are illustrated in **Fig. 1**. For maximum accuracy, these measurements should be made on posteroanterior (PA) and lateral films of the wrist, with the forearm in neutral rotation, and should be performed in a consistent manner with predictable landmarks.[1] Normal average values and ranges of these measurements[2–4] are given in **Table 1**.

Radial inclination is defined as the angle between the articular surface of the radius and the axial plane of the wrist in the PA view (see **Fig. 1**A). The orientation of the axial plane can be inferred from a line drawn perpendicular to the long axis of the radius. Although loss of radial inclination leads to an obvious cosmetic deformity of the wrist, it also has a direct correlation with a loss of grip strength.[5] In one long-term study, a rather marked decrease in radial inclination (to <5°) was

required before unsatisfactory results became significant.[4]

Radial tilt, also called volar tilt or palmar tilt, is defined as the angle between the articular surface of the radius and the axial plane in the lateral view (see **Fig. 1**B). For the typical Colles fracture, collapse is seen in the dorsal direction, resulting in a measurement less than the normal value of 11°. As angulation increases past the neutral (zero-degree) position and becomes dorsal in nature, this measurement is reported as dorsal tilt or as a negative number (representing reversal of the normal volar tilt). Most investigators agree that dorsal tilt up to 15° is acceptable,[4,6,7] although dorsal tilt of any degree is not found in the uninjured population.[3]

Malunions may also occur with abnormally increased volar tilt, whether due to initial volar displacement of the distal fragment, or because of overaggressive reduction of a Colles fracture. It is generally agreed that palmar tilt of more than 20° is unacceptable.[7]

Radial length is defined as the distance (typically reported in millimeters) that the radial styloid projects beyond the axial plane of the seat of the ulna, as measured in the PA view (see **Fig. 1**C). Ulnar variance is defined as the difference (in millimeters) between the axial plane of the ulnar edge of the lunate facet and that of the seat of the ulna, as measured in the PA view (see **Fig. 1**D).[8] This variance is reported as positive when the ulna is longer than the radius and negative when the ulna is shorter (eg, 2-mm negative ulnar

Section of Plastic Surgery, University of Michigan Medical School, 2130 Taubman Center, SPC 5340, 1500 East Medical Center Drive, Ann Arbor, MI 48109-5340, USA
* Corresponding author.
E-mail address: shaase@med.umich.edu

Hand Clin 28 (2012) 207–216
doi:10.1016/j.hcl.2012.03.008
0749-0712/12/$ – see front matter © 2012 Elsevier Inc. All rights reserved.

hand.theclinics.com

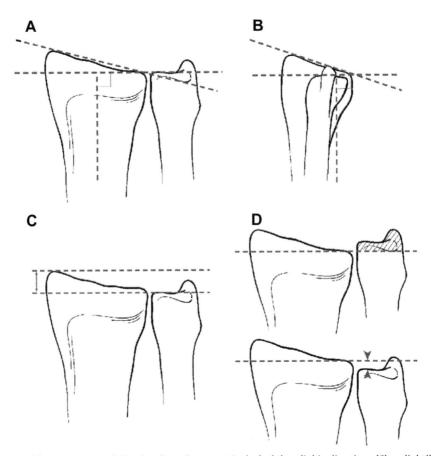

Fig. 1. Radiographic parameters of distal radius alignment include (*A*) radial inclination, (*B*) radial tilt, (*C*) radial height, and (*D*) ulnar variance. (*From* Sharpe F, Stevanovic M. Extra-articular distal radial fracture malunion. Hand Clin 2005;21(3):469–87.)

variance). Both radial length and ulnar variance are measurements related to radial shortening, and disturbance of these parameters leads most notably to incongruity of the distal radioulnar joint (DRUJ) and loss of forearm rotation.[9] Most investigators agree that a loss of more than 5 mm of radial length constitutes a malunion.[4,5,9,10]

Although many investigators have published articles related to these radiographic measurements, parameters to define an unstable fracture, or the ensuing malunion, have not been firmly established.[11] Based on a review of the literature and expert opinion, Margaliot and colleagues[12] defined unstable distal radius fractures by the following radiographic criteria:

1. Radial inclination <15°
2. Volar tilt >15°, dorsal tilt >10°
3. Radial height <9 mm
4. Intra-articular step or gap >2 mm

These criteria are very similar to those put forth by Graham for "acceptable healing of a distal radius fracture"[7]:

1. Radial inclination ≥15°
2. Volar tilt <20°, dorsal tilt <15°
3. Radial shortening <5 mm at DRUJ
4. Intra-articular incongruity ≤2 mm

Table 1
Distal radius radiographic parameters: normal values

Parameter	Normal Value	Range
Radial inclination	22°	12.9°–35°
Radial tilt	11°	3°–20°
Radial length	12.3 mm	8–17 mm
Ulnar variance	0.4 mm	−2.5 to +3.1 mm

Based on the existing literature, expert opinion, and their own experience, the authors use the following criteria to define malunion of the distal radius:

1. Radial inclination <10°
2. Volar tilt >20°, dorsal tilt >20°
3. Radial height <10 mm
4. Ulnar variance >2+
5. Intra-articular step or gap >2 mm

INCIDENCE

In Colles' initial description of this fracture, he reported that patients treated with splinting "all recovered without the smallest defect or deformity of the limb."[13] However, beginning in the early part of the twentieth century, several investigators began to recognize and treat symptomatic malunions of the distal radius. Based on several historical case series, the malunion rate after simple cast immobilization of distal radius fractures has been reported to be as high as 23.6%.[14] As advances in fracture fixation technology have continued to develop, surgeons have become more aggressive in the surgical treatment of these fractures. The pooled average malunion rate after surgical treatment was reported to be approximately 10.6% in the late twentieth century.[14] This analysis included several different techniques, namely percutaneous pinning, external fixation, and internal fixation. A more recent meta-analysis of multiple clinical trials reports the rate of loss reduction after internal or external fixation as around 4%.[12]

ETIOLOGY, INJURY PATTERNS, PATHOGENESIS

The most common fracture deformity seen in distal radius injuries is a dorsally displaced distal fragment (Colles fracture, **Fig. 2**). When reduction is incomplete, or when early failure of reduction occurs, the most common pattern of deformity observed is apex-volar angulation at the fracture site with radial shortening, leading to a more positive ulnar variance and radioulnar joint incongruity (**Fig. 3**). Occasionally this deformity is referred to as a dinner-fork deformity, because of the abnormal position of the hand on the forearm when viewed from the lateral position (**Fig. 4**). When the distal radius articular surface is dorsally tilted, adaptive carpal instability may develop as a result of the abnormal position of the proximal carpal row.[15,16] In addition to angulation and shortening, a significant number of malunions have a rotational deformity, either supinated or pronated at the malunion site.[17]

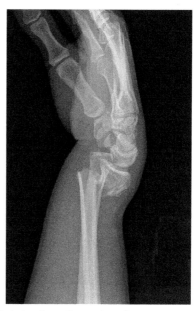

Fig. 2. Lateral radiograph of an extra-articular, dorsally displaced distal radius fracture (Colles fracture).

Malunion can be predicted in a patient with a Colles type fracture when the volar cortex, which is the strongest portion of the metaphysis, is not in contact (**Fig. 5**). In these situations any significant dorsal comminution is more likely to collapse as the thin bone fragments are resorbed, due to the loss of the buttress of an intact volar cortex. When the volar cortex is intact, it appears to help resist the collapse of this dorsal comminution.

INDICATIONS

Established malunions of the distal radius do not require surgical correction in the absence of symptoms. Many studies have shown that malunion results in decreased grip strength, decreased mobility, increased pain, difficulties with activities of daily living, and worsened cosmetic appearance.[5,18,19] Furthermore, increased severity of malunion can be directly correlated with worse DASH (disabilities of arm, shoulder, and hand) scores.[20]

However, many patients have no clinical symptoms and minimal functional deficit, despite measurable radiographic changes. This finding is most evident in elderly patients, in whom radiographic outcomes after distal radius fracture have not been associated with subjective or objective functional outcomes.[21,22] These studies are reinforced by a recent systematic review that demonstrated no difference in functional outcomes between cast immobilization and surgical fixation

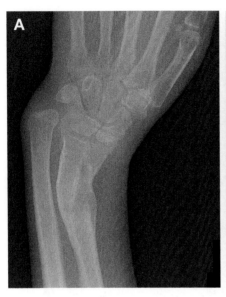
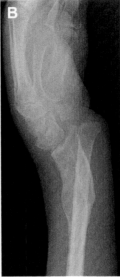

Fig. 3. (A) Posteroanterior and (B) lateral radiographs of a distal radius malunion with apex-volar angulation, shortening, and complete disruption of the distal radioulnar joint.

in patients aged 60 years and older, despite worse radiographic outcomes in the casted group.[23] Even in the often cited work of Knirk and Jupiter,[16] although radiographic progression of arthritis in young adults was associated with articular incongruity, it did not correlate well with symptoms, particularly pain.

Patients presenting with radiographic evidence of malunion, combined with clinical symptoms consistent with that diagnosis, should be strongly considered for surgical correction of the deformity. In addition to the symptoms of decreased strength, decreased range of motion, and pain, patients may complain of poor appearance of the wrist and/or carpal tunnel syndrome.[19] Many of these symptoms can be relieved by correcting the deformity, although if the patient's pain is secondary to degenerative arthritis, correction of the bony deformity may not successfully relieve all of their pain.

TIMING

The preferred timing for treatment of malunions has been the subject of some debate. Proponents of delayed treatment suggest that waiting for complete fracture consolidation and resolution of osteopenia may make bony distraction and fixation easier at the time of osteotomy. However, the authors believe that the potential disadvantages far outweigh the benefits of this approach. In these cases, fracture collapse is followed quickly by tightening of the soft-tissue envelope. As the tendons, nerves, and other structures become foreshortened, distraction becomes more and more difficult, especially if one waits upward of a year after the injury.

The authors prefer to treat malunions as soon as they are detected. If discovered within 4 to 8 weeks, the early fracture callus is easily distinguished from

Fig. 4. Lateral view of a patient with a dinner-fork deformity.

preferred approach, allowing one to elevate the dorsally displaced fracture fragment directly into the desired position and correcting the radial tilt to normal. The dorsal opening wedge osteotomy was then typically filled with a corticocancellous iliac crest bone graft and secured with internal fixation (dorsal plates).[26] Early on it was realized that Kirschner wires, although simple and readily available, may not suffice to support the bone graft against collapse. This shortcoming is due to the tendency of the soft tissues to recoil after this bone-lengthening procedure as well as the tendency of the bone graft to become friable during the subsequent period of revascularization and incorporation. For this reason, even some of the earliest articles on this topic preferred the use of rigid internal fixation over other methods.[26,27]

The use of dorsal plates for the correction of distal radius malunions, much like the use of these plates in primary fracture fixation, can lead to tendon irritation and rupture, and frequently require hardware removal.[28] With the development of volar locked plating systems for distal radius fractures, however, new approaches to malunion correction using these plates have been described. The fixed-angle plates available today allow for a distal-first plate placement, followed by osteotomy and simple derotation of the distal fragment in straightforward cases.[29] These plates can solidly purchase the sturdy volar cortex and buttress the osteotomy site sufficiently so that a large, corticocancellous graft is rarely required. Many of these cases have been successful with cancellous graft alone,[29,30] bone graft substitutes,[31] or bone cement.[32] In the case of nascent malunions, sometimes the incipient healing callus can be used in lieu of these other options.[33] In most of these cases, prolonged cast immobilization is also not required, because of the early stability provided by these plates.

When the malunion involves significant shortening (1 cm or more) as well as angulation, it becomes more difficult to treat. In these severe malunions, if chronic in nature, the soft tissues will be difficult to distract back to their native position. These cases can often be approached from the volar surface, as already described, and the osteotomy site can be distracted intraoperatively with a lamina spreader to help stretch the soft tissues. In these cases, rigid volar plating should be combined with structural corticocancellous autograft to provide the best protection against collapse. If the length discrepancy between the radius and ulna is too great, an ulnar-shortening osteotomy might be required to restore DRUJ congruity.[34] If alignment of the DRUJ cannot be obtained with these maneuvers, or if the DRUJ

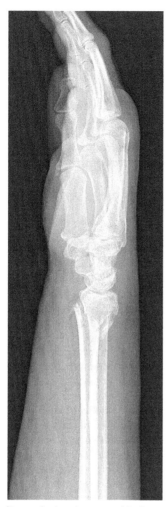

Fig. 5. Radiograph showing unstable fracture due to inadequate cortical contact.

the firmer cortical bone and can be readily removed, and anatomic alignment restored. By treating these problems early, the difficulties of soft-tissue contracture can be avoided or minimized. In a study comparing early (average 8 weeks from injury) to late (average 40 weeks from injury) malunion reconstruction, Jupiter and Ring[24] found that earlier reconstruction was both technically easier and resulted in a shorter period of disability.

TREATMENT OF DORSALLY DISPLACED MALUNIONS (COLLES FRACTURES)

The earliest treatments described for correction of distal radius malunion after Colles fracture consisted of a lateral or dorsal approach, osteotomy at the malunion site, and use of intramedullary bone pegs or onlay bone grafts to achieve healing.[25] As the technique evolved, the dorsal approach became the succumbs to painful arthritis, the distal ulna may need to be excised[35] or the DRUJ arthritis ablated by other means (eg, Sauvé-Kapandji procedure, Bowers hemiresection interposition arthroplasty, and so forth).

Complex malunions requiring correction in multiple planes and/or significant lengthening may be made easier by using a device specifically engineered to help with this operation, such as the RAYHACK Radial Malunion Distraction System (Wright Medical Technology, Inc, Arlington, TN). This system uses a specially engineered cutting guide and positioning device to accurately correct the malunion in multiple planes. The high-profile dorsal plate acts as a powerful strut to resist collapse, even when significant distraction is required. This plate may lead to significant tendon irritation, and is often removed after the osteotomy is completely healed (typically 1 year after surgery). In their case series using this device the authors saw reasonable results, although the outcomes are never spectacular given the severity of the deformity being addressed.[36]

In the elderly patient, osteoporosis predisposes the fracture to collapse, and the resulting malunion can often be significantly shortened. When this deformity proves to be symptomatic, it can be a challenging reconstruction. There may be legitimate concerns regarding how much manipulation (distraction, fixation, and so forth) the patient's fragile skeleton can tolerate. In patients suffering from this bone disease, a closing wedge osteotomy may seem preferable to an opening wedge technique. Wada and colleagues[37] described a series of 5 patients in whom a closing wedge osteotomy of the radius was performed simultaneously with an ulnar shortening osteotomy. Ulnar shortening of 6 to 11 mm was required in these cases to bring the DRUJ into congruity. All osteotomies healed within 3 months, and significant improvements in pain, function, grip strength, and range of motion were noted.

TREATMENT OF VOLARLY DISPLACED MALUNIONS (SMITH FRACTURES)

A volarly displaced malunion, such as may occur after a Smith fracture, is often easier to correct.[38] Typically the volar cortex has not been impacted or resorbed as much as is typical of the thin dorsal cortex. It is often possible to realign the volar cortex without the need for bone graft. In the case of small, intra-articular fractures (also called a volar Barton fracture), the carpus may have slipped palmarly as a fracture-dislocation event. If no angular correction is required, the corrective osteotomy can be conceptualized as a sliding

osteotomy, as described by Thivaios and McKee.[39] Using a volar exposure, and precise osteotomy technique to recreate the fracture pattern, Thivaios and McKee were able to reduce these nonunions easily by sliding the articular surface distally and dorsally, often without the need for any bone grafting. This technique can be used for both extra-articular and intra-articular fractures. Application of a volar buttress plate allows patients to undergo early wrist mobilization without concern for hardware failure.

TREATMENT OF INTRA-ARTICULAR MALUNIONS

Correction of intra-articular malunions is certainly desirable, as it is well known that significant step or gap deformities of the articular surface lead to increasing arthrosis and potentially worse function.[40] In isolation, correction of articular incongruity seems like a reasonably challenging case, and the challenge is compounded in patients with shortening, angulation, and an intra-articular component to their malunion (**Fig. 6**). As the complexity of the osteotomy increases and with multiple smaller fragments to consider, concerns about avascular necrosis and nonunion may arise, and the potential benefits of intervention weighed against the risk to the patient.

Despite these challenges, many investigators have reported case series on this topic with admirable outcomes. Ring and colleagues[41,42] have published an elegant description of their technique and results for these challenging cases. In all they treated 23 patients, and reduced the average articular incongruity from 4 to 0.4 mm. Their results show that this procedure can be both safe and effective, leading to improved wrist function. Ruch and colleagues[43] examined a particular subgroup of intra-articular malunions: those patients with a malunion of the palmar lunate facet. In their study, they demonstrated that early corrective osteotomy (average of 5.4 months from injury) can lead to improved range of motion, grip strength, and DASH scores, as well as correction of radiographic abnormalities.

Other adjunctive procedures have been described to aid in this operation. For instance, arthroscopy can be used to confirm accurate reduction of the intra-articular surface.[44] In cases when a portion of the articular surface cannot be salvaged, one group has described filling the void with an osteochondral graft from the seventh, eighth, or ninth rib. In a series of 7 patients, Obert and colleagues[45] showed an improvement in grip strength and DASH scores, along with pain reduction. Although intra-articular malunions can be

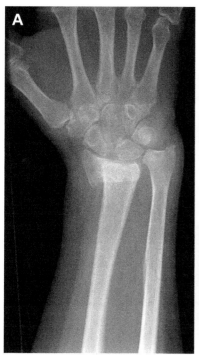 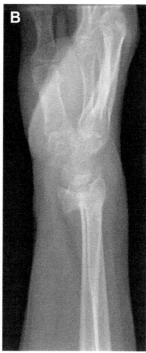

Fig. 6. (*A*) Posteroanterior and (*B*) lateral radiographs of an intra-articular malunion with severe shortening and intra-articular incongruity.

challenging cases, reconstruction can offer patients improvement in their symptoms in select cases (**Fig. 7**).

OUTCOMES OF MALUNION RECONSTRUCTION

A study in 2000 retrospectively evaluated 45 patients with an average 5.7-year follow-up and came to the conclusion that reconstructive procedures in patients with distal radius malunion may not completely restore normal function.[28] This concept needs to be understood by patients. Once a malunion has been established it is very difficult, if not impossible, to restore normal function to that patient.

Sammer and colleagues[36] evaluated 5 patients with severe malunion (radial shortening by more than 1 cm) using the RAYHACK device and showed a significant improvement in volar tilt, but other radiographic parameters changed only slightly and did not reach significance. Likewise, although Michigan Hand Outcomes Questionnaire scores improved significantly in some domains, grip and range-of-motion improvements did not reach statistical significance. Although not significant, ulnar wrist motion was noted to increase

from 9° to 21.8°, due to the decrease in ulnar positive variance.

Van Cauwelaert de Wyels and De Smet[46] reported on malunion correction in a group of 21 young and middle-aged patients (average age 38 years). There were statistically significant improvements in several radiographic parameters, and postoperative grip strength was 70% of the contralateral side. Postoperative DASH scores were 25.8 at almost 4 years' follow-up (no preoperative DASH score was reported). In another short-term study, Kiliç and colleagues[30] showed improvements in quick-form DASH scores, functional outcomes, and radiographic measures in a series of 17 patients at mean follow-up of 20 months.

In a long-term follow-up study, Lozano-Calderón and colleagues reported results on a series of 22 patients (average age 62 years) with a mixture of extra-articular and intra-articular malunion corrections. At an average of 13 years' follow-up, grip strength was 71% of the contralateral side and DASH scores were 16, suggesting only mild perceived disability.[47]

Correction of distal radius malunion may have a beneficial effect on the remainder of the wrist as well. In cases of radiocarpal and midcarpal instability resulting from distal radius malunion,

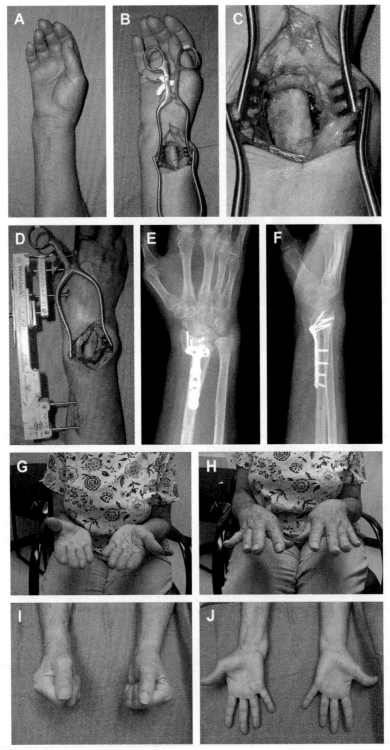

Fig. 7. (*A*) Preoperative deformity of the wrist is evident in this patient with intra-articular malunion (same patient as **Fig. 6**). (*B, C*) Volar exposure of the distal radius reveals the abrupt step-off on the volar cortex. (*D*) Dorsal exposure was also required in this complex case, to confirm the articular congruity was restored. External fixation was used to further off-load and protect the tenuous internal fixation. (*E, F*) Follow-up radiographs reveal significant correction of several parameters. (*G–J*) The patient was very satisfied with her final result, which included dramatic improvements in forearm rotation and cosmesis.

both forms of instability can be corrected by malunion reconstruction.[48]

SUMMARY

Despite encouraging results from small case series, correction of distal radius malunion remains a challenging procedure with uncertain outcomes. It is the authors' strong belief that the most appropriate treatment for a distal radius malunion is prevention. Comminuted fractures in osteoporotic individuals will predictably collapse if not treated. With rigid fixation techniques, specifically with volar, fixed-angle, locking-plate technology, none of these fractures should go on to malunion if treated promptly and efficiently. When considering the risk/benefit ratio for surgical treatment, one must not discount the impact a malunion can have on a patient's functional outcome, whether he or she is young or old.

If a symptomatic malunion is discovered, correction should be undertaken as early as possible. It is recommended that action be taken within 6 months of the primary injury to decrease the negative impact of soft-tissue contracture on the eventual reconstruction. Many patients still complain about residual problems after malunion surgery, but corrective surgery has been shown to improve both radiographic and functional outcomes, and may prevent secondary problems for these patients in the future.

REFERENCES

1. Kreder HJ, Hanel DP, McKee M, et al. X-ray film measurements for healed distal radius fractures. J Hand Surg Am 1996;21(1):31–9.
2. Friberg S, Lundstrom B. Radiographic measurements of the radio-carpal joint in normal adults. Acta Radiol Diagn (Stockh) 1976;17(2):249–56.
3. Mann FA, Kang SW, Gilula LA. Normal palmar tilt: is dorsal tilting really normal? J Hand Surg Br 1992;17(3):315–7.
4. Altissimi M, Antenucci R, Fiacca C, et al. Long-term results of conservative treatment of fractures of the distal radius. Clin Orthop Relat Res 1986;206:202–10.
5. Jenkins NH, Mintowt-Czyz WJ. Mal-union and dysfunction in Colles' fracture. J Hand Surg Br 1988;13(3):291–3.
6. Sharpe F, Stevanovic M. Extra-articular distal radial fracture malunion. Hand Clin 2005;21(3):469–87.
7. Graham TJ. Surgical correction of malunited fractures of the distal radius. J Am Acad Orthop Surg 1997;5(5):270–81.
8. Palmer AK, Glisson RR, Werner FW. Ulnar variance determination. J Hand Surg Am 1982;7(4):376–9.
9. Adams BD. Effects of radial deformity on distal radioulnar joint mechanics. J Hand Surg Am 1993;18(3):492–8.
10. Bronstein AJ, Trumble TE, Tencer AF. The effects of distal radius fracture malalignment on forearm rotation: a cadaveric study. J Hand Surg Am 1997;22(2):258–62.
11. Waters PM, Mintzer CM, Hipp JA, et al. Noninvasive measurement of distal radius instability. J Hand Surg Am 1997;22(4):572–9.
12. Margaliot Z, Haase SC, Kotsis SV, et al. A meta-analysis of outcomes of external fixation versus plate osteosynthesis for unstable distal radius fractures. J Hand Surg Am 2005;30(6):1185–99.
13. Colles A. On the fracture of the carpal extremity of the radius. Edinb Med Surg J 1814;10:182–6.
14. McGrory BJ, Amadio PC. Malunion of the distal radius. In: Cooney WP, Linscheid RL, Dobyns JH, editors. The wrist: diagnosis and operative treatment. St Louis (MO): Mosby; 1998. p. 356–84.
15. Linscheid RL, Dobyns JH, Beabout JW, et al. Traumatic instability of the wrist. Diagnosis, classification, and pathomechanics. J Bone Joint Surg Am 1972;54(8):1612–32.
16. Taleisnik J, Watson HK. Midcarpal instability caused by malunited fractures of the distal radius. J Hand Surg Am 1984;9(3):350–7.
17. Prommersberger KJ, Froehner SC, Schmitt RR, et al. Rotational deformity in malunited fractures of the distal radius. J Hand Surg Am 2004;29(1):110–5.
18. McQueen M, Caspers J. Colles fracture: does the anatomical result affect the final function? J Bone Joint Surg Br 1988;70(4):649–51.
19. Prommersberger KJ, Pillukat T, Muhldorfer M, et al. Malunion of the distal radius. Arch Orthop Trauma Surg 2012. [Epub ahead of print].
20. Brogren E, Hofer M, Petranek M, et al. Relationship between distal radius fracture malunion and arm-related disability: a prospective population-based cohort study with 1-year follow-up. BMC Musculoskelet Disord 2011;12:9.
21. Synn AJ, Makhni EC, Makhni MC, et al. Distal radius fractures in older patients: is anatomic reduction necessary? Clin Orthop Relat Res 2009;467(6):1612–20.
22. Arora R, Gabl M, Gschwentner M, et al. A comparative study of clinical and radiologic outcomes of unstable Colles type distal radius fractures in patients older than 70 years: nonoperative treatment versus volar locking plating. J Orthop Trauma 2009;23(4):237–42.
23. Diaz-Garcia RJ, Oda T, Shauver MJ, et al. A systematic review of outcomes and complications of treating unstable distal radius fractures in the elderly. J Hand Surg Am 2011;36(5):835.e2.
24. Jupiter JB, Ring D. A comparison of early and late reconstruction of malunited fractures of the distal

end of the radius. J Bone Joint Surg Am 1996;78(5): 739–48.

25. Speed JS, Knight RA. The treatment of malunited Colles's fractures. J Bone Joint Surg Am 1945; 27(3):361–7.

26. Fernandez DL. Correction of post-traumatic wrist deformity in adults by osteotomy, bone-grafting, and internal fixation. J Bone Joint Surg Am 1982; 64(8):1164–78.

27. Cooney WP 3rd, Dobyns JH, Linscheid RL. Complications of Colles' fractures. J Bone Joint Surg Am 1980;62(4):613–9.

28. Flinkkila T, Raatikainen T, Kaarela O, et al. Corrective osteotomy for malunion of the distal radius. Arch Orthop Trauma Surg 2000;120(1–2):23–6.

29. Del Pinal F, Garcia-Bernal FJ, Studer A, et al. Sagittal rotational malunions of the distal radius: the role of pure derotational osteotomy. J Hand Surg Eur Vol 2009;34(2):160–5.

30. Kilic A, Kabukcuoglu YS, Gul M, et al. Fixed-angle volar plates in corrective osteotomies of malunions of dorsally angulated distal radius fractures. Acta Orthop Traumatol Turc 2011;45(5):297–303.

31. Luchetti R. Corrective osteotomy of malunited distal radius fractures using carbonated hydroxyapatite as an alternative to autogenous bone grafting. J Hand Surg Am 2004;29(5):825–34.

32. Lozano-Calderon S, Moore M, Liebman M, et al. Distal radius osteotomy in the elderly patient using angular stable implants and Norian bone cement. J Hand Surg Am 2007;32(7):976–83.

33. Tarng YW, Yang SW, Hsu CJ. Palmar locking plates for corrective osteotomy of latent malunion of dorsally tilted distal radial fractures without structural bone grafting. Orthopedics 2011;34(6):178.

34. Oskam J, Bongers KM, Karthaus AJ, et al. Corrective osteotomy for malunion of the distal radius: the effect of concomitant ulnar shortening osteotomy. Arch Orthop Trauma Surg 1996;115(3–4):219–22.

35. Coulet B, Id El Ouali M, Boretto J, et al. Is distal ulna resection influential on outcomes of distal radius malunion corrective osteotomies? Orthop Traumatol Surg Res 2011;97(5):479–88.

36. Sammer DM, Kawamura K, Chung KC. Outcomes using an internal osteotomy and distraction device for corrective osteotomy of distal radius malunions requiring correction in multiple planes. J Hand Surg Am 2006;31(10):1567–77.

37. Wada T, Isogai S, Kanaya K, et al. Simultaneous radial closing wedge and ulnar shortening osteotomies for distal radius malunion. J Hand Surg Am 2004;29(2):264–72.

38. Sato K, Nakamura T, Iwamoto T, et al. Corrective osteotomy for volarly malunited distal radius fracture. J Hand Surg Am 2009;34(1):27–33, e1.

39. Thivaios GC, McKee MD. Sliding osteotomy for deformity correction following malunion of volarly displaced distal radial fractures. J Orthop Trauma 2003;17(5):326–33.

40. Knirk JL, Jupiter JB. Intra-articular fractures of the distal end of the radius in young adults. J Bone Joint Surg Am 1986;68(5):647–59.

41. Ring D, Prommersberger KJ, Gonzalez del Pino J, et al. Corrective osteotomy for intra-articular malunion of the distal part of the radius. J Bone Joint Surg Am 2005;87(7):1503–9.

42. Prommersberger KJ, Ring D, Gonzalez del Pino J, et al. Corrective osteotomy for intra-articular malunion of the distal part of the radius. Surgical technique. J Bone Joint Surg Am 2006;88(Suppl 1 Pt 2): 202–11.

43. Ruch DS, Wray WH 3rd, Papadonikolakis A, et al. Corrective osteotomy for isolated malunion of the palmar lunate facet in distal radius fractures. J Hand Surg Am 2010;35(11):1779–86.

44. Gobel F, Vardakas DG, Riano F, et al. Arthroscopically assisted intra-articular corrective osteotomy of a malunion of the distal radius. Am J Orthop (Belle Mead NJ) 2004;33(6):275–7.

45. Obert L, Lepage D, Sergent P, et al. Post-traumatic malunion of the distal radius treated with autologous costal cartilage graft: a technical note on seven cases. Orthop Traumatol Surg Res 2011; 97(4):430–7.

46. Van Cauwelaert de Wyels J, De Smet L. Corrective osteotomy for malunion of the distal radius in young and middle-aged patients: an outcome study. Chir Main 2003;22(2):84–9.

47. Lozano-Calderón SA, Brouwer KM, Doornberg JN, et al. Long-term outcomes of corrective osteotomy for the treatment of distal radius malunion. J Hand Surg Eur Vol 2010;35(5):370–80.

48. Verhaegen F, Degreef I, De Smet L. Evaluation of corrective osteotomy of the malunited distal radius on midcarpal and radiocarpal malalignment. J Hand Surg Am 2010;35(1):57–61.

The Use of Bone Grafts and Substitutes in the Treatment of Distal Radius Fractures

Kagan Ozer, MD[a],*, Kevin C. Chung, MD, MS[b]

KEYWORDS

- Autogenous • Bone graft • Distal radius • Fracture
- Malunion

The interest in developing biomaterials to augment fracture healing continues to grow. This trend is in part fueled by the high market value of these products, but also associated with an increased incidence of fractures related to aging and osteoporosis. New products coming to the market promise early return to function with minimal morbidity; however, indications to use these products, particularly in the treatment of distal radius fractures, remain unclear.

An ideal bone graft material stimulates bone healing and provides structural stability while being biocompatible, bioresorbable, easy to use, and cost-effective. Commercially available products offer various combinations of those features, but not all. Moreover, it is important to understand that different anatomic locations have varying levels of bone forming activity and stability. Therefore, a single study validating the use of a bone graft material in 1 location may not predict its performance in another anatomic site. In distal radius fractures, the risk of nonunion is minimal. Consequently, bone graft substitutes are primarily used to provide structural stability and perhaps early return to function. Structural stability is directly affected by the

method of fixation, with each fixation technique providing a different level of structural support. Although minimally invasive methods of fixation (pins and external fixation) could effectively be supplemented with bone graft substitutes for added stability, advances in plate design and technology, such as locking plates, make bone graft substitutes perhaps not as essential. This article reviews the biology of bone grafts and the clinical evidence in the use of bone graft substitutes for the treatment of distal radius fractures.

BONE GRAFT PROPERTIES

There are 4 essential elements for bone healing: (1) osteogenic cells (eg, osteoblasts or progenitor cells); (2) osteoinductive signals provided by growth factors; (3) an osteoconductive matrix; and (4) adequate blood and nutrient supply.[1] Bone graft materials are described on the basis of osteogenicity (presence of bone forming cells), osteoconductivity (ability to function as a scaffold) and osteoinductivity (ability to stimulate bone formation). Following trauma, the resultant fracture hematoma provides a source of hematopoietic cells that produce

Supported in part by grants from the National Institute on Aging and National Institute of Arthritis and Musculoskeletal and Skin Diseases (R01 AR062066) and from the National Institute of Arthritis and Musculoskeletal and Skin Diseases (2R01 AR047328-06) and a Midcareer Investigator Award in Patient-Oriented Research (K24 AR053120) (to Kevin C. Chung, MD).

[a] Department of Orthopaedic Surgery, University of Michigan Health System, 2098 South Main Street, Ann Arbor, MI 48103, USA
[b] Section of Plastic Surgery, Department of Surgery, The University of Michigan Health System, 2130 Taubman Center, 1500 East Medical Center Drive, Ann Arbor, MI 48109, USA
* Corresponding author.
E-mail address: kozer@umich.edu

Hand Clin 28 (2012) 217–223
doi:10.1016/j.hcl.2012.02.004

secreting growth factors (eg, bone morphogenic proteins [BMP], transforming growth factor [TGF]-β, insulinlike growth factor [IGF]-II, platelet-derived growth factor [PDGF]) that stimulate osteoblasts and differentiation of progenitor cells.[2] This results inmetaplasia of mesenchymal cells to produce collagen and proteoglycans and cartilage matrix and differentiate into osteoblasts. Every step of this process is regulated by a number of signaling pathways.

TYPES OF BONE GRAFTS

Based on their biologic and physical properties, bone grafts can be divided into 3 main categories (**Table 1**).[3]

Autograft

Autogenous bone grafts are considered the standard material, because they offer complete histocompatibility and provide the best osteoconductive, osteogenic, and osteoinductive properties.[2–4] Autografts usually contain osteogenic cells (viable up to 2 hours in normal saline) and bone matrix proteins. They offer structural support (if harvested with its cortical part) and are incorporated into surrounding bone through creeping substitution.[4] They also suffer from resorption and limited availability and viability. The most common source of these grafts is the iliac crest, but they can also be obtained in limited amounts from the tibial crest and olecranon. The iliac crest has frequently been used in the treatment of distal radius fractures[5–13] and for corrective osteotomies.[14–17] Although the outcomes based on radiographic

parameters and wrist function are satisfactory, iliac crest bone graft harvesting is associated with a number of complications, including donor site pain, hematoma, neuroma formation, chronic unexplained thigh pain, and local infection.[18–22] Depending on the series and the amount of bone harvested, the prevalence of 1 or more of these complications is reported to range from 9% to 49% in various series.[23–33] In addition, the procedure itself adds an average of 30 minutes to the operative time. Although iliac crest bone grafting was initially thought to be cost-effective, the direct and indirect costs (postoperative rehabilitation, cost of pain management, and time off work) were found to be substantially high.[34–37] Due to the high morbidity, increased operative time, and cost, surgeons are seeking alternative materials that can substitute for autogenous bone grafts.

Allograft

Allograft bone is osteoconductive and osteoinductive, but lacks the osteogenic properties of the autograft. Its major advantages include availability in various shapes and sizes and no donor site morbidity. However, it only partially retains the structural strength of the autograft. Although a few studies have shown disease transmission through allografts, recent advances in processing have likely made that a historical and theoretical concern.[38–41]

Allogenic bone is available in the form of demineralized bone matrix, morselized and cancellous chips, corticocancellous and cortical grafts, and osteochondral and whole-bone segments. Despite its low cost, there are only a few studies to date that

		Bone Grafts and Substitutes	OG	OI	OC	SS	Cost
Autograft			+	+	+	+[a]	+++/++++[b]
Allograft			-	+	+	+[a]	+/++
Substitutes	Biologic	Coral	-	+	+	-	++/+++
		Collagen type 1	-	+	+[c]	-	(No studies on DRFx)
		Demineralized bone matrix	-	±	+	-	+/++
	Synthetic	Factor-based (TGF-β, PDGF, FGF, BMP)	-	+	±	-	+++/++++[d]
		Cell-based (mesenchymal stem cells)	+	-	+[c]	-	(No studies on DRFx)
		Ceramic-based (calcium HA, tricalcium phosphate, calcium phosphate cement)	-	-	+	+	+/++
		Polymer-based	-	-	+	-	(No studies on DRFx)

Table 1
Modification of Laurencin's classification

Abbreviations: BMP, bone morphogenic proteins; DRF, distal radius fracture; FGF, fibroblast growth factor; HA, hydroxyapetite; OC, osteoconductive; OG, osteogenic; OI, osteoinductive; SS, structural support; TGF, transforming growth factor.
[a] If the graft includes cortical bone.
[b] Including direct and indirect costs, data based on studies of spinal fusion and tibial nonunions.
[c] If used with a carrier.
[d] Only Rh-BMP is tested on distal radius fractures.

have tested the performance of this graft on the treatment of distal radius fractures. Herrera and colleagues[42] treated 17 patients with an average age of 70 using cancellous bone chips and external fixation. This study did not include a control group, and the authors reported complete incorporation of the graft in 8 weeks with no loss of reduction. Rajan and colleagues[43] compared the performance of allograft bone chips with iliac crest bone graft in a randomized study of 90 patients with large metaphyseal defects. The overall functional outcome between the 2 groups showed no statistically significant difference. The iliac crest group had higher rates of donor site morbidity, longer operative and anesthesia times, and higher cost of treatment. Ryan and colleagues concluded that allograft was a reliable alternative to iliac crest bone grafting in the treatment of distal radius fractures. Ozer and colleagues[44] conducted a nonrandomized study on corrective osteotomies of the distal radius. Twenty-eight patients in 2 groups had corrective osteotomy and application of volar locking plate with and without allograft bone chips. In all patients, the thicker volar cortical contact was maintained or restored during the surgical procedure, which provided additional stability to the distal radius construct. Osteotomies in both groups healed uneventfully without significant difference in the functional outcome. The authors concluded that if the volar cortical contact was maintained with the volar locking plate, the use of the bone graft substitute did not have a negative effect on functional outcomes. Based on this limited number of studies, allograft seems to be a reliable alternative to autogenous bone grafts.

Substitutes

Biologic substitutes
Coral Corals have skeletons similar to cortical and cancellous bone. A hydrothermal exchange method converts the coral calcium phosphate to crystalline hydroxyapatite, which has a structure similar to human trabecular bone with a pore diameter of 200 and 500 μm. Despite its natural appearance, the product does not easily undergo osteoclastic resorption, and remains visible on radiographs for a long time. Although it has been used in different areas of the body, only in 1 study was this product tested in the treatment of distal radius fractures.[45] Wolfe and colleagues used coral hydroxyapatite bone graft along with external fixation and K-wires to treat distal radius fractures in 21 consecutive patients. Although the study did not have a control group, the authors reported comparable results to historical cohorts treated with autografts, but with significant cost savings

by using the hydroxyapatite. They concluded that coral was a safe and effective option as a bone graft substitute.

Demineralized bone matrix Demineralized bone matrix (DBM), also known as allograft bone matrix, is an osteoinductive and osteoconductive material that provides no structural support to the articular surface.[46–50] DBM also revascularizes quickly and acts as a suitable matrix for bone marrow cells. It does not induce an immunogenic reaction, because the antigenic surface structure of bone is destroyed during demineralization.[51] Consequently, its osteoinductive capacity can be affected by storage, processing, and sterilization methods and can vary from donor to donor and from batch to batch. It is commonly used in structurally stable bone defects to stimulate bone healing, and it is used in conjunction with autologous bone marrow. There are no clinical studies published to date to test the performance of this product in the treatment of distal radius fractures. Because nonunion is rarely a concern for distal radius fractures, indications to use a nonstructural bone graft substitute are limited.

Synthetic substitutes
Factor-based substitutes The family of TGF-β-like molecules and the related family of BMPs 2 through 10 have been shown to induce primitive mesenchymal stem cells to differentiate into chondrocytes and osteoblasts.[52] Among those, rhBMP-7, also called osteogenic protein-1 (OP-1), is an osteoinductive growth factor and is the only one used to treat distal radius fractures.[53] In a randomized study including 30 patients with distal radius malunions, Ekrol and colleagues[53] compared rhBMP-7 and iliac crest bone grafting following corrective osteotomies. Bony fixation was achieved either through nonbridging external fixation or the pi-plate. The authors concluded that rh-BMP7 does not confer the same stability as the iliac crest bone graft when used in conjunction with nonbridging external fixation, resulting in delayed union and osteolysis. Although healing has occurred when used with the pi-plate, overall healing at the osteotomy site was at a slower rate for the rh-BMP7 group than the iliac crest bone graft group.

Ceramic-based substitutes These are inorganic materials hardened by heat and subsequent cooling. Calcium hydroxyapatite (CaHA) is a biocompatible ceramic that is a highly crystalline form of calcium phosphate. Its composition of calcium-to-phosphate atomic ratio is 1.67, which makes it very similar to the mineralized phase of bone. The mineralized phase of bone is widely known for providing a rigid structure to support and protect the internal organs, but it is also responsible for the storage of ions such as calcium, magnesium, and sodium. This property makes it important in maintaining the proper concentrations of ions in the extracellular fluids. The unique similarity of CaHA to mineralized bone accounts for its osteoconductive potential and excellent biocompatibility.[54–56] Sakano and colleagues[57] tested CaHA on 25 patients with unstable distal radius fractures treated with external fixation. Despite a minor loss of radial height, they concluded that CaHA was a useful adjunct to external fixation and a reliable alternative for bone grafting. Later, Huber and colleagues[58] reported the results of 22 distal radius fractures of association for osteosynthesis types C2 and C3 fixated using a nonlocking palmar plate and CaHA. All patients had an uneventful healing with no loss of reduction. In a recent study of comminuted distal radius fractures fixated with volar locked plating in elderly patients, Goto and colleagues[59] reported increased ulnar variance in the group without bone graft compared with the group supplemented with CaHA. They concluded that a locking plate system would benefit from this bone substitute, especially in comminuted intra-articular fractures of the distal radius.

Tricalcium phosphate (TCP) is also a bioabsorbable and biocompatible material with a chemical composition and crystalline structure similar to that of the mineral phase of bone. Its rate of biodegradation is higher when compared with hydroxyapatite.[60] An inflammatory reaction and the resultant osteolysis around the graft material become visible on radiographs.[61–63] Scheer and Adolfsson reported on 17 patients who underwent corrective osteotomies of the distal radius fixated with 2 different kinds of plates (dorsal and volar locking) and supplemented with TCP. Although they noted a slight loss of height at the final follow-up, along with osteolysis around the graft in 10 out of 14 patients, they recommended TCP as an alternative to iliac crest bone grafting.[62] In a recent study on 39 patients with angular malunions of the distal radius, patients were randomized into 2 groups, those augmented with TCP and those without TCP, and then both fixated with a dorsal plate following corrective osteotomies.[63] The authors reported no advantage in using TCP as a bone substitute with regards to functional and radiographic outcome.

Finally, calcium phosphate (CaP) is the second most commonly tested material after autograft in the treatment of distal radius fractures.[64–69] CaP cement offers the advantage of being freely moldable and adaptable to bone defects, as well as having chemical and physical characteristics similar to the mineral phase of bone. In preparation for clinical use, calcium and phosphate are mixed with a buffer solution to form an injectable material. Sanchez-Sotelo and Munuera prospectively compared casting of acute fractures with and without CaP on 110 patients more than 50 years of age. They concluded that the CaP group showed better range of motion, grip strength, and reduction of pain, with significantly lower rates of malunion.[64] Two randomized prospective studies by Cassidy and colleagues[66] and Kopylov and colleagues[65] compared external fixation without bone graft and casting with CaP and showed improved grip strength and range of motion in the CaP groups at the 6- to 8-week interval. However, both studies reported no differences beyond 3 months.[65,66] CaP was found to accelerate rehabilitation. Other studies on the use of CaP in the treatment of distal radius fractures are uncontrolled case series to show it is a safe material and that it provides additional support at the fracture site.[67,68] One consistent issue was extraosseous distribution of the material, which in some series resulted in up to 70% of the subjects experiencing loss of reduction if no other method of fixation was used.

IMPLICATIONS ON CURRENT PRACTICE

The use of bone grafts in the treatment of distal radius fractures seems to be determined by tradition, training, and personal experience.[70] This is mostly due to the lack of robust evidence. A recent Cochrane Database analysis of randomized clinical trials concluded that there was insufficient evidence regarding the functional outcome and safety in the use of bone grafts and substitutes for the treatment of distal radius fractures.[71] In the absence of sufficient level 1 evidence, one can only form his or her opinion based on the best evidence available. As summarized in this article, autogenous bone grafts come associated with significant morbidity and cost. Bone graft substitutes do not cause donor site morbidity, but they can still be expensive and do not possess all of the features of an autogenous graft. In this case, perhaps, the first question that needs to be addressed is whether it is necessary to use bone grafts or substitute in every distal radius fracture with dorsal comminution? The quality of the bone, size of the bone defect, blood flow to the fracture site, and method of fixation/immobilization all affect the healing process and maintenance of reduction in distal radius fractures. Although it is not clear as to what constitutes a significant bone defect, in cases of open distal radius fractures with bone loss, or in corrective osteotomies requiring substantial lengthening, the use of iliac crest bone graft with cortical support is better justified. In case of a more common scenario when there is dorsal comminution without tricortical defect, if the fracture is amenable to be fixated with an angled locking plate and the thick volar cortex contact is restored, the use of a bone graft/substitute may not be necessary as long as the articular congruity is well-supported and maintained by the use of distal locking screws as it has been repeatedly shown in a number of previous reports.[72–77] Other minimally invasive and less rigid methods of fixation, such as external fixation, K-pin, and cast immobilizations, however, may still need to be supported by a graft/substitute,[64–66] which brings the second relevant question to be addressed. If the use of the bone graft or a substitute is deemed necessary, what is the ideal material? The authors advocate the use of iliac crest bone graft in cases of significant bone loss and nonunion. In all other conditions, the use of calcium phosphate and allograft bone chips, due to their ease of use, relatively low cost, and potential to provide structural support seem to provide satisfactory healing and functional recovery; additionally, they can be used as alternatives to autogenous bone grafting. However, no graft or substitute is ideal for all injuries. Indications and choice of graft substitute should be based on the needs of the individual patient until further comparative research clarifies the indications and most appropriate material for a given fracture and clinical situation.

REFERENCES

1. Einhorn TA. Enhancement of fracture-healing. J Bone Joint Surg Am 1995;77:940–56.
2. Khan SN, Cammisa FP Jr, Sandhu HS, et al. The biology of bone grafting. J Am Acad Orthop Surg 2005;13(1):77–86.
3. Laurencin C, Khan Y, El-Amin SF. Bone graft substitutes. Expert Rev Med Devices 2006;3:49–57.
4. Greenwald AS, Boden SD, Goldberg VM, et al, American Academy of Orthopaedic Surgeons. The Committee on Biological Implants. Bone-graft substitutes: facts, fictions, and applications. J Bone Joint Surg Am 2001;83(Suppl 2):98–103.
5. Axelrod TS, McMurtry RY. Open reduction and internal fixation of comminuted, intraarticular fractures of the distal radius. J Hand Surg Am 1990;15:1–11.
6. Jupiter JB, Lipton H. The operative treatment of intraarticular fractures of the distal radius. Clin Orthop 1993;292:48–61.
7. Missikian ML, Cooney WP, Amadio PC, et al. Open reduction and internal fixation for distal radius fractures. J Hand Surg Am 1992;17:745–55.
8. Fernandez DL, Geissler WB. Treatment of displaced articular fractures of the radius. J Hand Surg Am 1991;16:375–84.
9. Axelrod T, Paley D, Green J, et al. Limited open reduction of the lunate facet in comminuted intraarticular fractures of the distal radius. J Hand Surg Am 1988;13:372–7.
10. Leung KS, Shen WY, Tsang HK, et al. An effective treatment of comminuted fractures of the distal radius. J Hand Surg Am 1990;15:11–7.
11. Leung KS, So WS, Chiu VD, et al. Ligamentotaxis for comminuted distal radial fractures modified by primary cancellous grafting and functional bracing: long-term results. J Orthop Trauma 1991;5:265–71.
12. Rogachefsky RA, Ouellette EA, Sun S, et al. The use of tricorticocancellous bone graft in severely comminuted intra-articular fractures of the distal radius. J Hand Surg Am 2006;31(4):623–32.
13. Pennig DW. Dynamic external fixation of distal radius fractures. Hand Clin 1993;9:587–602.
14. Fernandez DL. Correction of post-traumatic wrist deformity in adults by osteotomy, bone-grafting, and internal fixation. J Bone Joint Surg Am 1982;64:1164–78.
15. Fernandez DL. Radial osteotomy and Bowers arthroplasty for malunited fractures of the distal end of the radius. J Bone Joint Surg Am 1988;70:1538–51.
16. Rogachefsky RA, Mendelsohn RB. Intraoperative use of an external fixator distraction device for corrective distal radius osteotomy. Tech Hand Up Extrem Surg 1999;3:203–9.
17. Ladd AL, Huene DS. Reconstructive osteotomy for malunion of the distal radius. Clin Orthop 1996;327:158–71.
18. Meads BM, Scougall PJ, Hargreaves IC. Wrist arthrodesis using a Synthes wrist fusion plate. J Hand Surg Br 2003;28(6):571–4.
19. O'Bierne J, Boyer MI, Axelrod TS. Wrist arthrodesis using a dynamic compression plate. J Bone Joint Surg Br 1995;77(5):700–4.
20. Sagerman SD, Palmer AK. Wrist arthrodesis using a dynamic compression plate. J Hand Surg Br 1996;21(4):437–41.
21. Moneim MS, Pribyl CR, Garst JR. Wrist arthrodesis. Technique and functional evaluation. Clin Orthop Relat Res 1997;341:23–9.
22. Zachary SV, Stern PJ. Complications following AO/ASIF wrist arthrodesis. J Hand Surg Am 1995;20(2):339–44.
23. Heary RF, Schlenk RP, Sacchieri TA, et al. Persistent iliac crest donor site pain: independent outcome assessment. Neurosurgery 2002;50:510–6.
24. Ahlmann E, Patzakis M, Roidis N, et al. Comparison of anterior and posterior iliac crest bone grafts in terms of harvest-site morbidity and functional outcomes. J Bone Joint Surg Am 2002;84:716–20.
25. Arrington ED, Smith WJ, Chambers HG, et al. Complications of iliac crest bone graft harvesting. Clin Orthop Relat Res 1996;329:300–9.

26. Banwart JC, Asher MA, Hassanein RS. Iliac crest bone graft harvest donor site morbidity. A statistical evaluation. Spine 1995;20:1055–60.

27. Canady J, Zeitler DP, Thompson SA, et al. Suitability of the iliac crest as a site for harvest of autogenous bone grafts. Cleft Palate Craniofac J 1993;30:579–81.

28. Cockin J. Autologous bone grafting: complications at the donor site. J Bone Joint Surg 1971;53:153.

29. Keller EE, Triplett WW. Iliac bone grafting: review of 160 consecutive cases. J Oral Maxillofac Surg 1987;45:11–4.

30. Sawin PD, Traynelis VC, Menezes AH. A comparative analysis of fusion rates and donor-site morbidity for autogeneic rib and iliac crest bone grafts in posterior cervical fusions. J Neurosurg 1998;88:255–65.

31. Summers B, Eisenstein SM. Donor site pain from the ilium. A complication of lumbar spine fusion. J Bone Joint Surg Br 1989;71:677–80.

32. Younger EM, Chapman MW. Morbidity at bone graft donor sites. J Orthop Trauma 1989;3:192–5.

33. Schwartz CE, Martha JF, Kowalski P, et al. Prospective evaluation of chronic pain associated with posterior autologous iliac crest bone graft harvest and its effect on postoperative outcome. Health Qual Life Outcomes 2009;7:49.

34. St. John TA, Vaccaro AR, Sah AP, et al. Physical and monetary costs associated with autogenous bone graft harvesting. Am J Orthop 2003;32:18–23.

35. Carreon LY, Glassman SD, Djurasovic M, et al. RhBMP-2 versus iliac crest bone graft for lumbar spine fusion in patients over 60 years of age: a cost–utility study. Spine (Phila Pa 1976) 2009;34(3):238–43.

36. Dahabreh Z, Calori GM, Kanakaris NK, et al. A cost analysis of treatment of tibial fracture nonunion by bone grafting or bone morphogenetic protein-7. Int Orthop 2009;33(5):1407–14.

37. Buttermann GR. Prospective nonrandomized comparison of an allograft with bone morphogenic protein versus an iliac-crest autograft in anterior cervical discectomy and fusion. Spine J 2008;8(3):426–35.

38. Kakaiya R, Miller WV, Gudino MD. Tissue transplant-transmitted infections. Transfusion 1991;31:277–84.

39. Shutkin NM. Homologous-serum hepatitis following the use of refrigerated bone–bank bone. J Bone Joint Surg Am 1954;36:160–2.

40. Conrad EU, Gretch DR, Obermeyer KR, et al. Transmission of the hepatitis-C virus by tissue transplantation. J Bone Joint Surg Am 1995;77:214–24.

41. Simonds RJ, Holmberg SD, Hurwitz RL, et al. Transmission of human immunodeficiency virus type 1 from a seronegative organ and tissue donor. N Engl J Med 1992;326:726–32.

42. Herrera M, Chapman CB, Roh M, et al. Treatment of unstable distal radius fractures with cancellous allograft and external fixation. J Hand Surg Am 1999;24(6):1269–78.

43. Rajan GP, Fornaro J, Trentz O, et al. Cancellous allograft versus autologous bone grafting for repair of comminuted distal radius fractures: a prospective, randomized trial. J Trauma 2006;60(6):1322–9.

44. Ozer K, Kiliç A, Sabel A, et al. The role of bone allografts in the treatment of angular malunions of the distal radius. J Hand Surg Am 2011;36(11):1804–9.

45. Wolfe SW, Pike L, Slade JF 3rd, et al. Augmentation of distal radius fracture fixation with coralline hydroxyapatite bone graft substitute. J Hand Surg Am 1999;24(4):816–27.

46. Peterson B, Whang PG, Iglesias R, et al. Osteoinductivity of commercially available demineralized bone matrix. Preparations in a spine fusion model. J Bone Joint Surg Am 2004;86:2243–50.

47. Wang JC, Alanay A, Mark D, et al. A comparison of commercially available demineralized bone matrix for spinal fusion. Eur Spine J 2007;16:1233–40.

48. McKee MD. Management of segmental bony defects: the role of osteoconductive orthobiologics. J Am Acad Orthop Surg 2006;14:S163–7.

49. Pietrzak WS, Perns SV, Keyes J, et al. Demineralized bone matrix graft: a scientific and clinical case study assessment. J Foot Ankle Surg 2005;44:345–53.

50. Katz JM, Nataraj C, Jaw R, et al. Demineralized bone matrix as an osteoinductive biomaterial and in vitro predictors of its biological potential. J Biomed Mater Res B Appl Biomater 2009;89:127–34.

51. Tuli SM, Singh AD. The osteoinductive property of decalcified bone matrix. An experimental study. J Bone Joint Surg Br 1978;60:116–23.

52. Vaibhav B, Nilesh P, Vikram S, et al. Bone morphogenic protein and its application in trauma cases: a current concept update. Injury 2007;38(11):1227–35.

53. Ekrol I, Hajducka C, Court-Brown C, et al. A comparison of RhBMP-7 (OP-1) and autogenous graft for metaphyseal defects after osteotomy of the distal radius. Injury 2008;39(Suppl 2):S73–82.

54. Erbe EM, Marx JG, Clineff TD, et al. Potential of an ultraporous ß-tricalcium phosphate synthetic cancellous bone void filler and bone marrow aspirate composite graft. Eur Spine J 2001;10(Suppl 2):S141–6.

55. Nandi SK, Kundu B, Ghosh SK, et al. Efficacy of nano-hydroxyapatite prepared by an aqueous solution combustion technique in healing bone defects of goat. J Vet Sci 2008;9:183–91.

56. Ghosh SK, Nandi SK, Kundu B, et al. In vivo response of porous hydroxyapatite and ß-tricalcium phosphate prepared by aqueous solution combustion method and comparison with bioglass scaffolds. J Biomed Mater Res B Appl Biomater 2008;86:217–27.

57. Sakano H, Koshino T, Takeuchi R, et al. Treatment of the unstable distal radius fracture with external fixation and a hydroxyapatite spacer. J Hand Surg Am 2001;26(5):923–30.

58. Huber FX, Hillmeier J, Herzog L, et al. Open reduction and palmar plate-osteosynthesis in combination with a nanocrystalline hydroxyapatite spacer in the treatment of comminuted fractures of the distal radius. J Hand Surg Br 2006;31(3):298–303.

59. Goto A, Murase T, Oka K, et al. Use of the volar fixed angle plate for comminuted distal radius fractures and augmentation with a hydroxyapatite bone graft substitute. Hand Surg 2011;16(1):29–37.

60. Daculsi G, LeGeros RZ, Heughebaert M, et al. Formation of carbonate apatite crystals after implantation of calcium phosphate ceramics. Calcif Tissue Int 1990;46:20–7.

61. Leroux T, Perez-Ordonez B, von Schroeder HP. Osteolysis after the use of a silicon-stabilized tricalcium phosphate-based bone substitute in a radius fracture: a case report. J Hand Surg Am 2007;32(4): 497–500.

62. Scheer JH, Adolfsson LE. Tricalcium phosphate bone substitute in corrective osteotomy of the distal radius. Injury 2009;40(3):262–7.

63. Jakubietz MG, Gruenert JG, Jakubietz RG. The use of beta-tricalcium phosphate bone graft substitute in dorsally plated, comminuted distal radius fractures. J Orthop Surg Res 2011;6:24.

64. Sanchez-Sotelo J, Munuera L, Madero R. Treatment of fractures of the distal radius with a remodellable bone cement. A prospective randomized study using norian SRS. J Bone Joint Surg Br 2000;82: 856–63.

65. Kopylov P, Runnqvist K, Jonsson K, et al. Norian SRS versus external fixation in redisplaced distal radial fractures. A randomized study in 40 patients. Acta Orthop Scand 1999;70(1):1–5.

66. Cassidy C, Jupiter JB, Cohen M, et al. Norian SRS cement compared with conventional fixation in distal radial fractures. A randomized study. J Bone Joint Surg Am 2003;85(11):2127–37.

67. Zimmermann R, Gabl M, Lutz M, et al. Injectable calcium phosphate bone cement Norian SRS for the treatment of intra-articular compression fractures of the distal radius in osteoporotic women. Arch Orthop Trauma Surg 2003;123(1):22–7.

68. Lozano-Calderón S, Moore M, Liebman M, et al. Distal radius osteotomy in the elderly patient using angular stable implants and Norian bone cement. J Hand Surg Am 2007;32(7):976–83.

69. Kopylov P, Adalberth K, Jonsson K, et al. Norian SRS versus functional treatment in redisplaced distal radial fractures: a randomized study in 20 patients. J Hand Surg Br 2002;27(6):538–41.

70. Tosti R, Ilyas AM. The role of bone grafting in distal radius fractures. J Hand Surg Am 2010;35(12): 2082–4.

71. Handoll HH, Watts AC. Bone grafts and bone substitutes for treating distal radial fractures in adults. Cochrane Database Syst Rev 2008;2:CD006836.

72. Orbay JL, Fernandez DL. Volar fixed-angle plate fixation for unstable distal radius fractures in the elderly patient. J Hand Surg Am 2004;9:96–102.

73. Orbay JL, Fernandez DL. Volar fixation for dorsally displaced fractures of the distal radius: a preliminary report. J Hand Surg Am 2002;27:205–15.

74. Rozental TD, Blazar PE. Functional outcome and complications after volar plating for dorsally displaced, unstable fractures of the distal radius. J Hand Surg Am 2006;31:359–65.

75. Wong KK, Chan KW, Kwok TK, et al. Volar fixation of dorsally displaced distal radial fracture using locking compression plate. J Orthop Surg 2005;13: 153–7.

76. Jupiter JB, Marent-Huber M, LCP Study Group. Operative management of distal radial fractures with 2.4-millimeter locking plates. A multicenter prospective case series. J Bone Joint Surg Am 2009;91:55–65.

77. Osada D, Kamei S, Masuzaki K, et al. Prospective study of distal radius fractures treated with a volar locking plate system. J Hand Surg Am 2008;33: 691–700.

Management of Soft-Tissue Injuries in Distal Radius Fractures

Fraser J. Leversedge, MD*, Ramesh C. Srinivasan, MD

KEYWORDS

- Distal radius fracture • Soft-tissue injury
- Compartment syndrome • Wrist ligament injury

Distal radius fractures account for approximately 15% of all fractures in adults, and are the most common fractures seen in the emergency department with an incidence of 640,000 per year in the United States alone.[1] Previous estimates of soft-tissue injuries associated with distal radius fractures have been reported to be as high as 31%.[2] These injuries may influence strategies for the acute management of the fracture but also may be a source of persisting pain and/or disability despite fracture healing. Although some soft-tissue injuries may be recognized at the time of initial evaluation of the injury, the diagnosis of a concomitant soft-tissue injury is often delayed until the completion of a secondary survey, during intraoperative inspection at the time of fracture repair, or during evaluation for the source of ongoing pain or dysfunction despite fracture union. In a previous *Hand Clinics* issue, Davis and Baratz described soft-tissue complications associated with distal radius fractures both before and after surgical treatment.[3] This review describes soft-tissue injuries and considerations for treatment associated with distal radius fractures, including injuries to the skin, tendon and muscle, ligaments, the triangular fibrocartilage complex (TFCC), neurovascular structures, and related conditions such as compartment syndrome and complex regional pain syndrome.

SOFT-TISSUE INJURIES ASSOCIATED WITH DISTAL RADIUS FRACTURES

Skin

Because many distal radius fractures occur in the elderly population, the potential for both fragility fracture and injury to the delicate soft-tissue envelope increases with age and with more complex medical comorbidities. Skin compromise may be caused by the injury directly or may be associated with the initial phases of treatment, such as fracture manipulation and splint/cast application. Careful evaluation of the extremity is advised to establish the presence or absence of an open fracture, as this will influence operative indications. Open fractures are treated with early wound debridement and irrigation, intravenous antibiotics, tetanus update, wound management, and fracture reduction and stabilization. Skin tears without an open fracture may be treated with local wound care and fracture management; avoiding complications of skin fragility during closed fracture manipulation may be facilitated by the use of regional or general anesthesia. Proper splint or cast application, paying particular attention to avoid pressure points from improper molding, is important in minimizing the risks of secondary skin compromise. Other steps that help decrease this risk include patient education emphasizing a reduction in limb swelling or edema, and the recognition of signs or symptoms related to complications of splinting.

Tendon and Muscle

Tendon injury after a distal radius fracture is rare. Primary tendon injury occurs at the time of the fracture and is due to tendon laceration from a sharp fracture fragment or fracture site incarceration, in contradistinction to secondary tendon injury, which may present late as a delayed rupture

Department of Orthopaedic Surgery, Duke University, DUMC Box 2836, Durham, NC 27710, USA
* Corresponding author.
E-mail address: fraser.leversedge@duke.edu

Hand Clin 28 (2012) 225–233
doi:10.1016/j.hcl.2012.03.005

or as restricted tendon excursion caused by peritendinous adhesions.

Rupture of the extensor pollicis longus (EPL) has been reported to occur in 0.07% to 0.88% of distal radius fractures treated nonoperatively.[4,5] EPL tendon rupture usually occurs within 8 weeks of the initial injury, although delayed rupture, occurring years later, has been reported.[4,5] Two causes of delayed EPL rupture have been proposed: (1) attritional injury caused by mechanical impingement of the EPL tendon during excursion over irregularities in the dorsal cortex of the displaced distal radius fracture (**Fig. 1**); and (2) vascular compromise of the tendon resulting from increased pressure from hematoma and/or fracture displacement or callous within the third extensor compartment at the wrist (**Fig. 2**).[6] EPL tendon rupture is diagnosed clinically by the inability to actively hyperextend the thumb interphalangeal joint in combination with a loss of passive tenodesis of the EPL with wrist motion on physical examination. Treatment options include extensor indicis proprius (EIP) to EPL transfer,[7] EPL reconstruction with intercalary tendon grafting,[8] or thumb interphalangeal joint arthrodesis.[9] Other extensor tendon injuries have been described, including

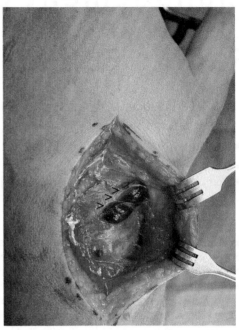

Fig. 2. The protruding hematoma (*arrowheads*) contained within the third dorsal extensor compartment is visualized in this dorsal approach to the left distal radius for surgical repair of a distal radius fracture. Increased intracompartmental pressure is thought to be a contributing cause of delayed ruptures of the EPL tendon. (© 2010, Leversedge F.J.)

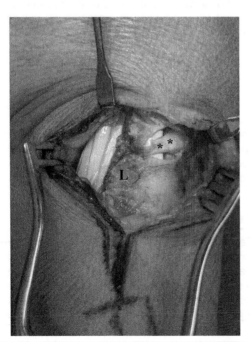

Fig. 1. Dorsal view of the left wrist of a patient who sustained a delayed rupture of the EPL tendon (*asterisks*), just distal to the Lister tubercle (L), following closed management of a comminuted distal radius fracture. (© 2010, Leversedge F.J.)

extensor digitorum communis (EDC) tendon rupture, intersection syndrome, and extensor tenosynovitis. Incarceration of the extensor carpi ulnaris (ECU) within the fracture site may be detected clinically by the presence of a vacant ECU sulcus over the distal ulna, and a widened distal radioulnar joint (DRUJ) on radiographic assessment.[10]

Flexor tendon injuries may be less common than extensor injuries, owing to the more protected anatomy of the flexor tendons. The pronator quadratus muscle provides a relative anatomic barrier to direct injury, and the tendons are less constrained within the flexor canal compared with the more intimate positioning of the extensor tendons within their dorsal compartments immediately dorsal to the distal radius.[3] Flexor carpi radialis (FCR), flexor pollicis longus (FPL), flexor digitorum superficialis (FDS), and flexor digitorum profundus (FDP) tendon ruptures have all been reported in the acute or delayed setting.[11] The senior author (F.J.L.) has described a case report involving the entrapment of multiple flexor tendons within a distal radius fracture site and associated fracture nonunion (Leversedge FJ, unpublished case report, 2012) (**Fig. 3**).

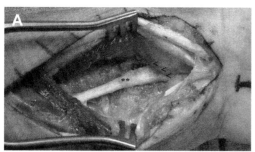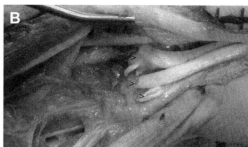

Fig. 3. (A) Volar exposure of the right distal forearm in a patient found to have entrapment and associated rupture of the flexor digitorum profundus tendons (*asterisks*) within the distal radius fracture site (*arrowheads*), contributing to dysfunction and fracture nonunion. (B) Volar exposure of the same patient, highlighting the distal flexor tendon stumps (*arrowheads*). (© 2010, Leversedge F.J.)

Triangular Fibrocartilage Complex

The incidence of TFCC injury associated with distal radius fracture has been reported to range between 35% and 78%.[12–14] Although the incidence may be overestimated in some studies because of the potential for preexisting TFCC lesions, Geissler and colleagues[12] demonstrated arthroscopically that 64% of patients with concomitant ulnar styloid fractures also had a tear of the TFCC. This finding suggests a strong association between these 2 types of injury. Radial shortening, dorsal angulation, fracture pattern, and magnitude of displacement on radiographic examination have been shown to be predictive of TFCC injury.[13,15–17]

In 1989, Palmer[18] described a classification system for TFCC tears. These injuries may be classified as being partial or complete, central or peripheral, and may be further classified by location. When present, up to 87.5% of TFCC injuries are peripheral in nature based on arthroscopic examination (ulnar/type B or radial/type D).[12] Certain peripheral TFCC tears may be associated with DRUJ instability and, therefore, stability of the DRUJ should be assessed. Unrecognized DRUJ instability caused by disruption of the volar and/or dorsal distal radioulnar ligaments may be a source of residual pain and disability after distal radius fractures.[19] The incidence of persistent symptomatic DRUJ instability after distal radius fracture treatment ranges from 6.7% to 25.4%.[17,20,21] However, this association is variable and depends on several factors, including the method by which DRUJ instability is assessed, the age of the patient, and the method of treatment of the distal radius fracture. Injury to the TFCC that causes DRUJ instability may be treated with bony stabilization or ligamentous repair via arthroscopic or open means. Mikic[22] reported 70% excellent and 30% fair or poor results in 35 patients with TFCC injury associated with DRUJ instability who were treated with DRUJ reduction and pin stabilization or open repair of the TFCC soft tissue or bony avulsion.

Favorable patient outcomes have been shown after acute repair of complete ulnar-sided TFCC tears in the setting of an acute distal radius fracture. Ruch and colleagues[23] retrospectively reviewed 13 patients treated with arthroscopic TFCC repair at the time of arthroscopic-assisted external fixation of distal radius fractures. Indications for TFCC repair included: (1) evidence of displacement of the radius relative to the ulna greater than 5 mm, (2) absence of an ulnar styloid base fracture, and (3) a complete peripheral tear of the TFCC; 92% of patients in this series achieved an excellent or good result. The investigators demonstrated functional wrist motion 2 years after surgery, with average grip strength of 78% on the uninjured side and Disabilities of the Shoulder, Arm, and Hand (DASH) outcomes scores notable for a mean functional score of 13 and a mean athletic score of 12. No increase in translation for the DRUJ was noted on physical examination or radiographically for any patient postoperatively. Fujitani and colleagues[17] reported successful treatment of intraoperatively and clinically determined DRUJ instability in the setting of distal radius fractures repaired via an open-FCR approach with locked volar plating. These investigators described a separate ulnar incision and volar distal radioulnar ligament reattachment using a bone-anchoring system. Although they did not report functional outcomes, Fujitani and colleagues reported no occurrence of clinical or radiographic DRUJ instability. The superiority of bony repair versus soft-tissue ligamentous repair via arthroscopic or open means in the setting of DRUJ instability associated with distal radius fractures remains unknown at this time.

Ligament Injury

Scapholunate interosseous ligament injury

The incidence of scapholunate interosseous ligament (SLIL) injury associated with distal radius fractures has been reported to be as high as 54% in patients with a displaced distal radius fracture.[14] The SLIL is C-shaped and attaches along the dorsal, proximal, and volar margins of the articulating surfaces of the scaphoid and lunate. The dorsal component of the ligament is the thickest, strongest, and most critical portion of this ligament.[24,25] SLIL injuries may be classified as partial or complete, and not all SLIL injures cause carpal instability.

Diagnosis of SLIL disassociation in the setting of distal radius fractures may be challenging because of the swelling, deformity, and pain associated with the fracture. Clinical examination emphasizes localized tenderness at the scapholunate interval, and a positive Watson maneuver may be present. Indirect assessment of the SLIL on plain radiographs includes evaluation of the following parameters: (1) scapholunate interosseous distance, (2) scapholunate angle, and (3) scaphoid morphology. Previous studies have shown that abnormal widening of the SLIL interval secondary to an SLIL dissociative injury may be greater than 2 to 5 mm (**Fig. 4**).[26–30] Kwon and Baek[31] recently demonstrated that an SLIL gap of greater than 2 mm via fluoroscopy was associated with a high-grade SLIL tear (grade III or IV), as confirmed by arthroscopy. A scapholunate angle outside of the normal range of 30° to 60° may indicate SLIL injury also, and this increased scaphoid flexion is observed to correlate with a cortical ring sign on the posteroanterior

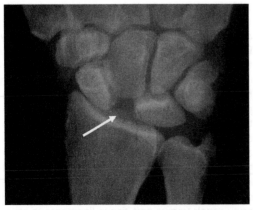

Fig. 4. Posteroanterior radiograph of the right wrist, demonstrating characteristic scapholunate dissociation with a gap of greater than 6 mm (*arrow*) and a cortical ring sign.

radiographic view of the wrist, caused by the excessive flexion of the scaphoid following dissociation from the lunate. The cortical ring sign highlights the greater proportion of the scaphoid cortex paralleling the x-ray beam as the scaphoid flexes. The ring-to-pole sign measurement of 7 mm or less, suggestive of increased scaphoid flexion, is consistent with scapholunate dissociation. Partial or complete SLIL tears may not demonstrate such characteristic radiographic findings on static radiographs, although radiographs augmented by a directed load or dynamic views may be useful. Recently, Kwon and colleagues[32] described the modified carpal stretch test in which traction is applied across the wrist during fluoroscopic evaluation. A step-off or incongruity in the alignment of the scaphoid and lunate is appreciated as a disruption of the Gilula arc at the proximal carpal row.[33] Evaluation of the modified carpal stretch test using arthroscopy as a reference standard demonstrated an average sensitivity of 78%, specificity of 72%, positive predictive value of 60%, and negative predictive value of 87% for determining Geissler grade III or IV SLIL injuries. Arthroscopy and arthrotomy remain the standard for confirmation of both partial and complete SLIL tears.

Treatment of SLIL injuries should be individualized depending on the age and expectations of the patient. Forward and colleagues[34] prospectively followed 51 patients with an SLIL injury confirmed arthroscopically at the time of treatment of a distal radius fracture; however, no treatment was rendered for the SLIL injury. Patients with grade III injuries were noted to have a greater amount of static and dynamic scapholunate dissociation, greater SLIL angle, as well as worse subjective complaints of pain at 1 year after injury compared with patients with grade I or II injuries. Tang and colleagues[35] prospectively followed 20 of 424 patients with distal radius fractures who presented with evidence of SLIL dissociation on radiographs and/or with a positive modified carpal stretch test. Eighteen of these 20 patients treated with cast immobilization had fair or poor wrist function 1 year after injury as measured by Green and O'Brien scores. The results of these studies indicate that in younger patients with concomitant SLIL injury and radiographic evidence of dissociation, consideration should be given to early operative ligamentous repair or reconstruction at the time of distal radius repair. This step is crucial, given the potential for development of scapholunate advanced collapse arthrosis of the wrist.

Outcomes of the arthroscopic treatment of SLIL, TFCC, and lunotriquetral interosseous ligament (LTIL) tears in the setting of distal radius fractures treated with arthroscopically assisted reduction with external fixation and pinning has been reported. Varitimidis and colleagues[36] demonstrated improved supination and flexion at all time points compared with patients who were treated without arthroscopy. DASH questionnaire scores were similar for both groups at 24 months. In comparison, the difference in mean modified Mayo wrist scores remained statistically significant, with improved scores noted in the arthroscopic treatment group. Injuries to the SLIL were demonstrated in 9 (45%) of the patients in this study group; 7 patients had grade II tears, and 2 patients had grade III tears. The investigators hypothesized that multiple factors contributed to the improved outcomes in the arthroscopy group, including improved articular reduction, removal of joint debris/hematoma, and the concomitant treatment of soft-tissue ligamentous injury.[36]

Recently, Tang and colleagues[37] evaluated 40 patients with an acute, displaced distal radius fracture. The investigators performed a diagnostic wrist arthroscopy at the time of operative fracture repair, but did not treat any of the identified ligamentous injuries. There were no differences reported DASH scores, pain (visual analog scale) or postoperative range of motion for each of the following groups: no associated injury, TFCC injury, SLIL injury, or TFCC and SLIL injury. These results suggest that treatment of stable injuries of the TFCC and SLIL associated with distal radius fractures requiring surgical treatment does not affect short-term outcomes; however, the effect on long-term outcomes is not known.

Lunotriquetral interosseous ligament injury

LTIL injuries are difficult to confirm, despite improved diagnostic accuracy with subjective complaints of localized pain, and clinical findings positive for localized tenderness at the LTIL with positive lunotriquetral shear and ballottement tests. The incidence of LTIL injury associated with a distal radius fracture is less than that of injuries to the TFCC or SLIL. Geissler and colleagues[12] reported an overall incidence of 15% for partial or complete tears of the LTIL after distal radius fracture. When comparing extra-articular and intra-articular distal radius fractures, Roberts and colleagues[13] showed that 13.3% of extra-articular fractures and 6.7% of intra-articular fractures had concomitant injury to the LTIL. Combined SLIL and LTIL ligamentous injuries were demonstrated arthroscopically in 5.6% of patients with intra-articular distal radius fractures.[13] The study methodology precluded determination of the age of injury, therefore it is possible that there was an overestimation of acute injury incidence. In a separate study, Varitimidis and

colleagues[36] arthroscopically demonstrated LTIL tears in 4 of 16 patients. All of these tears were stable to probing and were treated with arthroscopic debridement only; however, no treatment controls were identified in this small series.

At present, there are no well-controlled outcomes studies that confirm improved outcomes with surgical treatment of acute or chronic LTIL ligament injury in the setting of distal radius fractures. Direct LTIL repair or LTIL reconstruction, such as temporary pin stabilization, capsulorrhaphy, and arthrodesis, have all produced inconsistent outcomes.[38,39]

Dorsal capsular/extrinsic wrist ligament injury

Avulsion, or "chip" fracture, from the dorsal aspect of the triquetrum has been associated with disruption of the dorsal radiocarpal ligament insertion into the triquetrum. Several studies have implicated this fracture pattern as occurring secondary to impaction/compression of the ulnar styloid into the triquetrum with axial loading of the wrist (**Fig. 5**).[40]

Nerve Injury

The unique anatomy of the median, ulnar, and radial nerves presents a risk for direct and indirect nerve injury inherent to trauma affecting the distal radius. In the distal forearm, the median nerve typically emerges from the FDS-FDP interval to course distally between the FDS and the FCR. Vance and Gelberman[41] demonstrated that the distance between the median nerve and the radius decreases as it courses distally in the forearm, from 1 cm at mid-forearm to 3 mm at wrist level. The ulnar nerve travels deep to the flexor carpi ulnaris in the forearm and volar to the transverse carpal ligament in the distal ulnar tunnel. The radial nerve bifurcates into the posterior interosseous

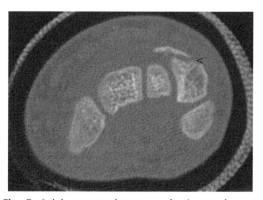

Fig. 5. Axial computed tomography image demonstrating a dorsal fracture of the triquetrum (*arrowhead*). (© 2010, Leversedge F.J.)

nerve and the superficial branch of the radial nerve approximately 3.6 cm proximal to the leading edge of the supinator muscle. The superficial branch of the radial nerve descends in the forearm deep to the brachioradialis (BR) muscle and pierces the fascia between the BR and extensor carpi radialis longus tendons, approximately 9 cm proximal to the radial styloid. It branches near the wrist, providing sensation to the dorsoradial hand. The posterior interosseous nerve courses through the supinator to lie in the interval between the abductor pollicis longus/ECU and the extensor digiti minimi/EDC, before terminating as afferent fibers into the wrist capsule volar to the fourth dorsal extensor compartment.

Median neuropathy may be present acutely or have a delayed onset following a distal radius fracture. Nerve dysfunction may be secondary to neuropraxia associated with fracture displacement, or be due to the development of elevated intracarpal tunnel pressures as a consequence of fracture displacement or hematoma. The incidence of acute median neuropathy requiring urgent decompression following distal radius fracture is estimated to be 4% to 9%.[42,43] Dyer and colleagues[43] reported that the amount of fracture translation (>35%) was a statistically significant predictor of acute carpal tunnel syndrome.

The development of a median nerve problem may be adversely influenced by the positioning of the injured wrist in excessive flexion during closed reduction and splint or cast application. Gelberman and colleagues[44] demonstrated that carpal tunnel pressures increased to an average of 47 mm Hg at 40° of flexion, compared with 18 mm Hg when the wrist was at neutral. Initial treatment of acute carpal tunnel syndrome should include placement of the wrist into a neutral position, limb elevation, and the removal of all constrictive dressings and/or splints. If median nerve function does not improve on serial examinations, the nerve should be decompressed urgently. A delay in treatment may correlate with worse outcomes related to nerve recovery, as Bauman and colleagues[45] found when they reported early return of median nerve function in only 1 of 4 (25%) patients when decompression was performed at 36 to 96 hours following the onset of median neuropathy.

Although laceration to the radial nerve has not been reported after distal radius fracture, superficial radial nerve neuritis or neuropraxic injury can occur. Careful manipulation with closed or open reduction techniques and protective splint application are crucial for minimizing nerve irritation. In addition, an emphasis on a reduction of swelling with strict elevation of the injured limb may help avoid this complication.

Injuries of the ulnar nerve associated with distal radius fracture are rare. Soong and Ring[46] reported on 5 patients with acute, complete motor and sensory ulnar nerve palsy associated with a distal radius fracture. All fractures were high-energy with wide displacement; 3 had an associated ulna fracture and 2 patients had open fractures. The ulnar nerve was found to be intact in 3 patients who underwent exploration and decompression of the distal ulnar tunnel. Four of the patients had complete or near-complete recovery of ulnar nerve function; one patient had residual moderate motor and sensory dysfunction. Complete transection of the ulnar nerve has been reported,[47] and case reports of DRUJ entrapment and dorsal displacement of the nerve relative to the ulnar styloid have been described.[48–51] Initial treatment of ulnar nerve dysfunction in the setting of distal radius fracture is closed fracture reduction and serial observation of nerve function. If ulnar nerve function does not improve, consideration should be given to nerve exploration with formal release of the distal ulnar tunnel to minimize the possibility of permanent nerve dysfunction.[41]

Vascular Injury

Acute vascular injuries associated with distal radius fractures are rare. Case reports of ulnar artery entrapment, dorsal displacement of the ulnar artery relative to the ulnar styloid, and radial artery pseudoaneurysm with subsequent microembolism to the thumb have been reported.[50–52] The outcomes of arterial injury associated with distal radius fractures in 6 patients were reported by de Witte and colleagues,[53] who described 2 partial lacerations of the radial artery, 1 complete radial artery, 1 complete ulnar artery, 1 thrombosed radial artery, and 1 thrombosed ulnar artery. Three of these fractures were open and 3 had an associated distal ulna fracture, consistent with a higher-energy injury mechanism. Direct arterial repair was performed in 2 patients and 1 patient had vein graft reconstruction of the radial artery, whereas arterial ligation was performed in the remaining 3 patients. All patients had well-perfused hands at an average follow-up of 9 months (range 5–16 months). In general, a careful and documented vascular examination of all patients with distal radius fractures is imperative. For patients with a dysvascular limb following distal radius fracture, emergent angiography, vascular exploration and repair or reconstruction, as well as fracture reduction and stabilization are indicated.

Compartment Syndrome

Although compartment syndrome complicating a distal radius fracture has a prevalence of less than 1%,[2] distal radius fracture is the most common cause of forearm compartment syndrome in adults.[54] A global injury assessment should include the evaluation and documentation of the condition of both the hand and forearm compartments. Traditionally, 10 separate osteofascial compartments of the hand have been described: dorsal interosseous (4), volar interosseous (3), adductor pollicis brevis, thenar, and hypothenar muscle groups.[55] The forearm has traditionally been described as having 3 separate compartments: the volar, dorsal, and mobile wad. However, anatomic dissections have confirmed variations in subcompartmentalization of each and also that the volar compartment may be considered as 3 separate subcompartments: superficial volar, deep volar, and the pronator quadratus.[56] In the setting of compartment syndrome, particularly following a higher-energy injury, each compartment and subcompartment should be evaluated carefully for indications of emergent surgical decompression.[57]

Pertinent physical examination findings suggesting compartment syndrome may include swollen or tense compartments, pain out of proportion to the injury, pain with passive stretch of the compartmental structures, neurologic disturbance, and vascular compromise. When compartment syndrome is suspected, patients should be monitored closely with documented serial examinations as indicated. Intracompartmental pressure measurements using a needle manometer may be used as a confirmatory test, or for diagnostic purposes in the obtunded patient.

Management of an injury with a potential risk for compartment syndrome or an incipient compartment syndrome includes the immediate removal of all potentially compressive circumferential dressings/casts/splints, elevation of the injured extremity to the level of the heart, and serial examinations. If symptoms do not improve quickly, emergent operative fasciotomies of the involved compartments are mandatory, in conjunction with operative fracture reduction and stabilization. A recent systematic review reported that after fasciotomy skin grafting was required in 61% of forearm compartment syndrome cases with 21% of patients experiencing a persistent neurologic deficit.[54]

Complex Regional Pain Syndrome

Complex regional pain syndrome, also known as reflex sympathetic dystrophy or algodystrophy, is characterized by pain, hypersensitivity, swelling, vasomotor instability, and stiffness, and has been reported to have an incidence of 22% to 37% in prospective studies evaluating distal radius fractures.[58,59] Treatment may include pain medication, therapy, and sympathetic blocks. Davis and Baratz[3] recommended the following regimen: methylprednisolone (Medrol Dose Pack) and mild analgesic at first visit; amitriptyline (Elavil) may be added if sleep disturbances are noted. Patients are referred for daily therapy, and instructed to use the injured hand. If pain is refractory, the patient is referred for a sympathetic stellate ganglion block. Recently, Zollinger and colleagues[59,60] reported a decreased rate of complex regional pain syndrome in wrist-fracture patients treated with 500 mg per day of vitamin C for 50 days after injury.

SUMMARY

Soft-tissue injuries are commonly associated with distal radius fractures including injuries to the skin, musculotendinous units, intrinsic and extrinsic ligaments, the TFCC, and neurovascular structures, as well as compartment syndrome and complex regional pain syndrome. Although these injuries may be evident at the time of initial assessment or during intraoperative treatment, many soft-tissue injuries are detected at the time of delayed evaluation, because of persisting symptoms or dysfunction despite appropriate management of acute fracture. Unfortunately, there are few evidence-based outcomes studies from which to synthesize a systematic approach for the management of these injuries. Awareness of the potential for concomitant soft-tissue injury is crucial for the timely diagnosis and treatment, as is patient education as regards the prognosis for recovery. Careful pretreatment and posttreatment clinical evaluation and improved diagnostic capabilities for the detection of these soft-tissue injuries may provide a basis for a greater understanding of these common injuries along with the outcomes of the available treatment options.

REFERENCES

1. Chung KC, Spilson SV. The frequency and epidemiology of hand and forearm fractures in the United States. J Hand Surg Am 2001;26:908–15.
2. Cooney WP III, Dobyns JH, Linschied RL. Complications of Colles' fractures. J Bone Joint Surg Am 1980;62:613–9.
3. Davis DI, Baratz M. Soft tissue complications of distal radius fractures. Hand Clin 2010;26:229–35.
4. Heidermann J, Gausepohl T, Pennig D. Narrowing of the third extensor tendon compartment in minimal displaced distal radius fractures with impending

rupture of the EPL tendon. Handchir Mikrochir Plast Chir 2002;34:324–7.

5. Hove LM. Delayed rupture of the thumb extensor tendon: a 5 year study of 18 consecutive cases. Acta Orthop Scand 1994;65:199–203.

6. Engkvist O, Lundborg G. Rupture of the extensor pollicis longus tendon after fracture of the lower end of the radius: a clinical and microangiographic study. Hand 1979;11:76–86.

7. Magnussen PA, Harvey FJ, Tonkin MA. Extensor indicis proprius transfer for rupture of the extensor pollicis longus tendon. J Bone Joint Surg Br 1990; 72:881–3.

8. Hamlin C, Littler JW. Restoration of the extensor pollicis longus tendon by an intercalated graft. J Bone Joint Surg Am 1977;59(3):412–3.

9. Bonatz E, Kramer TD, Masear VR. Rupture of the extensor pollicis longus tendon. Am J Orthop 1996; 25(2):118–22.

10. Paley D, McMurtry RY, Murray JF. Dorsal dislocation of the ulnar styloid and extensor carpi ulnaris tendon into the distal radioulnar joint: the empty sulcus sign. J Hand Surg Am 1987;12:1029–32.

11. DiMatteo L, Wolf JM. Flexor carpi radialis tendon rupture as a complication of a closed distal radius fracture: a case report. J Hand Surg Am 2007; 32(6):818–20.

12. Geissler WB, Freeland AE, Savoie FH, et al. Intracarpal soft-tissue lesions associated with an intra-articular fracture of the distal end of the radius. J Bone Joint Surg Am 1996;78:357–65.

13. Roberts RS, Bennett JD, Roth JH, et al. Arthroscopic diagnosis of intra-articular soft tissue injuries associated with distal radial fractures. J Hand Surg Am 1997;22:772–6.

14. Lindau T, Arner M, Hagberg L. Intraarticular lesions in distal fractures of the radius in young adults: a descriptive arthroscopic study in 50 patients. J Hand Surg Br 1997;22:638–43.

15. Bombaci H, Polat A, Deniz G, et al. The value of plain X-ray in predicting TFCC injury after distal radial fractures. J Hand Surg Eur 2008;33:322–6.

16. May MM, Lawton JN, Blazar PE. Ulnar styloid fractures associated with distal radius fractures: incidence and implications for distal radioulnar joint instability. J Hand Surg Am 2002;27:965–71.

17. Fujitani R, Omokawa S, Akahane M, et al. Predictors of distal radioulnar joint instability in distal radial fractures. J Hand Surg Am 2011;36:1919–25.

18. Palmer AK. Triangular fibrocartilage complex lesions: a classification. J Hand Surg Am 1989;14:594–606.

19. Geissler WB, Fernandez DL, Lamey DM. Distal radioulnar joint injuries associated with fractures of the distal radius. Clin Orthop Relat Res 1996;327: 135–46.

20. Lindau T, Aldercruetz C, Aspenberg P. Peripheral tears of the triangular fibrocartilage complex cause distal radioulnar joint instability after distal radius fractures. J Hand Surg Am 2000;25:464–8.

21. Lindau T, Hagberg H, Aldercreutz C, et al. Distal radioulnar instability is an independent worsening factor in distal radius fractures. Clin Orthop Relat Res 2000;376:229–35.

22. Mikic ZD. Treatment of acute injuries of the triangular fibrocartilage complex associated with distal radioulnar joint instability. J Hand Surg Am 1995;20:319–23.

23. Ruch DS, Yang CC, Paterson Smith B. Results of acute arthroscopically repaired triangular fibrocartilage complex injuries associated with intra-articular distal radius fractures. Arthroscopy 2003;19:511–6.

24. Berger RA. The gross and histologic anatomy of the scapholunate interosseous ligament. J Hand Surg Am 1996;21:170–8.

25. Berger RA, Imeada T, Berglund L, et al. Constraint and material properties of the subregions of the scapholunate interosseous ligament. J Hand Surg Am 1999;24:953–62.

26. Belsole RJ. Radiography of the wrist. Clin Orthop Relat Res 1986;202:50–6.

27. Cautilli GP, Wehbe MA. Scapho-lunate distance and cortical ring sign. J Hand Surg Am 1991;16:501–3.

28. Kindynis P, Resnick D, Kang HS, et al. Demonstration of the scapholunate space with radiography. Radiology 1990;175:278–80.

29. Linscheid RL, Dobyns JH, Beaubout JW, et al. Traumatic instability of the wrist: diagnosis, classification, and pathomechanics. J Bone Joint Surg Am 1972; 54:1612–32.

30. Moneim MS. The tangential posteroanterior radiograph to demonstrate scapholunate dissociation. J Bone Joint Surg Am 1981;63:1324–6.

31. Kwon BC, Baek GH. Fluoroscopic diagnosis of scapholunate interosseous ligament injuries in distal radius fractures. Clin Orthop Relat Res 2008;466: 969–76.

32. Kwon BC, Choi SJ, Song SY, et al. Modified carpal stretch test as a screening tool for detection of scapholunate interosseous ligament injuries associated with distal radial fractures. J Bone Joint Surg Am 2011;93:855–62.

33. Peh WC, Gilula LA. Normal disruption of carpal arcs. J Hand Surg Am 1996;21:581–6.

34. Forward DP, Lindau TR, Melsom DS. Intercarpal ligament injuries associated with fractures of the distal part of the radius. J Bone Joint Surg Am 2007;89: 2334–40.

35. Tang JB, Shi D, Gu YQ, et al. Can cast immobilization successfully treat scapholunate dissociation associated with distal radius fractures? J Hand Surg Am 1996;21:583–90.

36. Varitimidis SE, Basdekis GK, Dailiana H, et al. Treatment of intra-articular fractures of the distal radius: fluoroscopic or arthroscopic reduction? J Bone Joint Surg Br 2008;90:778–85.

37. Tang P, Swart E, Ding A. Do wrist ligament injuries affect outcomes in operative distal radius fractures? Clinical Paper Session 10: Wrist Injuries. Las Vegas (NV): ASSH, September 10, 2011;9: 13–9:18am.

38. Omokawa S, Fujitani R, Inada Y. Dorsal radiocarpal ligament capsulodesis for chronic dynamic lunotriquetral instability. J Hand Surg Am 2009;34:237–43.

39. Shin AY, Weinstein LP, Berger RA, et al. Treatment of isolated injuries of the lunotriquetral ligament. A comparison of arthrodesis, ligament reconstruction, and ligament repair. J Bone Joint Surg Br 2001;83: 1023–8.

40. Garcia-Elias M. Dorsal fractures of the triquetrum—avulsion or compression fractures. J Hand Surg Am 1987;12:266–8.

41. Vance RM, Gelberman RH. Acute ulnar neuropathy with fractures at the wrist. J Bone Joint Surg Am 1978;60:962–5.

42. Arora R, Lutz M, Hennerbichler A, et al. Complications following internal fixation of unstable distal radius fracture with a palmar locking-plate. J Orthop Trauma 2007;21(5):316–22.

43. Dyer G, Lozano-Calderon S, Gannon C, et al. Predictors of acute carpal tunnel syndrome associated with fractures of the distal radius. J Hand Surg 2008;33(8):1309–13.

44. Gelberman RH, Szabo RM, Mortensen WW. Carpal tunnel pressures and wrist position in patients with Colles' fractures. J Trauma 1984;24(8):747–9.

45. Bauman TD, Gelberman RH, Mubarak SJ, et al. The acute carpal tunnel syndrome. Clin Orthop Relat Res 1981;156:151–6.

46. Soong M, Ring D. Ulnar nerve palsy associated with fracture of the distal radius. J Orthop Trauma 2007; 21(2):113–6.

47. Pazart F, Stindel E, Le Nen D. Fracture of the distal part of the radius associated with severed ulnar nerve. Chir Main 1999;18:197–201.

48. Clarke AC, Spencer RF. Ulnar nerve palsy following fractures of the distal radius: clinical anatomical studies. J Hand Surg Br 1991;16:438–40.

49. Poppi M, Padovani R, Martinelli P, et al. Fracture of the distal radius with ulnar nerve palsy. J Trauma 1978;18:278–9.

50. Sohal JK, Chia B, Catalano LW. Dorsal displacement of the ulnar nerve after a displaced distal radius fracture: a case report. J Hand Surg Am 2009;34: 432–5.

51. Fernandez DL. Irreducible radiocarpal fracture-dislocation and radioulnar dissociation with entrapment of the ulnar nerve, artery, and flexor profundus II-V—a case report. J Hand Surg Am 1981;6:456–61.

52. Dao KD, Venn-Watson E, Shin AY. Radial artery pseudoaneurysm complication from use of AO/ASIF volar distal radius plate: a case report. J Hand Surg Am 2001;26:448–53.

53. De Witte PB, Lozano-Calderon S, Harness N, et al. Acute vascular injury associated with fracture of the distal radius: a report of 6 cases. J Orthop Trauma 2008;22(9):611–4.

54. Kalyani BS, Fisher BE, Roberts CS, et al. Compartment syndrome of the forearm: a systematic review. J Hand Surg Am 2011;36:535–43.

55. DiFelice A Jr, Seiler JG 3rd, Whitesides TE Jr. The compartments of the hand: an anatomic study. J Hand Surg 1998;23A:682–6.

56. Leversedge FJ, Moore TJ, Peterson BC, et al. Compartment syndrome of the upper extremity—current concepts. J Hand Surg Am 2011;36:544–60.

57. Sotereanos DG, McCarthy DM, Towers JD, et al. The pronator quadratus: a distinct forearm space? J Hand Surg Am 1995;20:496–9.

58. Atkins RM, Duckworth T, Kanis JA. Features of algodystrophy after Colles' fracture. J Hand Surg 1989; 14B:161–4.

59. Zollinger PE, Tuinebreijer WE, Kreis RW, et al. Effect of vitamin C on reflex sympathetic dystrophy in wrist fracture trial. Lancet 1999;354:2025–8.

60. Zollinger PE, Tuinbreijer WE, Breederveld RS, et al. Can vitamin C prevent complex regional pain syndrome in patients with wrist fractures? A randomized, controlled multicenter dose-response study. J Bone Joint Surg Am 2007;89:1424–31.

Recovery After Fracture of the Distal Radius

Arjan G.J. Bot, MD[a], David C. Ring, MD, PhD[b],*

KEYWORDS

- Recovery • Distal radius fracture • Coaching • Exercises

DISABILITY AND IMPAIRMENT

Recovery from a fracture of the distal radius must address both impairment and disability. Impairment is measurable objective pathophysiology, such as limited motion or sensation. Disability, on the other hand, is the idea that one is incapable of an action. Patients with distal radius fractures often experience disability as inability to trust or depend on the hand. "It probably feels like you're not going to be able to rely on your hand the way you need to" is a statement that identifies the goal while communicating empathy regarding how difficult and counterintuitive recovery can be for the patient. During recovery from a fracture of the distal radius, as with most illnesses, symptom intensity and disability are determined more by mindset and circumstances than by pathophysiology or impairment.[1–4]

Impairment

Patients should expect slight to moderate impairment of motion after a fracture of the distal radius. Diaz-Garcia and colleagues'[5] review of published studies reported a mean arc of wrist flexion and extension of 116° to 133° and forearm rotation of 140° to 175° after recovery from a fracture of the distal radius in older patients, regardless of the treatment method. Six months after a conservatively treated distal radius fracture, the mean arc of flexion and extension and the forearm rotation were known to be 75% to 97% and 87% to 97%, respectively, compared with the uninjured side.[6–10] Six months after operative treatment the numbers were similar: mean flexion, 67% to 88%; extension, 72% to 93%; supination, 78% to 100%; and pronation, 87% to 100%.[6,8,11–17] Grip strength, which is partly volitional and therefore not strictly an objective impairment, averaged 53% to 86% after operative treatment[6–10] and 43% to 92% after nonoperative treatment, compared with the uninjured side 6 months after injury.[6,8,11–17]

Disability

Patients may have more influence over disability than impairment after fracture of the distal radius. In a study with 57 patients recovering from a wrist fracture and 13 from an ankle fracture, fear and catastrophic thinking were associated with pain intensity and recovery of muscle strength.[18] In another study of wrist, ankle, and hip fractures, pain intensity at baseline and postinjury anxiety were the most important predictors of pain intensity after the fracture.[2] Souer and colleagues[4] noted that at an average of 22 months after volar plate fixation, 71% of the variability in DASH scores (Disabilities of the Arm, Shoulder and Hand) was

Disclosures: (A.G.J.B.) Stichting Anna Fonds, VSBfonds, Prins Bernhard Cultuurfonds/Banning-de Jong Fonds. (D.C.R.) Study-specific grants: Skeletal Dynamics (pending); Consultant: Wright Medical, Skeletal Dynamics, Biomet; Honoraria: AO North America, AO International; Royalties received: Wright Medical; Royalties contracted: Biomet, Skeletal Dynamics; Stock options: Illuminos; Funding for Hand Surgery Fellowship: AO North America.

[a] Orthopaedic Hand and Upper Extremity Service, Massachusetts General Hospital, 55 Fruit Street, Boston, MA 02114, USA
[b] Orthopaedic Hand and Upper Extremity Service, Yawkey Center, Massachusetts General Hospital, Harvard Medical School, Suite 2100, 55 Fruit Street, Boston, MA 02114, USA
* Corresponding author.
E-mail address: dring@partners.org

Hand Clin 28 (2012) 235–243
doi:10.1016/j.hcl.2012.03.006

hand.theclinics.com

determined by pain and arc of forearm rotation, with 65% of this variability resulting from pain alone.

In a study of 120 patients recovering from a fracture of the distal radius, MacDermid and colleagues[3] found that 25% of the variation in the Patient-Related Wrist Evaluation (PRWE) score 6 months after injury was accounted for by workers compensation, education, and prereduction radial shortening, whereas 25% was accounted for by the arc of wrist flexion and extension, with the remaining 50% unaccounted for.

Grip strength is mainly influenced by depression, pain, and motivation.[19–24] Karnezis and Fragkiadakis found that 43% of the variation in PRWE 2 years after nonoperative treatment of a fracture of the distal radius was determined by grip strength, but motion was not significantly affected.[25] A study of 20 patients found that grip strength correlated with all tasks in the Jebsen Hand Test, but motion correlated only with lifting large objects.[26]

Chung and colleagues[1] assessed 49 patients 1 year after a distal radius fracture and found that only age and income were associated with disability, whereas radiographic outcomes had no association with disability. In a separate study, Chung and colleagues[17] found no significant differences in disability between younger and older patients 1 year after volar plate fixation of the distal radius using the Michigan Hand Questionnaire (MHQ). However, income and articular incongruities, but not motion, were found to be significant predictors of the MHQ in younger patients.[17]

In a study of 125 patients, Chung and Haas[27] plotted receiver operating characteristic (ROC) curves and identified the following thresholds for patient satisfaction: 65% of grip strength (sensitivity of 0.89, specificity of 0.63), 87% of pinch strength (sensitivity of 0.60, specificity of 0.86), and 95% of the arc of wrist flexion and extension (sensitivity of 0.47, specificity of 0.88).

Disproportionate Pain and Disability

Finger stiffness is one of the most common sequelae following a fracture of the distal radius. Patients with stiff fingers usually have greater pain intensity and disability than would normally be expected. This disproportionate pain and disability has many labels, some of which are cultural (eg, algodystrophy in Britain) and others historical (eg, causalgia, reflex sympathetic dystrophy). The International Association for the Study of Pain currently favors the label complex regional pain syndrome (CRPS) because implication of the sympathetic nervous system contributed to overutilization of costly and ineffective stellate ganglion blocks and other treatments.[28,29] Two Cochrane

reviews on spinal cord stimulation and local anesthetic sympathetic blockade in the treatment of CRPS I concluded that there is not enough evidence to support the use of either treatment.[29,30] The diagnostic criteria currently available for CRPS are subjective and imprecise. The lack of a plausible explanation for the signs and symptoms associated with CRPS is one of the diagnostic criteria for this condition. Therefore, it can be argued that the diagnosis of CRPS is never appropriate after a fracture of the distal radius. A fracture of the distal radius is associated with ecchymosis and swelling in the hand that leads to stiffness and pain if the patient is too protective to exercise the hand and use it for daily activities.

The reported prevalence of disproportionate pain and disability among patients recovering from a fracture of the distal radius varies widely, between 1% and 37% in published series,[31–37] perhaps in part because it is poorly defined, subjective, and unverifiable. Along these lines, it is difficult to interpret the trials suggesting that vitamin C limits the occurrence of CRPS, given that the diagnosis is subjective and variably defined, and the only published trials were performed by advocates of vitamin C.[36,38] A recent trial by McQueen and colleagues[39] showed no benefit of vitamin C on patients with CRPS.

In general, physicians ascribe disproportionate pain and disability to a poorly understood pathophysiologic process currently labeled CRPS, whereas psychologists emphasize the importance of psychological factors (catastrophic thinking in particular) and illness behavior (eg, pain avoidance).[28] Use of the term CRPS places emphasis on an elusive and possibly mythical pathophysiologic process; leads to medical and surgical treatments that, to date, are at best wishful thinking and at worst harmful; and distracts the patient and the provider from effective treatments such as cognitive behavior therapy.[28] In our opinion, until we have a better understanding of this illness, it should be referred to descriptively as disproportionate pain and disability, rather than using specific biomedical terms, and should be treated with an evidence-based approach based on cognitive behavior therapy.

TECHNIQUES FOR REDUCING IMPAIRMENT
Edema

The most important preventive measure a patient can use to reduce swelling is to use the hand as normally as possible. Using the hand for light daily tasks (writing, typing, washing) is safe and should be encouraged. Patients often ask "should I squeeze a ball," which we believe reflects the tendency to feel passive about recovery ("the ball will heal my hand"). We counter with, "I want you to squeeze your hand into a tight ball, over and over again, as much as you can." We demonstrate the blanching that occurs when the hand is squeezed into a tight fist and use the analogy of squeezing out a sponge. The same is true for opening the hand into rigid extension, which is also encouraged: "tight open, tight fist." Elevation is also useful but difficult to maintain if the hand is used for daily tasks. The role of passive treatments such as massage, wrapping, or using gloves[40,41] is debatable, and passive approaches should be used with caution to optimize patients' active role in their own recovery (self-efficacy).

Tessman and Schmidt[42] found better absolute reduction in swelling measured with volume displacement with gloves compared with elastic bandages in a very small randomized trial. Härén and colleagues[43] compared manual lymph drainage as described by Vodder (12 patients) with usual exercises (14 patients) after fracture of the distal radius treated with an external fixator. The investigators documented significantly less edema measured volumetrically shortly after removal of the fixator but no differences at later time points. A randomized trial comparing modified manual edema mobilization with the standard technique in 30 patients who underwent plating, external fixation, or cast fixation of the distal radius showed no differences in edema, pain, or motion.[44]

Motion

Finger and forearm motion exercises should be initiated immediately after injury or treatment, with finger motion taking priority. The easiest finger exercise for patients to understand is a composite fist with self-assist using the other hand, which also addresses edema. There is value to keeping it simple. Using an uninjured hand to push and stretch an injured hand can be counterintuitive and typically feels unsafe to start, because pain can trigger protection and preparation for the worst (catastrophic thinking). It is important to normalize this and show empathy by discussing this normal human response: "It probably feels like the wrong thing to do"; "Patients often tell me it feels like they will pop the sutures or dislodge the plate. Is that how it feels"; "Exercises after fracture or surgery are counterintuitive." Providers should emphasize that patients need to get the arm moving themselves to limit passive attitudes toward recovery.

The key is to help patients change from a "protective" to that of a "healthy stretch" mindset, which is not an easy task to accomplish.

Regularly performing finger and forearm exercises enables the patients to experience a return of motion to the hand, making the process feel more natural and allowing the patients to make the transition themselves. It is important for the provider to empathize, teach, and be patient, while avoiding words or actions that might reinforce a protective mindset. For instance, the common phrases "work to pain, but not beyond" or "don't over do it" are unhelpful for patients who are struggling to control their catastrophic thinking. The phrase "no pain, no gain" is also not helpful because it implies that the patient is "a wimp" or should be ashamed, when in fact their protectiveness is entirely normal and expected.

Analogies can help make complex concepts understandable and, like stories, often communicate counterintuitive concepts more effectively. The "smoke alarm in the kitchen" analogy is useful to help normalize a protective response to pain. The pain is like the smoke or grease created during cooking; it sets the alarm off, but it is not a fire. Most fire alarms while cooking in the kitchen are false alarms, but this does not mean that the alarm is broken. It is actually working perfectly and just as it is designed. Patients need to realize that humans are programmed and evolved to respond protectively to pain and to prepare for the worst, so we should not be surprised or ashamed to feel that painful exercises are the wrong thing to do and might cause harm.

Patients find it very convincing that the pain alarm is a true alarm. Human intelligence collects all the things that prove our theory (rationalization, pattern forming) while tending to disregard the evidence that our theory may be incorrect. That is how the magician fools us, through our intelligence and our strengths, not through the weaknesses of our brain. Just like it may seem very convincing that the lady in the box is sawed in half, it can seem convincing that stretching exercises will cause harm—again, given the way our brain works that is to be expected. This phenomenon is nothing to be ashamed of, but it is necessary to be prepared for it. Patients will ask, "Should I ignore the pain?" and the answer would be, "No. You have to be prepared for how the pain will make you feel protective and prepare for the worst, and how it will convince you that the exercises are not a good idea." Psychologists call this act of preparation mindfulness. Patients need to be very mindful of how their body works and be prepared for the counterintuitive nature of the recovery process. They should be prepared for the alarm and, just as in the kitchen, expect it to nearly always be a false alarm. They should be prepared to manage the alarm (open the window or disconnect the alarm) and keep stretching (keep cooking).

As stated earlier, the goal is to get into a healthy stretch mindset. We know that when we stretch or do yoga the discomfort we feel is healthy. We know that we are not stretching properly until we feel the discomfort. Once patients "filter" the alarm as we do with workouts, sports, and yoga, they will be able to do much more effective stretches and will feel they are healthy. This change in mindset takes time, and each patient must reach this mindset in his or her own way and at his or her own pace. The health provider should understand how long this process can take (months) and encourage the patient that everything will work out—there is no rush.

With nonbridging external fixators and internal plate and screw fixation, it is safe to initiate wrist flexion and extension exercises as soon as possible; however, when patients are in pain, wrist motion exercises are particularly counterintuitive early on. There is now very good evidence that final wrist motion does not depend on early initiation of wrist stretches.

Lozano-Calderon and colleagues,[12] in a randomized trial including 60 patients, compared the initiation of wrist stretches 2 weeks after volar plate fixation with initiation after 6 weeks. They found no differences in pain, Gartland and Werley score, Mayo Wrist score, and range of motion 3 and 6 months after the fracture.[12] Two studies also documented similar findings in patients treated with percutaneous pinning.[45,46]

McQueen[13] compared nonbridging fixators with external fixators in a randomized trial with 60 patients. After 1 year, flexion and grip strength were significantly better in the nonbridging group (87% vs 69% of the uninjured side) but extension was not, findings consistent with the greater residual dorsal angulation of the fracture in the bridging fixator group.[13] Atroshi and colleagues[47] randomized 38 patients to bridging or nonbridging external fixation and found no differences in pain, DASH, grip strength, or range of motion. Krishnan and colleagues[48] randomized 60 patients to bridging or nonbridging external fixation and found no differences in grip strength and pain, but the group treated with bridging external fixation had more flexion (60° vs 50°) and radial deviation. McQueen and colleagues,[8] in a study including 120 patients, compared open reduction internal fixation, casting, early motion after external fixator, and late motion after treatment with external fixation and found no significant differences in outcome. Jenkins and colleagues[49] randomized 106 adults to bridging or nonbridging external fixator and noted that the patients in the nonbridging group had more grip strength but motion comparable to that in patients in the bridging group. Franck and colleagues[50] randomized 40 patients treated with Kirschner wires (K-wires) to nonbridging external fixators and found significantly better ulnar deviation in the external fixation group but no other differences in outcome measures.

Wilcke and colleagues[16] randomized 63 patients to volar plating or bridging external fixation. After a year, disability was the same, but the patients in the plating group had significantly better (but probably not clinically relevant) extension (94% vs 85% of the uninjured side), supination (99% vs 89%), and pronation (99% vs 92%).[16]

Davis and Buchanan[51] compared early motion with late motion in patients treated with a cast. After 1 week of treatment with a cast, 55 patients were randomized to 3 weeks additional casting or tubigrip.[51] The patients in the tubigrip group had better Gartland and Werley score, but all other outcome measures were comparable.[51] Two other similar studies had the same findings.[10,52] Dias and colleagues[53] randomized 97 patients with nondisplaced fractures to conventional casting for 5 weeks or crepe bandage and 90 patients with displaced fractures to casting or modified casting (where a strap could be loosened volarly so motion was possible). For the patients in the nondisplaced group, outcomes were comparable, but the patients with displaced fractures treated with a modified cast had more grip strength (76% vs 58%) than the patients with a conventional cast.[53] Abbaszadegan and colleagues[54] randomized 68 patients to 4 weeks of plaster cast or elastic bandage and found better grip strength (78%–94%), arc of wrist flexion and extension (89% vs 98%), and radial and ulnar deviation in the group treated with a bandage.

We prefer to see full finger and forearm motion before we initiate wrist flexion and extension exercises. Patients and therapists often emphasize strengthening exercises, but strength returns with normal use, and strengthening exercises should not be initiated until motion is well established to avoid distracting the patients from the more important stretching exercises. Scar massage might help reduce adhesions of the skin to the tendons.[55] There is no evidence that other scar treatments are effective. When patients are not gaining satisfactory function, dynamic or progressive splinting is sometimes considered,[40,56] although these are passive treatments and there is no evidence that they are more effective than active self-assisted stretching. We prefer to help patients get comfortable with exercises in which they use objects such as a tabletop to create a fulcrum to obtain a better stretch of the wrist capsule.

Formal Physical or Occupational Therapy

It is not infrequent for a patient with a fracture of the distal radius to inquire, "will I need therapy?" at the first office visit. Again, we think this reflects the tendency of many patients to take a passive role in their recovery. Our answer is, "You will need to do lots of stretching exercises to get yourself recovered." We emphasize that our role and that of a therapist is teaching, coaching, and camaraderie.

In a retrospective study, Oskarsson and colleagues[57] documented that the 40 patients who requested physiotherapy had less motion and weaker grip 35 weeks after fracture than the 70 patients who did not. Lyngcoln and colleagues[58] found that adherence to the prescribed regimen of physiotherapy correlated with less pain but not greater motion. Taylor and Bennell concluded that there were no differences in range of motion when 30 patients were randomized to passive mobilization or to sham passive mobilization (soft tissue massage) in addition to normal treatment.[59,60]

Souer and colleagues[15] randomized 46 patients to formal occupational therapy and 48 to independent exercises after volar plating. After 6 months, the group randomized to independent exercises had better motion, although the differences were small. Among a group treated with volar plating, Krischak and colleagues[61] randomized 23 patients to home exercises and 23 to formal physiotherapy. The patients assigned to home exercises had better grip strength and motion and less disability than the patients randomized to formal therapy. Another study found no differences between exercises/advice and formal physiotherapy in 42 patients treated with cast or K wires.[7] In a group treated with K wires or a cast, Kay and colleagues[62] randomized 28 patients to formal physiotherapy and 28 to independent exercises. After 6 weeks, the group treated with physiotherapy had less pain, but all other outcomes were comparable with outcomes in the other group.[62] Another study by Kay and colleagues[63] found that patients randomized to passive mobilization techniques in addition to physiotherapy and home exercises had slightly more flexion but no differences in motion, pain, or grip strength.

Among patients treated nonoperatively, Christensen and colleagues[64] found no differences between exercise instructions alone and exercise instructions and formal occupational therapy. In a very small, randomized trial (9 patients per group), Watt and colleagues[65] found formal physiotherapy to be better than independent exercises in patients treated with a cast. Pasila and colleagues[66] found no differences between patients rehabilitating with home exercises and those with physiotherapy. Wakefield and McQueen[9] randomized 96 older patients (87 women; mean age, 72 years) to formal physiotherapy or home exercises. Among the 66 patients who were analyzed, the patients randomized to physiotherapy had more range of wrist motion; all other results were comparable.[9] Gronlund and colleagues compared 17 patients undergoing early occupational therapy with 23 patients with usual care and found no difference in results at 3 months.[59,67] Bache and colleagues, in an older group of 98 patients (mean age of 69 years), compared formal physiotherapy with home exercises and found that after 12 weeks, supination was better in the home exercises group, but other motions, pain, and grip strength were all comparable.[59,68]

TECHNIQUES FOR REDUCING DISABILITY

Studies have shown that depressive symptoms and posttraumatic stress disorder are common after orthopedic trauma.[69,70] In patients recovering from a fracture of the distal radius, Gong and colleagues[71] found that symptoms of depression correlated with pain and disability but not operative or nonoperative treatment.

Coping strategies, symptoms of depression, catastrophic thinking, heightened illness concern, cultural factors, circumstantial sources of stress, and social factors (such as secondary gain) are all very responsive to treatment with techniques based on cognitive behavioral therapy.[72] Cognitive behavioral therapy in its simplest form implies learning to distinguish thought from fact. The cognitive errors and pain-avoidant behavior to which humans are prone during injury or illness can become fixed or habitual, particularly among patients accustomed to trusting their gut feelings.

Occupational and physical therapists have some formal training in psychology and can develop these aspects of their expertise. All health providers need to work on effective communication skills, empathy in particular, and avoid using words and concepts that reinforce catastrophic thinking. In the future, psychologists, or at least cognitive and behavioral treatments, will likely be part of the treatment regimen for patients recovering from fractures of the distal radius. For now, health care providers should learn from experts about the cognitive and emotional aspects of human illness behavior and try to incorporate the treatment strategies that are firmly based on evidence.

For example, patients with disproportionate pain and disability tend to present their hand as if it is separate from them, almost as if they brought it in to drop off for repair and pick up later. This dissociation and passivity are part of the normal human protective response to injury and pain, just taken a bit too far. Mirror therapy is a behavioral treatment that helps patients reincorporate their hand and arm as an integral part of themselves, which gets them back on track for recovery.[73-78]

Perhaps the most common cognitive error (misconception) in a hand surgeon's office is, "these fingers won't bend until the swelling is gone." With enough empathy and coaching, a physician can get the patient to make a full fist within a few minutes. Seeing that the patient's gut feeling was inaccurate can be empowering, but it can also be very uncomfortable, so this should not be attempted until the physician is sure the patient is ready. Intuitive people do not particularly like magic shows, it is difficult for an intuitive person to experience such a divide between their thoughts (the woman is sawed in half) and the fact that it is just sleight of hand when they are used to trusting their thoughts. Physicians need to be patient and see the patient every week or so initially if necessary (in practice this is rarely necessary but can be helpful when patients find exercises particularly counterintuitive).

We have noticed that patients tend to "turn the corner" in achieving the "healthy stretch" mindset as they begin to use the hand for anything that is important to them. At this stage, patients are finally convinced that they will recover and that the pain alarm is a false alarm. It can be very beneficial to encourage patients to try things that are important to them. Advise them that "it will definitely hurt, but it is definitely safe." Just plant that seed without trying to convince them, and then give them a week or two to try to get up the courage to go against their gut feeling.

SUMMARY

Disability after a distal radius fracture is determined as much or more by mindset and circumstances than by pathophysiology or impairment. Active self-assisted exercises are the most important part of the recovery process, and the health care providers' role is primarily empathy and coaching patients through the normal protective response to pain and injury. Our job is to guide patients toward the healthy stretch mindset, using empathy and encouraging them to return to activities that are important to them. The stretches themselves are straightforward, but they will not be done well until the patient is ready to fully participate in the recovery process.

REFERENCES

1. Chung KC, Kotsis SV, Kim HM. Predictors of functional outcomes after surgical treatment of distal radius fractures. J Hand Surg Am 2007;32(1):76–83.
2. Jelicic M, Kempen GI. Do psychological factors influence pain following a fracture of the extremities? Injury 1999;30(5):323–5.
3. MacDermid JC, Donner A, Richards RS, et al. Patient versus injury factors as predictors of pain and disability six months after a distal radius fracture. J Clin Epidemiol 2002;55(9):849–54.
4. Souer JS, Lozano-Calderon SA, Ring D. Predictors of wrist function and health status after operative treatment of fractures of the distal radius. J Hand Surg Am 2008;33(2):157–63.
5. Diaz-Garcia RJ, Oda T, Shauver MJ, et al. A systematic review of outcomes and complications of treating unstable distal radius fractures in the elderly. J Hand Surg Am 2011;36(5):824–835.e2.
6. Egol KA, Walsh M, Romo-Cardoso S, et al. Distal radial fractures in the elderly: operative compared with nonoperative treatment. J Bone Joint Surg Am 2010;92(9):1851–7.
7. Maciel JS, Taylor NF, McIlveen C. A randomised clinical trial of activity-focussed physiotherapy on patients with distal radius fractures. Arch Orthop Trauma Surg 2005;125(8):515–20.
8. McQueen MM, Hajducka C, Court-Brown CM. Redisplaced unstable fractures of the distal radius: a prospective randomised comparison of four methods of treatment. J Bone Joint Surg Br 1996;78(3):404–9.
9. Wakefield AE, McQueen MM. The role of physiotherapy and clinical predictors of outcome after fracture of the distal radius. J Bone Joint Surg Br 2000;82(7):972–6.
10. Millett PJ, Rushton N. Early mobilization in the treatment of Colles' fracture: a 3 year prospective study. Injury 1995;26(10):671–5.
11. Hove LM, Krukhaug Y, Revheim K, et al. Dynamic compared with static external fixation of unstable fractures of the distal part of the radius: a prospective, randomized multicenter study. J Bone Joint Surg Am 2010;92(8):1687–96.
12. Lozano-Calderon SA, Souer S, Mudgal C, et al. Wrist mobilization following volar plate fixation of fractures of the distal part of the radius. J Bone Joint Surg Am 2008;90(6):1297–304.
13. McQueen MM. Redisplaced unstable fractures of the distal radius. A randomised, prospective study of bridging versus non-bridging external fixation. J Bone Joint Surg Br 1998;80(4):665–9.
14. Sommerkamp TG, Seeman M, Silliman J, et al. Dynamic external fixation of unstable fractures of the distal part of the radius. A prospective, randomized comparison with static external fixation. J Bone Joint Surg Am 1994;76(8):1149–61.

15. Souer JS, Buijze G, Ring D. A prospective randomized controlled trial comparing occupational therapy with independent exercises after volar plate fixation of a fracture of the distal part of the radius. J Bone Joint Surg Am 2011;93(19):1761–6.

16. Wilcke MK, Abbaszadegan H, Adolphson PY. Patient-perceived outcome after displaced distal radius fractures. A comparison between radiological parameters, objective physical variables, and the DASH score. J Hand Ther 2007;20(4):290–8 [quiz: 9].

17. Chung KC, Squitieri L, Kim HM. Comparative outcomes study using the volar locking plating system for distal radius fractures in both young adults and adults older than 60 years. J Hand Surg Am 2008;33(6):809–19.

18. Linton SJ, Buer N, Samuelsson L, et al. Pain-related fear, catastrophizing and pain in the recovery from a fracture. Scand J Pain 2010;1(1):38–42.

19. van Milligen BA, Lamers F, de Hoop GT, et al. Objective physical functioning in patients with depressive and/or anxiety disorders. J Affect Disord 2011; 131(1–3):193–9.

20. van Lier AM, Payette H. Determinants of handgrip strength in free-living elderly at risk of malnutrition. Disabil Rehabil 2003;25(20):1181–6.

21. Rantanen T, Penninx BW, Masaki K, et al. Depressed mood and body mass index as predictors of muscle strength decline in old men. J Am Geriatr Soc 2000; 48(6):613–7.

22. Phillips HJ, Biland J, Costa R, et al. Five-position grip strength measures in individuals with clinical depression. J Orthop Sports Phys Ther 2011;41(3):149–54.

23. Payette H, Hanusaik N, Boutier V, et al. Muscle strength and functional mobility in relation to lean body mass in free-living frail elderly women. Eur J Clin Nutr 1998;52(1):45–53.

24. Morrey BF, Adams RA. Semiconstrained arthroplasty for the treatment of rheumatoid arthritis of the elbow. J Bone Joint Surg Am 1992;74A:479–90.

25. Karnezis IA, Fragkiadakis EG. Association between objective clinical variables and patient-rated disability of the wrist. J Bone Joint Surg Br 2002; 84(7):967–70.

26. Tremayne A, Taylor N, McBurney H, et al. Correlation of impairment and activity limitation after wrist fracture. Physiother Res Int 2002;7(2):90–9.

27. Chung KC, Haas A. Relationship between patient satisfaction and objective functional outcome after surgical treatment for distal radius fractures. J Hand Ther 2009;22(4):302–7.

28. Ring D, Barth R, Barsky A. Evidence-based medicine: disproportionate pain and disability. J Hand Surg Am 2010;35(8):1345–7.

29. Cepeda MS, Carr DB, Lau J. Local anesthetic sympathetic blockade for complex regional pain syndrome. Cochrane Database Syst Rev 2005;4: CD004598.

30. Mailis-Gagnon A, Furlan AD, Sandoval JA, et al. Spinal cord stimulation for chronic pain. Cochrane Database Syst Rev 2004;3:CD003783.

31. Atkins RM, Duckworth T, Kanis JA. Algodystrophy following Colles' fracture. J Hand Surg Br 1989; 14(2):161–4.

32. Atkins RM, Duckworth T, Kanis JA. Features of algodystrophy after Colles' fracture. J Bone Joint Surg Br 1990;72(1):105–10.

33. Dijkstra PU, Groothoff JW, ten Duis HJ, et al. Incidence of complex regional pain syndrome type I after fractures of the distal radius. Eur J Pain 2003;7(5):457–62.

34. Field J, Warwick D, Bannister GC. Features of algodystrophy ten years after Colles' fracture. J Hand Surg Br 1992;17(3):318–20.

35. McKay SD, MacDermid JC, Roth JH, et al. Assessment of complications of distal radius fractures and development of a complication checklist. J Hand Surg Am 2001;26(5):916–22.

36. Zollinger PE, Tuinebreijer WE, Breederveld RS, et al. Can vitamin C prevent complex regional pain syndrome in patients with wrist fractures? A randomized, controlled, multicenter dose-response study. J Bone Joint Surg Am 2007;89(7):1424–31.

37. Bickerstaff DR, Kanis JA. Algodystrophy: an underrecognized complication of minor trauma. Br J Rheumatol 1994;33(3):240–8.

38. Zollinger PE, Tuinebreijer WE, Kreis RW, et al. Effect of vitamin C on frequency of reflex sympathetic dystrophy in wrist fractures: a randomised trial. Lancet 1999;354(9195):2025–8.

39. McQueen MM, Court-Brown CM, Ralston S. Do antioxidants modulate the outcome of fractures? A prospective randomized controlled trial [abstract]. J Hand Surg 2011;36E(Suppl 1):S112.

40. MacDermid JC. Hand therapy management of intra-articular fractures with open reduction and pi plate fixation: a therapist's perspective. Tech Hand Up Extrem Surg 2004;8(4):219–23.

41. Michlovitz SL, LaStayo PC, Alzner S, et al. Distal radius fractures: therapy practice patterns. J Hand Ther 2001;14(4):249–57.

42. Tessmann UJ, Schmidt J. New aspects in rehabilitation after distal radius fractures. Akt Traumatol 2006; 36(3):113–7.

43. Härén K, Backman C, Wiberg M. Effect of manual lymph drainage as described by Vodder on oedema of the hand after fracture of the distal radius: a prospective clinical study. Scand J Plast Reconstr Surg Hand Surg 2000;34(4):367–72.

44. Knygsand-Roenhoej K, Maribo T. A randomized clinical controlled study comparing the effect of modified manual edema mobilization treatment with traditional edema technique in patients with a fracture of the distal radius. J Hand Ther 2011;24(3):184–93 [quiz: 94].

45. Allain J, le Guilloux P, Le Mouel S, et al. Transstyloid fixation of fractures of the distal radius. A

prospective randomized comparison between 6- and 1-week postoperative immobilization in 60 fractures. Acta Orthop Scand 1999;70(2):119–23.

46. Milliez PY, Dallaserra M, Defives T, et al. Effect of early mobilization following Kapandji's method of intrafocal wiring in fractures of the distal end of the radius. Results of a prospective study of 60 cases. Int Orthop 1992;16(1):39–43 [in French].

47. Atroshi I, Brogren E, Larsson GU, et al. Wrist-bridging versus non-bridging external fixation for displaced distal radius fractures: a randomized assessor-blind clinical trial of 38 patients followed for 1 year. Acta Orthop 2006;77(3):445–53.

48. Krishnan J, Wigg AE, Walker RW, et al. Intra-articular fractures of the distal radius: a prospective randomised controlled trial comparing static bridging and dynamic non-bridging external fixation. J Hand Surg Br 2003;28(5):417–21.

49. Jenkins NH, Jones DG, Mintowt-Czyz WJ. External fixation and recovery of function following fractures of the distal radius in young adults. Injury 1988; 19(4):235–8.

50. Franck WM, Dahlen C, Amlang M, et al. Distal radius fracture—is non-bridging articular external fixator a therapeutic alternative? A prospective randomized study. Unfallchirurg 2000;103(10):826–33 [in German].

51. Davis TR, Buchanan JM. A controlled prospective study of early mobilization of minimally displaced fractures of the distal radial metaphysis. Injury 1987;18(4):283–5.

52. Jensen MR, Andersen KH, Jensen CH. Management of undisplaced or minimally displaced Colles' fracture: one or three weeks of immobilization. J Orthop Sci 1997;2(6):424–7.

53. Dias JJ, Wray CC, Jones JM, et al. The value of early mobilisation in the treatment of Colles' fractures. J Bone Joint Surg Br 1987;69(3):463–7.

54. Abbaszadegan H, Conradi P, Jonsson U. Fixation not needed for undisplaced Colles' fracture. Acta Orthop Scand 1989;60(1):60–2.

55. Smith DW, Brou KE, Henry MH. Early active rehabilitation for operatively stabilized distal radius fractures. J Hand Ther 2004;17(1):43–9.

56. Slutsky DJ, Herman M. Rehabilitation of distal radius fractures: a biomechanical guide. Hand Clin 2005; 21(3):455–68.

57. Oskarsson GV, Hjall A, Aaser P. Physiotherapy: an overestimated factor in after-treatment of fractures in the distal radius? Arch Orthop Trauma Surg 1997;116(6–7):373–5.

58. Lyngcoln A, Taylor N, Pizzari T, et al. The relationship between adherence to hand therapy and short-term outcome after distal radius fracture. J Hand Ther 2005;18(1):2–8 [quiz: 9].

59. Handoll HH, Madhok R, Howe TE. Rehabilitation for distal radial fractures in adults. Cochrane Database Syst Rev 2006;3:CD003324.

60. Taylor NF, Bennell KL. The effectiveness of passive joint mobilization on the return of active wrist extension following Colles' fracture. A clinical trial. New Zeal J Physiother 1994;22(1):24–8.

61. Krischak GD, Krasteva A, Schneider F, et al. Physiotherapy after volar plating of wrist fractures is effective using a home exercise program. Arch Phys Med Rehabil 2009;90(4):537–44.

62. Kay S, McMahon M, Stiller K. An advice and exercise program has some benefits over natural recovery after distal radius fracture: a randomised trial. Aust J Physiother 2008;54(4):253–9.

63. Kay S, Haensel N, Stiller K. The effect of passive mobilisation following fractures involving the distal radius: a randomised study. Aust J Physiother 2000;46(2):93–101.

64. Christensen OM, Kunov A, Hansen FF, et al. Occupational therapy and Colles' fractures. Int Orthop 2001;25(1):43–5.

65. Watt CF, Taylor NF, Baskus K. Do Colles' fracture patients benefit from routine referral to physiotherapy following cast removal? Arch Orthop Trauma Surg 2000;120(7–8):413–5.

66. Pasila M, Karaharju EO, Lepisto PV. Role of physical therapy in recovery of function after Colles' fracture. Arch Phys Med Rehabil 1974;55(3):130–4.

67. Gronlund B, Harreby MS, Kofoed R, et al. The importance of early exercise therapy in the treatment of Colles' fracture. A clinically controlled study. Ugeskr Laeger 1990;152(35):2491–3 [in Danish].

68. Bache SJ, Ankcorn L, Hiller L, et al. Two different approaches to physiotherapeutic management of patients with distal radial fractures [abstract]. Physiotherapy 2000;86(7):383.

69. Crichlow RJ, Andres PL, Morrison SM, et al. Depression in orthopaedic trauma patients. Prevalence and severity. J Bone Joint Surg Am 2006; 88(9):1927–33.

70. Glynn SM, Asarnow JR, Asarnow R, et al. The development of acute post-traumatic stress disorder after orofacial injury: a prospective study in a large urban hospital. J Oral Maxillofac Surg 2003;61(7):785–92.

71. Gong HS, Lee JO, Huh JK, et al. Comparison of depressive symptoms during the early recovery period in patients with a distal radius fracture treated by volar plating and cast immobilisation. Injury 2011; 42(11):1266–70.

72. Vranceanu AM, Barsky A, Ring D. Psychosocial aspects of disabling musculoskeletal pain. J Bone Joint Surg Am 2009;91(8):2014–8.

73. Altschuler EL, Wisdom SB, Stone L, et al. Rehabilitation of hemiparesis after stroke with a mirror. Lancet 1999;353(9169):2035–6.

74. Cacchio A, De Blasis E, Necozione S, et al. Mirror therapy for chronic complex regional pain syndrome type 1 and stroke. N Engl J Med 2009;361(6):634–6.

75. Chan BL, Witt R, Charrow AP, et al. Mirror therapy for phantom limb pain. N Engl J Med 2007;357(21): 2206–7.

76. McCabe CS, Haigh RC, Ring EF, et al. A controlled pilot study of the utility of mirror visual feedback in the treatment of complex regional pain syndrome (type 1). Rheumatology (Oxford) 2003;42(1):97–101.

77. Moseley GL. Graded motor imagery is effective for long-standing complex regional pain syndrome: a randomised controlled trial. Pain 2004;108(1–2): 192–8.

78. Ramachandran VS, Rogers-Ramachandran D, Cobb S. Touching the phantom limb. Nature 1995;377(6549): 489–90.

Future Treatment and Research Directions in Distal Radius Fracture

Jesse Jupiter, MD

KEYWORDS

• Distal radius • Future • Fracture • Treatment • Economics

Dr Harold Horowitz, writing in the *Journal of the American Medical Association* in 1999, presented an apocryphal story of an intern's admission note, dated November 17, 2150. The patient being admitted is a 150-year-old woman with a urinary tract infection. Along with many chronic medical disorders, her surgical history is noteworthy and may be a small window into our future. She had a coronary artery bypass grafting 80 years prior with follow-up prophylactic gene therapy 40 years later; bilateral corneal transplants 75 years ago; a kidney-pancreas transplant 60 years ago; bilateral knee replacements 47 years ago; and a femoral head excision with regrowth by osteophyte-stimulating factor for osteoarthritis of her left hip 35 years prior. Unfortunately, despite all of these medical advances, the patient was confined to a nursing home for the past 55 years and was bedridden. The cost of this fictional 2-day hospitalization for the urinary tract infection was estimated to be 340,000 dollars.[1]

Although apocryphal, this story presents several provocative issues that will have some relevance to the discussion of the possible future directions in the management of fractures of the distal end of the radius. This article attempts to project what we might encounter in the future with regard to epidemiology, risk and prevention, fracture assessment and treatment, and the ever increasing concern for the economic impact of this prevalent injury.

EPIDEMIOLOGY

Whether or not people will have their lives dramatically extended in the next few decades, it is clear that people are living longer, healthier, and more active lives. The 2 peak incidences of distal radius fracture will remain within the pediatric and geriatric age groups, with the latter experiencing a substantial increase in the coming years.[2,3] In a recent systematic review by Diaz-Garcia and colleagues,[4] it was estimated using Medicare data that as many as 372,000 individuals 65 years and older will sustain a distal radius fracture during the next year. This high incidence rate will most likely increase as the Baby Boomer generation continues to age. We will also certainly witness an increase in the number of outcomes evaluations, not simply of functional and radiographic parameters but of quality of life and cost-analysis data.[5]

RISK FACTORS

Given the recognized prevalence and economic impact of fragility fractures such as those seen in the hip and distal radius, research into the mechanism as well as the treatment of osteoporosis will have increasing importance. In the immediate future, there will be greater emphasis on diagnosis followed by pharmacologic treatment, albeit currently unpredictable.[6] Systematic reviews and meta-analyses will be found more and more in the literature, which is very likely to result in diagnosis and treatment algorithms that, it is hoped, are based on best evidence.[7] Electronic medical records will automatically flag postmenopausal women and even men older than 50 years, creating pathways to obtain dual-energy x-ray absorptiometry (DXA) scans.[8] Very likely this will also be evident when the diagnosis of a distal radius

Orthopaedic Surgery, Harvard Medical School, Massachusetts General Hospital, Yawkey 2 Suite 2100, Boston, MA 02114, USA
E-mail address: JJUPITER1@PARTNERS.ORG

Hand Clin 28 (2012) 245–248
doi:10.1016/j.hcl.2012.02.006
0749-0712/12/$ – see front matter © 2012 Published by Elsevier Inc.

fracture is placed on the "problem list." It remains to be seen whether tools such as the World Health Organization's Fracture Risk Assessment (FRAX) tool will become standard practice or will simply be replaced by a more predictable method of objectively assessing the probability of a patient being at risk for a fragility fracture.[9]

Most of the pharmacologic agents currently available are antiresorptive, but the future holds promise for more active drugs and genetic analysis, leading to far earlier treatment and preventive measures. Of interest in Horowitz's fictional intern's admission note, his index patient had slow-cyclic release estrogen implants replaced annually. There is every reason to believe that in the future we will see the use of this type of prophylaxis that is used to enhance the metaphyseal regions of the hip or wrist, especially after a contralateral fracture.[10] These and other advanced treatment protocols, such as injectable forms of growth factors and bone morphogenic proteins, are discussed in further detail in the following sections of this article.

Can the risk of a fracture from a fall from a standing height be better understood and even minimized? Studies have implicated postural instability or "sway" as an important risk factor for the development of a distal radius fracture[11] Postural instability can be tested by the ability of a subject to maintain his or her balance on a tilt board with a progressive decrease in the ambient light. Crilly and colleagues[11] identified a subset of women with a fracture of the distal radius with diminished postural stability when compared with control patients matched for age, gender, and associated medical illnesses. It was suggested that medication interactions could be one of the contributing factors. If a device could be developed and maintained in the office of every primary care physician to test postural instability coupled with a DXA scan, it could become part of every annual physical examination for at-risk populations.

FRACTURE ASSESSMENT

The concept that function will follow form as an outcome of an osteoporotic associated distal radius fracture has long been an accepted tenet of treatment. Ng and McQueen[12] made a series of recommendations regarding radiologic articular congruity in a recent review of studies involving distal radius fractures. These investigators recommended that articular reconstruction be achieved with less than 2 mm of gap or step-off, that the radius be restored to within 2 mm of its normal length, and that carpal alignment be restored,

with the ultimate aim of treatment being a pain-free wrist joint without functional limitations.

Although there is historical evidence of functional recovery treated with limited fracture reduction and early functional use of the hand and arm both in the Chinese literature and through the work of Lucas-Champonniere,[13,14] the need for a more perfect fracture alignment is once again being challenged. In a recent retrospective case-controlled study, Egol and colleagues[15] compared surgical treatment with cast immobilization in elderly patients who suffered a distal radius fracture. The study revealed no significant difference in function or overall outcomes between the operative and nonoperative groups, despite poorer radiographic alignment in the nonoperative group. A prospective randomized study by Arora and colleagues[16] comparing volar locking plates with cast treatment in elderly patients found a similar result. What does this mean for the near future? The American Academy of Orthopedic Surgery recently attempted to create a clinical practice guideline for the treatment of distal radius fractures, yet after extensive reviews of outcome studies and despite the experience of the investigative task force, nearly all the recommendations were thought to be inconclusive.[17] It is clear that additional efforts, both within our specialties as well as those entities responsible for payment, will be ongoing in attempts to establish more precise guidelines leading to best-practice algorithms.

Shauver and colleagues[18] evaluated current and future costs to Medicare in the United States, and estimated that based on current trends in the use of internal fixation, the cost will reach $240 million within a few years for the treatment of distal radius fractures. This figure is largely attributable to the fact that the newer plate technology costs Medicare nearly 3 times more than the traditional treatment options. Thus the burden of proof will increasingly be on our specialties to use more clearly defined outcome tools and evidence-based level I studies if we wish to continue to use surgical treatment with costly implants.

TREATMENT

Years of experience using percutaneous pins or Kirschner wires with or without casts or external fixation have realized the problems with such methods, and have led to the development of the angular stable plate. Will the current enthusiasm for volar locking plates remain, or will it be yet another example of Scott's parabola illustrating the rise and fall of a new surgical technique?[19] A remarkable amount of energy and effort is being directed toward the development of minimally invasive treatment techniques for all fractures except, it seems, for those of the distal radius. The direction of treatment protocols seems to be the opposite for this fracture, even with the high incidence associated with this injury. Despite favorable outcome studies, there remain substantial complications related to both the techniques and implants used during internal fixation.[20]

What, then, might be some of the future percutaneous methods that will offer fracture stability, functional restoration, and patient safety? The early experience with percutaneous injectable calcium phosphate bone cement was promising, hampered only by a lack of a predictable method of creating a metaphyseal void to accept an adequate quantity of the cement.[21] This procedure can and should be readily improved on by the development of inexpensive balloon technology, although it may well be the case that the medical-industry complex is reluctant to search for a less profitable treatment method.

Along these lines, we are seeing some developments of new technologies such as percutaneous expandable balloons made of tantalum metal that will also accept screws. Although there is currently no evidence available validating this as a superior treatment option, clinical experience is encouraging. It is this author's belief that the enthusiasm of the volar locking plates for dorsally displaced metaphyseal plates in the older patient will be challenged by alternative percutaneous methods in the near future, and may end up as another example of Scott's parabola. In the somewhat distant future we are likely to see the application of injectable orthobiologics to rapidly enhance the development of sufficient callous that would allow the use of only a removable splint for the treatment of distal radius fractures. The relatively subcutaneous location of the distal radius will make this a likely location to investigate such a technology.

Will there be improvements in the management of higher-velocity intra-articular fractures? Current techniques of internal fixation, external fixation, and even bridge plating are not always effective in terms of outcomes, at times even resulting in malalignment with loss of wrist mobility. Arthroscopically assisted reduction has had some support, but as yet has proved to be somewhat less applicable for many who are not facile with the techniques of wrist arthroscopy. Perhaps as surgeons become more trained in wrist arthroscopy, and with the advancement of imaging and reduction tools, we may see a resurgence of interest in this technology.[22,23] Yet another technological advance that will see a role in severely disrupted articular fractures will be metal hemiarthroplasties that resurface the distal end of the radius. Current experience is extremely limited, but this technology may well be applicable in the future.[24]

ECONOMICS

In view of an increase in health care spending, we are all becoming more challenged to use the most cost-effective method of treatment for our patients, and this will surely become a more integral part of our decision analyses for determinants of best practices. As the incidence of distal radius fractures continues to increase, it will be increasingly important for surgeons to provide valid and appropriate data regarding cost and outcomes as we move toward future treatment options that provide better care for this prevalent injury.

REFERENCES

1. Horowitz HW. Millennial child. Intern's admission note, November17, 2150. JAMA 1999;282:1799.
2. Bailey DA, Wedge JH, McCulloch RG, et al. Epidemiology of fractures of the distal end of the radius in children as associated with growth. J Bone Joint Surg Am 1989;71:1225–31.
3. McQueen MM. Epidemiology of fractures of the radius and ulna. In: McQueen MM, Jupiter JB, editors. Radius and ulna. Oxford (United Kingdom): Butterworth; 2000. p. 1–12.
4. Diaz-Garcia RJ, Oda J, Shauver MJ, et al. A systematic review of outcomes and complications of treating unstable distal radius fractures in the elderly. J Hand Surg 2011;36A:824–35.
5. Quigley L, Sprague S, Michlau T. Economic analysis. In: Bhandari M, editor. Evidence based orthopaedics. Oxford (United Kingdom): Wiley Blackwell; 2012. p. 30–4.
6. Kaufman JD, Bolander ME, Bunta AD, et al. Barriers and solutions to osteoporosis care in patients with a hip fracture. J Bone Joint Surg Am 2003;85:1837–43.
7. Chung KC, Burns PB, Kim MH. A practical guide to metaanalysis. J Hand Surg 2006;31:1671–8.
8. Feldstein A, Elmer PJ, Smith DH, et al. Electronic medical record reminder improves osteoporosis management after a fracture: a randomized controlled trial. J Am Geriatr Soc 2006;54:450–7.
9. Kanis JA, Johnell O, Oden A, et al. FRAX and the assessment of fracture probability in men and women from the UK. Osteoporos Int 2008;19:385–97.
10. Einhorn TA, Majeska RJ, Mahaideen A, et al. A single percutaneous injection of recombinant human bone morphogenic protein-2 accelerates fracture repair. J Bone Joint Surg Am 2003;85:1425–35.

11. Crilly RG, Delaguerriere-Richardson LD, Roth JH. Postural instability and Colles fracture. Age Ageing 1987;16:133–8.

12. Ng CY, McQueen MM. What are the radiologic predictors of functional outcome following fractures of the distal radius. J Bone Joint Surg Br 2011;93: 145–50.

13. Futami T, Yamamoto M. Chinese external fixation treatment of fractures of the distal end of the radius. J Hand Surg Am 1989;14:1028–32.

14. Lucas-Champonniere J. Traitement des fractures du radius et du péroné par le massage: traitement des fractures pararticulaires simples et compliquées de plaie sans immobilisation, mobilisation et massage. Bull Mem Soc Chir Paris 1886;12:560 [in French].

15. Egol KA, Walsh M, Romo-Cardoso S, et al. Distal radius fractures in the elderly: operative compared with non-operative treatment. J Bone Joint Surg Am 2010;92:1851–7.

16. Arora R, Lutz M, Deml C, et al. A prospective randomized trial comparing non-operative treatment with volar locking plate fixation for displaced and unstable distal radius fracture in patients sixty-five years of age and older. J Bone Joint Surg Am 2011;93:2146–53.

17. AAOS Now. Chicago (IL): American Academy of Orthopaedic Surgeons; 2009.

18. Shauver MJ, Yin H, Banergee M, et al. Current and future national costs to Medicare for the treatment of distal radius fractures in the elderly. J Hand Surg Am 2011;36:1282–7.

19. Scott JW. The rise and fall of a new surgical technique. Br Med J 2001;323:1477.

20. Rozental TD, Blazar PE. Functional outcome and complications after volar plating for dorsally displaced unstable fractures of the distal radius. J Hand Surg Am 2006;31:359–65.

21. Cassidy C, Jupiter JB, Cohen M, et al. Norian SRS versus conventional therapy in distal radius fractures: multicenter study of 323 patients. J Bone Joint Surg Am 2003;85:2127–37.

22. Doi K, Hattori Y, Otsuka K, et al. Intraarticular fractures of the distal aspect of the radius: arthroscopy assisted reduction compared to open reduction and internal fixation. J Bone Joint Surg Am 1999;81:1093–110.

23. dePinal F. Dry arthroscopy of the wrist; its role in the management of articular distal radius fracture. Scand J Surg 2008;97:298–304.

24. Adams B. Total wrist arthroplasty. Tech Hand Up Extrem Surg 2004;8:130–7.

Index

Note: Page numbers of article titles are in **boldface** type.

Hand Clin 28 (2012) 249–252
doi:10.1016/S0749-0712(12)00027-3
0749-0712/12/$ – see front matter © 2012 Elsevier Inc. All rights reserved.

hand.theclinics.com

Moving?

Make sure your subscription moves with you!

To notify us of your new address, find your **Clinics Account Number** (located on your mailing label above your name), and contact customer service at:

Email: journalscustomerservice-usa@elsevier.com

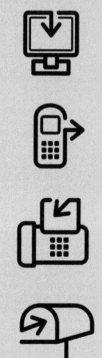

800-654-2452 (subscribers in the U.S. & Canada)
314-447-8871 (subscribers outside of the U.S. & Canada)

Fax number: 314-447-8029

Elsevier Health Sciences Division
Subscription Customer Service
3251 Riverport Lane
Maryland Heights, MO 63043

*To ensure uninterrupted delivery of your subscription, please notify us at least 4 weeks in advance of move.

Printed and bound by CPI Group (UK) Ltd, Croydon, CR0 4YY

03/10/2024

01040356-0020